Atlas of Psychiatric Pharmacotherapy

Atlas of Psychiatric Pharmacotherapy

Roni Shiloh, MD
Geha Psychiatric Hospital
Sackler Faculty of Medicine
Tel-Aviv University
Israel

David Nutt, DM, MRCP, FRCPsych
Professor of Psychopharmacology
School of Medical Sciences
University of Bristol, UK

Abraham Weizman, MD
Director of Research
Geha Psychiatric Hospital
Professor of Psychiatry
Sackler Faculty of Medicine
Tel-Aviv University
Israel

MARTIN DUNITZ

© Martin Dunitz Ltd 1999

First published in the United Kingdom in 1999 by

Martin Dunitz Ltd
The Livery House
7—9 Pratt Street
London NW1 0AE

Revised edition 2000

A CIP record for this book is available from the British Library.

ISBN 1- 85317-934-5

Distributed in the United States by:
Blackwell Science Inc.
Commerce Plac, 350 Main Street
Malden, MA 02148, USA
Tel: 1-800-215-1000

Distributed in Canada by:
Login Brothers Book Company
324 Salteaux Crescent
Winnipeg, Manitoba, R3J 3T2
Canada
Tel: 204-224-4068

Distributed in Brazil by:
Ernesto Reichmann Distribuidora de Livros, Ltda
Rua Coronel Marques 335, Tatuape 03440-000
São Paulo, Brazil

Composition by Scribe Design, Gillingham, Kent, UK
Printed and bound in Spain by Grafos, S.A.

Contents

Introduction

This book was written, first and foremost, for the clinician who is required to know, understand, and decide efficiently about options for biological treatments. It is also hoped that it will be useful to students in other fields, e.g. pharmacology, psychology and neuroscience. The purpose of this book is to give the reader a comprehensive perspective of existing knowledge, without engaging in speculations or theories that are insufficiently grounded. This book has been written in order to enable the reader to reach clear decisions based on the most up-to-date literature.

To this end, we present a number of topics:

1. Basic aspects related to mechanisms of drug action, including the spectrum of potential pharmacological and biological treatments available in psychiatric medicine; the qualitative and quantitative differences between the optional treatments; their side effects and the latest known data regarding their operative mechanisms.

   Treatments that are not biological in nature (psychotherapies, for example) are often referred to concisely, when they constitute the primary treatment modality.

2. Treatment strategies regarding the main psychiatric diagnostic entities, based on the bank of research published recently. The focus is on providing the reader with guidelines based on the proven efficacy of the various treatment options, rather than prescribing a definite treatment algorithm.

3. Interactions, mainly pharmacokinetic, between drugs/other substances and the aforementioned biological treatments. We believe that this issue is of utmost importance, in light of the fact that a substantial proportion of psychiatric patients take a wide range of drugs concomitantly (including drugs prescribed for non-psychiatric conditions). It has been our clinical experience that information of this type is insufficiently accessible to the clinician in the field, and this book should serve to help the clinician make better and more efficient decisions.

The majority of the information in this book is based on evidence-based published literature during the last five years, with emphasis on the latest data. We have tried to categorize the written and graphic data given by the quantity of the evidence:

Well-established data: is that which is based on a number of research studies, at least some of which were well controlled (double-blind, cross over, placebo-controlled); the size of the sample group was significantly large, and the central message of the research was replicated for substantiation.

Partially-established data: is that based on open-labeled research produced from small samplings, or which has not been replicated.

Not well established data: is that based on small case series or on anecdotal reports.

In order to simplify the reader's use of the material, we have categorized the main subjects in psychiatry to extremely concise sub-topics. Each specific issue is presented, at most, on a two-page spread, so that all the material is set before the reader in a self-contained fashion. The majority of the text is aimed to explain and expand on the graphic presentations.

Another consideration during the preparation of this book was its potential use in various academic spheres, and we believe that the format adopted for the book is the most efficient for such use as well.

This book is not a substitute for textbooks; supplementary and more in-depth reading of psychiatric and pharmacological literature is, of course, required. The concept and format of the book have been designed primarily for readers with a basic knowledge of psychiatry. Nevertheless, medical students, psychiatric and neurological residents, as well as general practitioners, should find this book useful in their search for data on specific issues.

Roni Shiloh
David Nutt
Abraham Weizman

SECTION A

BASIC PRINCIPLES OF PSYCHIATRIC PHARMACOTHERAPY

1.1 Principles of drug action – presynaptic nerve
Control and modulation of neurotransmitter release

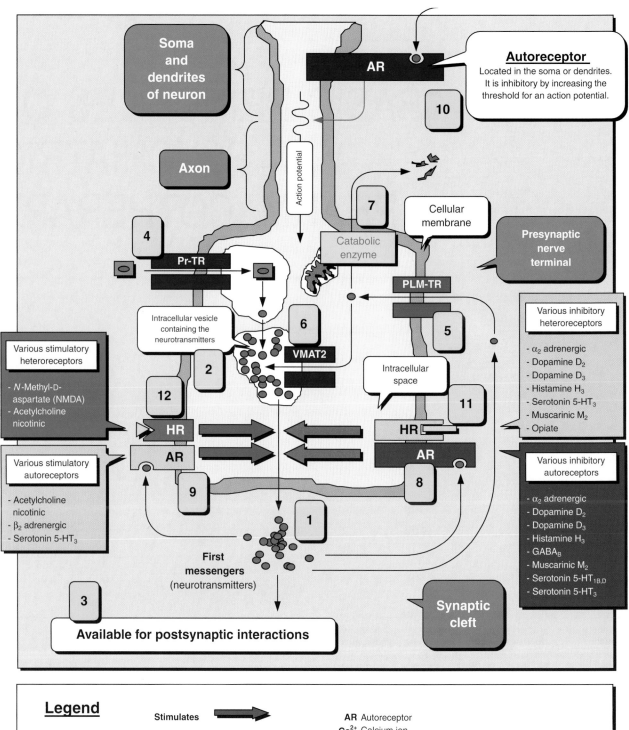

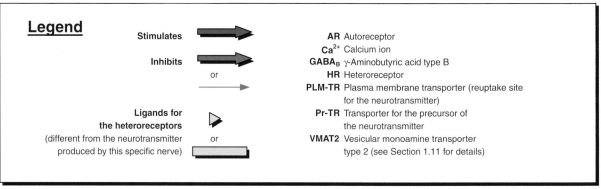

A comprehensive understanding of neuronal functioning and the various mechanisms of drug action is a key factor for achieving proper mastery of psychiatric pharmacotherapy. Practically all our ideas about the therapeutic effects of the major psychotropic drugs is based on their action at pre- and postsynaptic receptors or on transporters. First messengers; these are substances such as neurotransmitters that interact with postsynaptic receptors to induce consequent intracellular changes. Following their interactions with receptors, they are either metabolized or taken for re-use. Research in recent years has focused on the better understanding of these receptor interactions and the intracellular changes attributable to drug administration.

Notes about the numbered items in the scheme

1–3. In the central nervous system, information is transferred via electrical impulses (action potentials) originating in the soma of neurons and progressing along the nerve's axon and up to its terminal regions, where it is transformed into chemical information in the form of neurotransmitters (**1**). Most nerves release one neurotransmitter, although some nerves can release two (generally a non-peptide and a peptide). They can be modulated by numerous other neurotransmitters. Neurotransmitters are stored in intracellular vesicles (**2**), and following the arrival of an action potential, they undergo exocytosis (a calcium-dependent process) into the synaptic cleft where they are available for postsynaptic interactions (**3**). There are several hundred known neurotransmitters; those most relevant to psychiatric pharmacotherapy are listed in Table 1.1

4–7. The amount of neurotransmitters available for exocytosis depends on several intact mechanisms.

a. Availability of precursor for the neurotransmitter and proper functioning of its uptake site into the presynaptic nerve (the precursor transporter ; Pr-TR) (**4**).

b. Proper reuptake of the neurotransmitters into the presynaptic nerve terminal by the plasma membrane transporter (PLM-TR) (**5**) and intact transport of the neurotransmitter from the cell's cytoplasm into the storage vesicle by the vesicular monoamine transporter type 2 (VMAT2) (**6**).

c. An appropriate metabolism of the neurotransmitter by enzymes such as mitochondrial monoamine oxidases (**7**).

8–12. There are several main modulatory systems that together govern the rate of neurotransmitter release into the synaptic cleft:

a. Autoreceptors (ARs) which interact with the neurotransmitter produced by the same nerve, and consequently suppress (**8**) or stimulate (**9**) the release of neurotransmitters into the synaptic cleft. They are located in the presynaptic nerve terminals (**8,9**) or in the soma, dendrites and axons of central nervous system neurons (**10**).

b. Heteroreceptors (HRs) which can either suppress (**11**) or enhance (**12**) the release of the neurotransmitter. They are termed heteroreceptors since they are activated by neurotransmitters different from those produced by the nerve they are on. There might be numerous different heteroreceptors which bind various neurotransmitters on a single nerve.

Table 1.2 summarizes some of the main modulating mechanisms relevant to intact functioning of the presynaptic nerve.

Psychotropic medications can either enhance or suppress many of the major processes or modulatory events listed in 4–7 and 8–12 above.

Table 1.1

Biogenic amines	Amino acids	Peptides		Miscellaneous
Acetylcholine	Aspartate	Angiotensin	Oxcytocin	Adenosine
Dopamine	Glutamate	Bombesin	Prolactin	Adenosine triphosphate (ATP)
Histamine	Glycine	Bradykinin	Somatostatin	Nitric oxide
Norepinephrine	γ-Aminobutyric acid (GABA)	Cholecystokinin	Tachykinins	Carbon monoxide
(noradrenaline)	Homocysteate	Endorphins	Vasoactive intestinal peptide	
Serotonin		Melatonin		

Table 1.2

Nerve type	Inhibitory AR	Inhibitory HR	Stimulatory AR	Stimulatory HR
Cholinergic	Muscarinic type 2 (M_2)	α_2-adrenoreceptor; dopamine type D_2/D_3; serotonin type 5-HT_3	Nicotinic	N-methyl-D-aspartate (NMDA)
Dopaminergic	Dopamine type D_2/D_3	Muscarinic type 2 (M_2); serotonin type 5-HT_3 ?		Nicotinic; N-methyl-D-aspartate (NMDA)
GABAergic (releases γ-aminobutyric acid)	GABA type B ($GABA_B$)			
Histaminergic	Histamine type 3 (H_3)			
Noradrenergic	α_2-adrenoreceptor	Dopaminergic type D_2; histamine type 3 (H_3); muscarinic type 2 (M_2); opiate	β_2-adrenoreceptor	Nicotinic
Serotonergic	Serotonin type 5-$HT_{1B,D}$	α_2-adrenoreceptor;	Serotonin type 5-HT_3	

1.2 Principles of drug action – postsynaptic nerve

Postsynaptic interactions and consequent intracellular changes

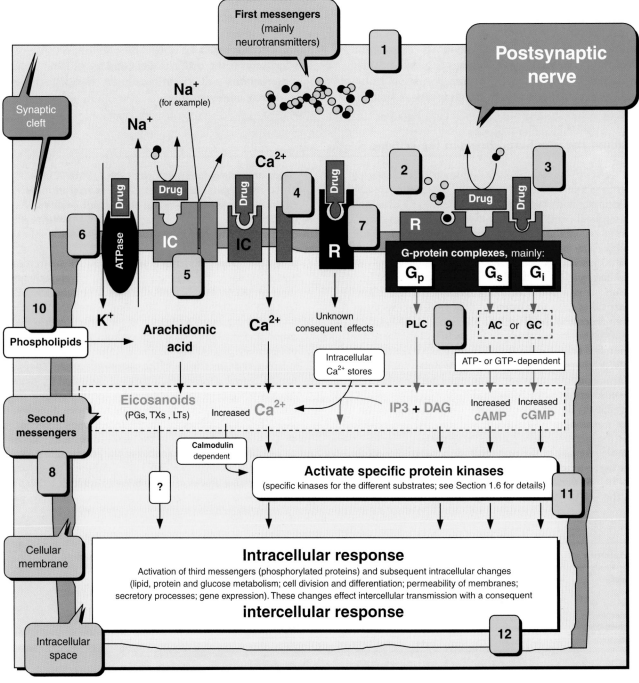

Legend

AC	Adenylate cyclase
ATP	Adenosine triphosphate
cAMP	Cyclic adenosine monophosphate
cGMP	Cyclic guanine monophosphate
DAG	Diacylglycerol
GC	Guanylate cyclase

G-proteins There are several types, characterized by different α subunits (see Sections 1.3-1.5 for further details):
G_i inhibits the activity of adenylate cyclase and activates phospholipase C, A_2 and potassium channels;
G_o modulates voltage-sensitive calcium channels and phospholipase C; G_p stimulates phospholipase C;
G_s Activates adenylate cyclase and calcium channels

IC	Ion channel
IP3	Inositol triphosphate
LTs	Leukotrienes
PGs	Prostaglandins
PLC	Phospholipase C
R	Receptor
TXs	Thromboxanes

Stimulates →
Inhibits →

Postsynaptic interactions are one of the major aspects of almost all drugs used in psychiatry. These interactions may account for the drug's therapeutic effects, or can cause its adverse side-effect profile. Most drugs in use are non-selective, meaning that they have interactions with multiple pre- and postsynaptic receptors or transporters. Most current knowledge about the mechanism of drug action is based on direct pre- and postsynaptic drug interactions and the subsequent modulation of intracellular components such as second, third and fourth messengers. Second messengers are specific intracellular components that are indirectly stimulated by the first messengers to activate certain enzymes called protein kinases. The most studied second messengers are calcium ion, inositol triphosphate (IP3), diacylglycerol (DAG),

cyclic adenosine monophosphate (cAMP) and cyclic guanine monophosphate (cGMP). Protein kinases modulate cellular activities by phosphorylating certain inactive proteins. The protein kinases are named after the second messengers that activate them (cAMP-dependent protein kinase for example). There are also other types of protein kinases that are not second-messenger-dependent. They include protein tyrosine kinases, which phosphorylate substrate proteins specifically on tyrosine residues, casein kinases and numerous others.

Following protein kinase activities the phosphorylated proteins (termed third messengers) are activated and then bring about subsequent modifications in cellular functioning.

Notes about the numbered items in the scheme

1. Normal neuronal activity requires intact pre- and postsynaptic interactions between first messengers (**1**) (e.g. neurotransmitters) and their target receptors or transporters located on the extracellular membrane.

2,3. Neurotransmitters bind with high affinity to postsynaptic receptors that are linked to either protein complexes termed G-proteins, or ion channels. G-proteins are so-termed because of their ability to bind the guanine nucleotides guanosine triphosphate (GTP) and guanosine diphosphate (GDP). G-proteins serve to couple receptors to specific intracellular effector systems. Three major types of G-proteins are involved in signal transduction: G_p, G_s and G_i. These protein complexes differ from one another in their α subunits (see Sections 1.3–1.5 for further details), which, in turn, gives rise to different and sometimes opposing effects on consequent intracellular functioning. Many of the drugs used in psychiatry can either antagonize the receptors linked to specific G-proteins (**2**) or stimulate them in a similar way to that of the endogenous first messenger (**3**). Synaptic responses mediated by receptor-gated channels and G-protein-linked receptors have considerably different time courses. The direct effects of ligand-gated channels are rapid and transitory, usually ending in less than one millisecond, whereas those mediated by G-protein-linked

receptors are slower in onset (requiring at least 100 ms to develop) and can be very long in duration (minutes). Some established examples of brain G-protein-linked receptors are presented in Section 1.5.

4-6. Some drugs or even the same drugs described previously can interact with ion channels such as calcium ion channels (**4**) or the sodium channels (**5**). They can affect membrane pumps such as – sodium-potassium ATPase (**6**). In all of these cases they can either suppress or enhance the permeability of these membrane structures.

7. Some drugs also bind with high affinity to receptors whose transmitters have not been identified as yet (orphan receptors).

8–10. Pharmacotherapy that alters first-messenger activities and interacts with various membrane receptors inevitably alter the functioning of second-messenger components (**8**). These are substances such as phospholipase C, adenylate cyclase, guanylate cyclase (**9**), phospholipids and arachidonic acid (**10**). They can also modify cellular functioning by changing the intracellular concentrations of major ions, especially calcium (**4**), which is also considered a second messenger.

11,12. The outcome of the altered second-messenger activities is a modification of protein kinase functioning (**11**), which is followed by enduring intra- and intercellular responses (**12**).

1.3 Signal transduction (I)

Receptor–G$_s$-protein interactions and activation of the second-messenger system

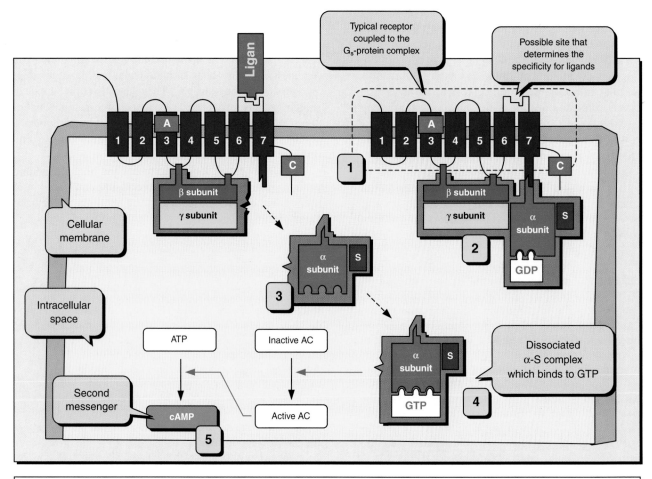

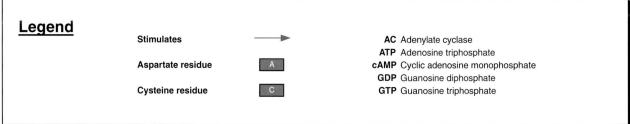

Notes about the numbered items in the scheme

1. Receptors that are coupled to the G-protein complex have a characteristic structure:

    a. Seven transmembrane domains (numbered from 1 to 7).

    b. The NH$_2$ terminal at the extracellular site and the COOH terminal intracellularly.

    c. All have an aspartate residue at the third domain (lettered A). This suggests that binding involves an ionic interaction between the carboxylate side-chain of the aspartate and the neurotransmitter amino group.

    d. Receptors that inhibit adenylate cyclase (e.g. G$_i$) have a longer third and shorter fourth cytoplasmatic loop. Stimulating receptors are coupled to G$_s$, as in the scheme, have a shorter third loop and a longer fourth loop.

    e. All receptors have a cysteine residue at similar points in the fourth cytoplasmatic loop (lettered C).

    f. The sixth and seventh domains are important in determining the specificity for the binding ligand.

2–5. *Mechanism of receptor regulation.* When a ligand binds to the receptor, the G$_s$-protein, which is in an inactive form [GDP component attached to α, β, γ and S sub-units (**2**)], is activated. This induces an allosteric change in the α subunit that makes it bind with much greater affinity to GTP than to GDP (**3**). At the same time, the activated complex dissociates into GTP plus an α–S complex (**4**), and a β–γ complex, which remains attached to the receptor. The active complex (the GTP plus an α–S complex, and especially the α-subunit) activates adenylate cyclase which converts adenosine triphosphate (ATP) to cyclic adenosine monophosphate (cAMP), which is a second messeneger (**5**) that increases the activities of several intracellular protein kinases, which in turn regulate many metabolic processes.

1.4 Signal transduction (II)

Receptor–G_p protein interactions and activation of the second-messenger system

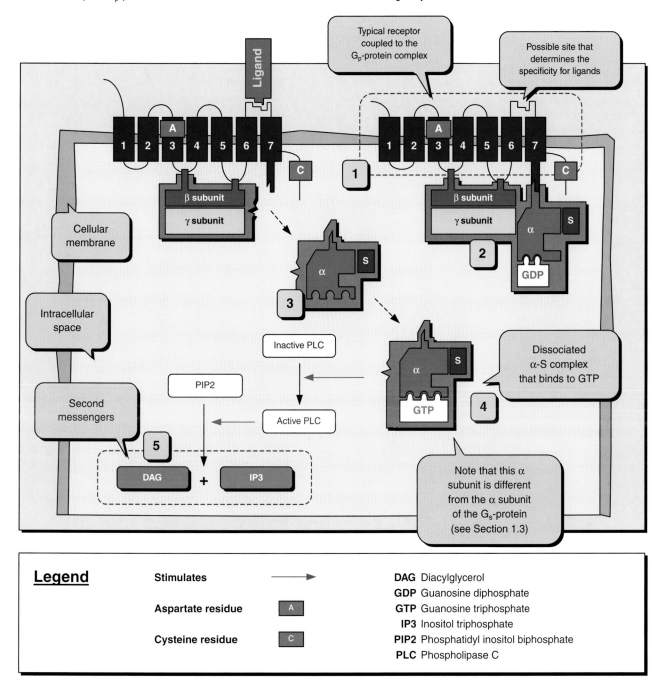

Legend

Stimulates →	**DAG** Diacylglycerol
	GDP Guanosine diphosphate
Aspartate residue [A]	**GTP** Guanosine triphosphate
	IP3 Inositol triphosphate
Cysteine residue [C]	**PIP2** Phosphatidyl inositol biphosphate
	PLC Phospholipase C

Notes about the numbered items in the scheme

1. Typical receptors that are coupled to the G-protein complex have a characteristic structure (see Section 1.3 for details).

2–5. *Mechanism of receptor regulation.* When a ligand binds to the receptor at the membrane binding site, the G_p-protein, which is in an inactive form [GDP component attached to α, β, γ and S subunits (**2**)], is activated. This activation induces an allosteric change in the α subunit that makes it bind with a much greater affinity to GTP than to GDP (**3**). At the same time, the activated complex dissociates into GTP plus an α–S complex (**4**), and a β–γ complex, which remains attached to the receptor. The active complex (the GTP plus an α–S complex, and especially the α subunit) activates phospholipase C, which converts phosphatidyl inositol biphosphate (PIP2) to inositol triphosphate (IP3) and diacylglycerol (DAG), both of which are second messengers (**5**). DAG enhances the activities of intracellular protein kinase C (which further regulates many cellular processes). IP3 stimulates the release of calcium ions (stored in vesicles of the endoplasmatic reticulum) into the cytoplasm.

1.5 Activation of receptors coupled to G-proteins, ion channels or other intracellular components
Cellular mediators and consequent changes in second messengers or other intracellular compounds

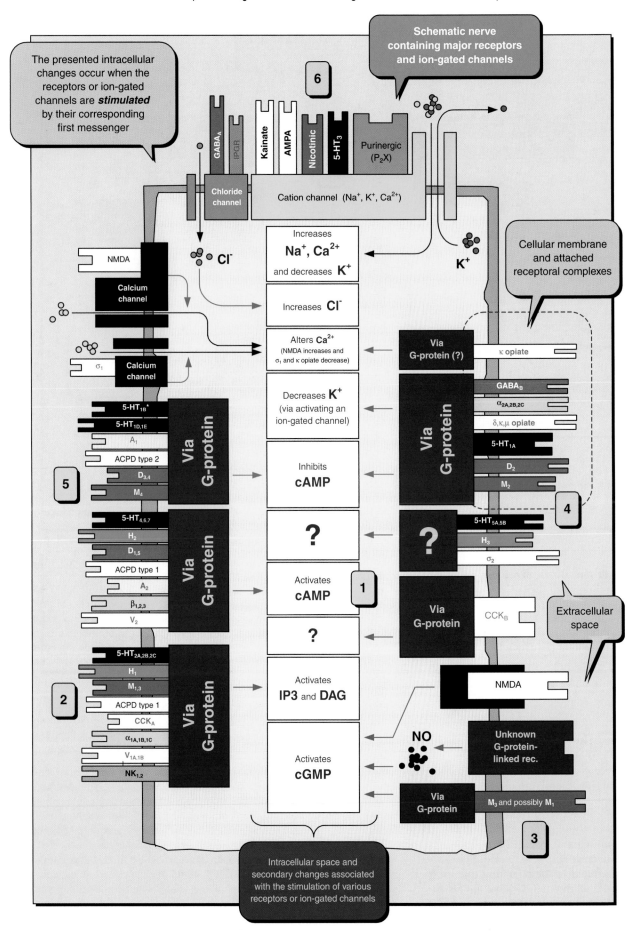

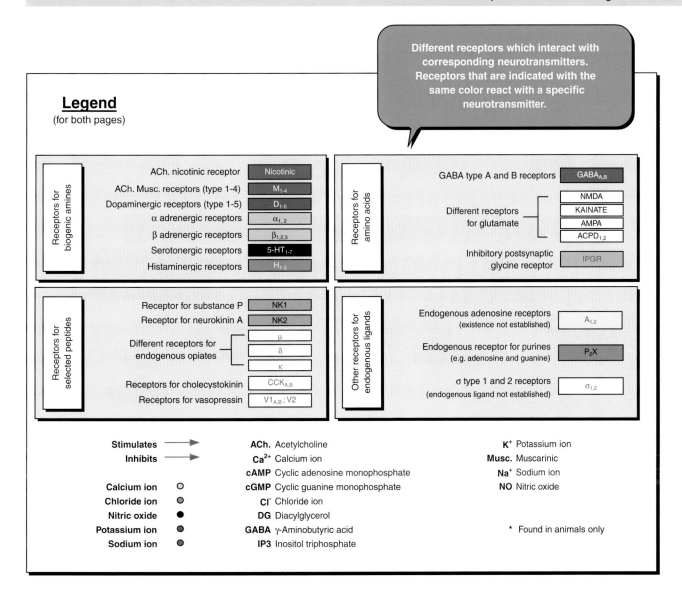

Different receptors which interact with corresponding neurotransmitters. Receptors that are indicated with the same color react with a specific neurotransmitter.

Legend
(for both pages)

Receptors for biogenic amines

ACh. nicotinic receptor	Nicotinic
ACh. Musc. receptors (type 1-4)	M_{1-4}
Dopaminergic receptors (type 1-5)	D_{1-5}
α adrenergic receptors	$\alpha_{1,2}$
β adrenergic receptors	$\beta_{1,2,3}$
Serotonergic receptors	5-HT_{1-7}
Histaminergic receptors	H_{1-3}

Receptors for amino acids

GABA type A and B receptors	$GABA_{A,B}$
Different receptors for glutamate	NMDA / KAINATE / AMPA / $ACPD_{1,2}$
Inhibitory postsynaptic glycine receptor	IPGR

Receptors for selected peptides

Receptor for substance P	NK1
Receptor for neurokinin A	NK2
Different receptors for endogenous opiates	μ / δ / κ
Receptors for cholecystokinin	$CCK_{A,B}$
Receptors for vasopressin	$V1_{A,B}; V2$

Other receptors for endogenous ligands

Endogenous adenosine receptors (existence not established)	$A_{1,2}$
Endogenous receptor for purines (e.g. adenosine and guanine)	P_2X
σ type 1 and 2 receptors (endogenous ligand not established)	$\sigma_{1,2}$

Stimulates →
Inhibits →

Calcium ion ○
Chloride ion ◐
Nitric oxide ●
Potassium ion ◐
Sodium ion ◐

ACh. Acetylcholine
Ca^{2+} Calcium ion
cAMP Cyclic adenosine monophosphate
cGMP Cyclic guanine monophosphate
Cl$^-$ Chloride ion
DG Diacylglycerol
GABA γ-Aminobutyric acid
IP3 Inositol triphosphate

K$^+$ Potassium ion
Musc. Muscarinic
Na$^+$ Sodium ion
NO Nitric oxide

* Found in animals only

Notes about the numbered items in the scheme:

Most brain receptors are either linked to G-proteins or located directly on ion channels. The scheme on the left attempts to simplify and integrate the current knowledge about the secondary intracellular changes which follow the stimulation of the various receptors.

There are two major ways in which to understand the scheme:
1. If one needs to know which type of receptors can elicit a certain response then one should look at the desired response [activated cyclic adenosine monophosphate (cAMP) for example] and then notice which receptors are associated with the stimulation of this second messenger. In this example it can be seen that the serotonergic receptors $5\text{-HT}_{4,6,7}$, the histaminergic receptor H_2, the D_1 and D_5 dopaminergic receptors, the A_2 endogenous receptor for adenosine, the ACPD type 1 receptor for glutamate, the $\beta_{1,2,3}$ adrenergic receptors and the V_2 receptor for vasopressin can all activate cAMP, and they do so via the G-protein mechanism.
2-5. If one needs to know what intracellular responses are estimated to occur when an activity of a certain neurotransmitter is altered (either enhanced or suppressed) then one should look at the different colors of the receptors. All the receptors that

have high affinity for a certain neurotransmitter are colored the same. For example, all the different acetylcholine receptors (nicotinic and the four types of muscarinic) are colored green. Therefore, when one administers a cholinergic drug such as pyridostigmine or tacrine, one expects an increase in the concentration of acetylcholine in the synaptic cleft. The acetylcholine will potentially interact with all the acetylcholine receptors, and the secondary effects of these interactions should be as follows:
a. Stimulated M_1 and M_3 receptors activate inositol triphosphate (IP3), discylglycerol (DAG) (**2**) and cyclic guanine monophophate (cGMP) (**3**).
b. Stimulating the M_2 receptors inhibits the activities of cAMP and decreases potassium concentration in the intracellular space (**4**).
c. Stimulating the M_4 receptors inhibits the activities of cAMP (**5**).
d. Stimulating the nicotinic receptors increases cation (mostly potassium) concentrations via a direct action on ion-gated channels (**6**).

These four responses are expected to occur, but there is little data concerning which of the four predominates, if at all.

1.6   Signal transduction (III)

Second messenger–protein kinase interactions and consequent activation of third messengers

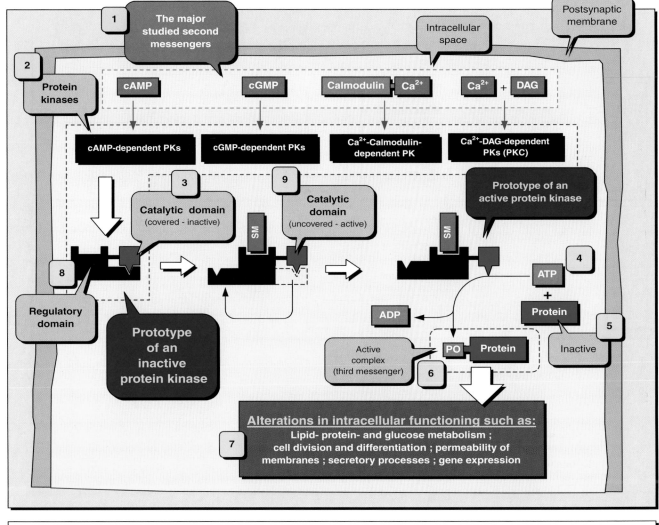

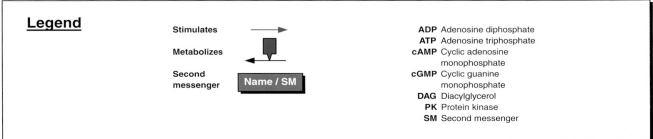

Notes about the numbered items in the scheme

1. Signal transduction refers to the cascade of intraneural interactions, beginning with extracellular first messengers (neurotransmitters, peptides), which affect the cell membrane receptors, the consequent activation of the second-messenger system, which in turn activates more intraneural messengers, leading to a specific cellular response. The major second messengers involved in signal transduction are cAMP, cGMP, calcium as part of a larger complex that contains four calcium molecules and a calcium-dependent regulatory protein called calmodulin, and calcium with the second messenger diacylglycerol.

2. Each of these second messengers has a specific affinity for another type of intracellular protein called protein kinase (PK).

The PKs are named according to the specific second messenger that stimulates them.

3-9. Most PKs have a similar mode of action. The typical PK has two major domains. A catalytic domain (**3**), when activated, can transfer a phosphate group (PO_4) from ATP (**4**) to a specific and inactive intracellular protein (**5**). The PO_4 group converts the protein into an active complex termed third messenger (**6**) which induces a specific cellular response (**7**). The second major domain of the typical PK is the regulatory domain (**8**). When the PK is inactive, the regulatory domain covers the catalytic site and suppresses its activities. When a second messenger binds to the regulatory domain (**9**), it induces a conformational change that uncovers the catalytic site and enables it to react with ATP.

1.7 Gene expression

Transcription, protein synthesis and consequent cellular changes

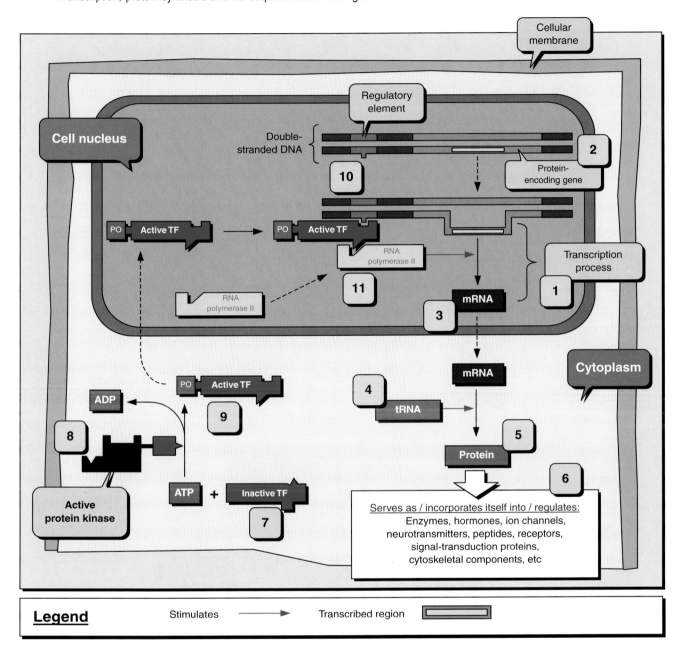

Notes about the numbered items in the scheme

1–5. The term 'transcription' (**1**) refers to the process of translating genetic information from a protein-encoding gene (**2**) located on a certain region of the single-stranded deoxyribonucleic acid (DNA) into a messenger ribonucleic acid (mRNA) (**3**). The mRNA is a template for a transfer RNA (tRNA) (**4**) which has the capacity to translate coded information on the mRNA into a protein chain (**5**). Specific tRNAs transport distinct amino acids to the protein-building site, where they bind to a complementary codon on the mRNA, thus directing the incorporation of the appropriate amino acid into a growing protein chain.

6. Once a new protein is synthesized, it can modulate cellular functioning via numerous ways. It can incorporate itself into various cellular structures, with consequent alterations in their

functioning. It can serve as an enzyme, neurotransmitter peptide or hormone that governs cellular activities. It can alter signal transduction mechanisms, receptor configurations and activities, ion channel permeability, and practically almost all of the major processes related to normal cell functioning.

7–11. Protein synthesis begins when an inactive protein termed a transcription factor (**7**) becomes activated by a certain protein kinase (**8**). The activated transcription factor (TF) (**9**) is then capable of identifying a unique sequence of the DNA, termed a regulatory element (**10**), which lies adjacent to the protein-encoding gene. Finally, the enzyme RNA polymerase II (**11**) binds to a site on the activated TF, where it begins transcribing DNA information into mRNA coding.

1.8 Neurotransmitters (synthesis and degradation)

Biogenic amines: NE, DA, 5-HT, ACh, epinephrine, histamine

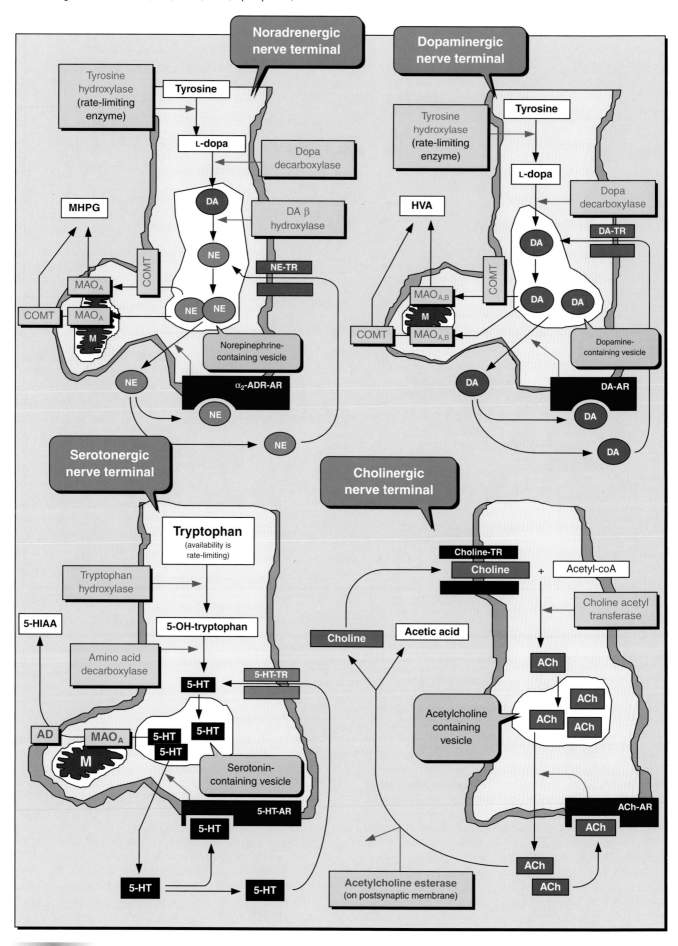

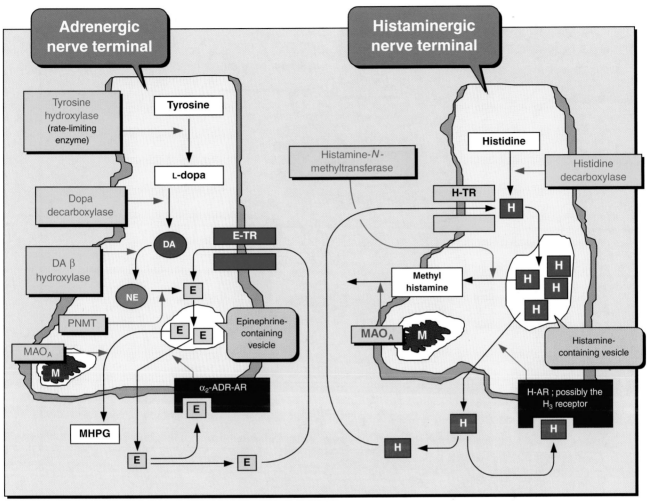

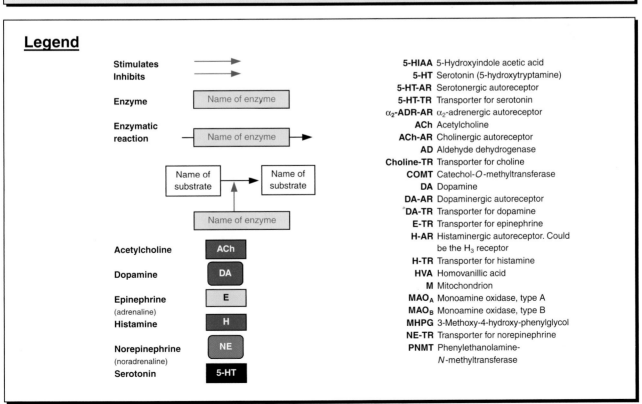

Legend

Stimulates	→
Inhibits	→
Enzyme	Name of enzyme
Enzymatic reaction	Name of enzyme →

Name of substrate → Name of substrate (Name of enzyme)

Acetylcholine	ACh
Dopamine	DA
Epinephrine (adrenaline)	E
Histamine	H
Norepinephrine (noradrenaline)	NE
Serotonin	5-HT

5-HIAA	5-Hydroxyindole acetic acid
5-HT	Serotonin (5-hydroxytryptamine)
5-HT-AR	Serotonergic autoreceptor
5-HT-TR	Transporter for serotonin
α₂-ADR-AR	α_2-adrenergic autoreceptor
ACh	Acetylcholine
ACh-AR	Cholinergic autoreceptor
AD	Aldehyde dehydrogenase
Choline-TR	Transporter for choline
COMT	Catechol-O-methyltransferase
DA	Dopamine
DA-AR	Dopaminergic autoreceptor
DA-TR	Transporter for dopamine
E-TR	Transporter for epinephrine
H-AR	Histaminergic autoreceptor. Could be the H₃ receptor
H-TR	Transporter for histamine
HVA	Homovanillic acid
M	Mitochondrion
MAO$_A$	Monoamine oxidase, type A
MAO$_B$	Monoamine oxidase, type B
MHPG	3-Methoxy-4-hydroxy-phenylglycol
NE-TR	Transporter for norepinephrine
PNMT	Phenylethanolamine-N-methyltransferase

1.9 Neurotransmitters
Glutamate; excitatory

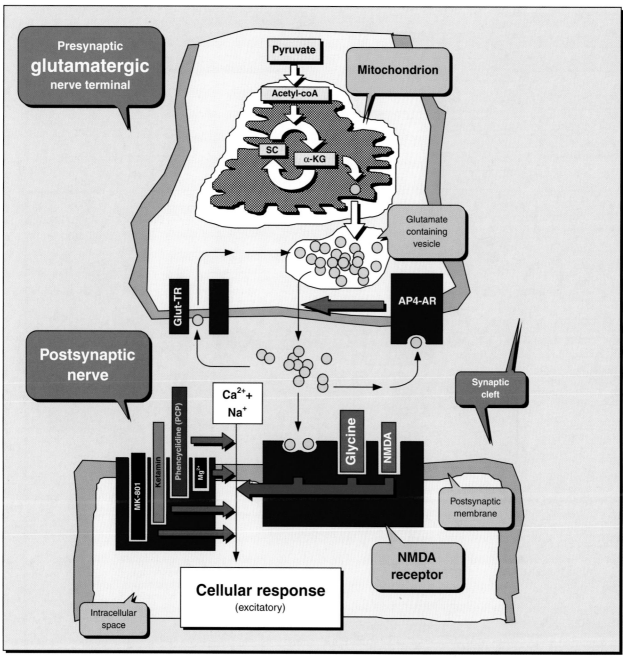

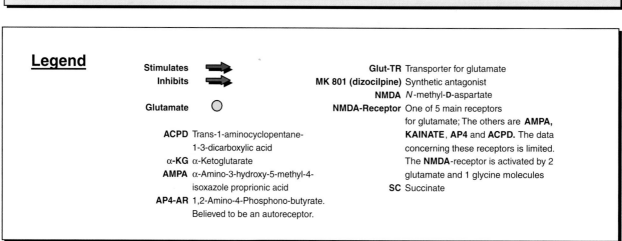

Legend

Stimulates	⇒	**Glut-TR**	Transporter for glutamate
Inhibits	⇒	**MK 801 (dizocilpine)**	Synthetic antagonist
		NMDA	N-methyl-D-aspartate
Glutamate	○	**NMDA-Receptor**	One of 5 main receptors

ACPD Trans-1-aminocyclopentane-1-3-dicarboxylic acid
for glutamate; The others are **AMPA**, **KAINATE**, **AP4** and **ACPD**. The data concerning these receptors is limited. The **NMDA**-receptor is activated by 2 glutamate and 1 glycine molecules

α-KG α-Ketoglutarate

AMPA α-Amino-3-hydroxy-5-methyl-4-isoxazole proprionic acid

AP4-AR 1,2-Amino-4-Phosphono-butyrate. Believed to be an autoreceptor.

SC Succinate

1.10 Neurotransmitters

γ-Aminobutyric acid (GABA); inhibitory

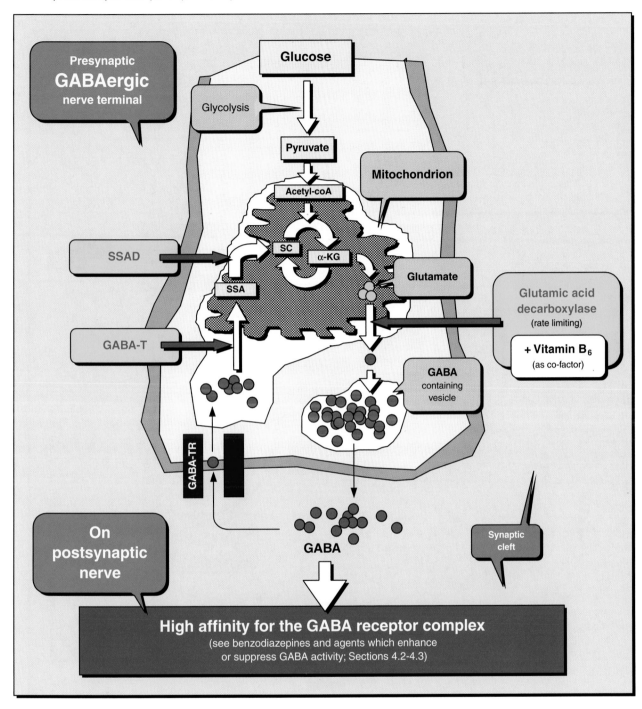

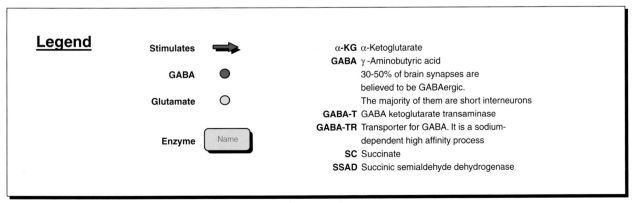

1.11 Vesicular monoamine transporter

Vesicular monoamine transporter type 2 (VMAT2)

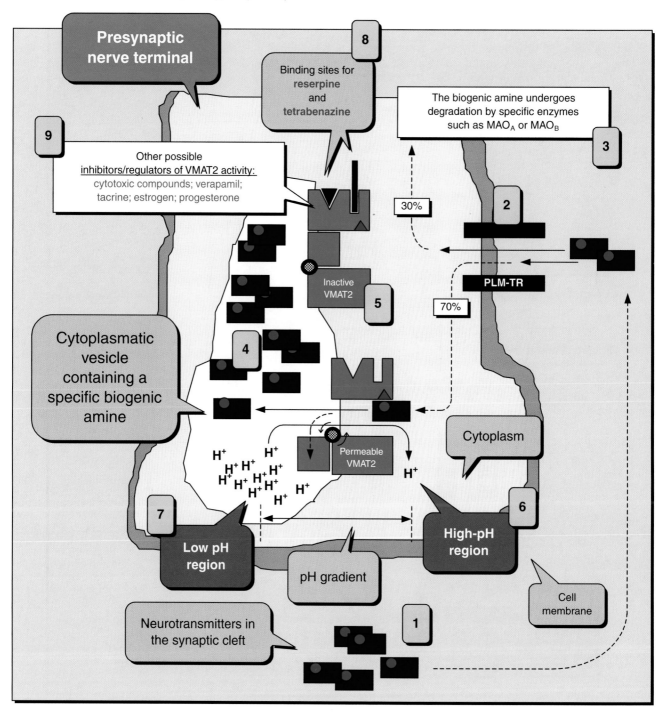

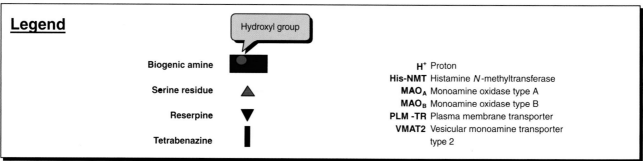

Notes about the numbered items in the scheme

1,2. A neurotransmitter, once released from the presynaptic nerve into the synaptic cleft, can be involved in several processes. Some fraction of the released neurotransmitter can affect the corresponding post- or presynaptic receptors, with a consequent secondary intracellular changes. Following this, it disengages from the specific receptor back into the synaptic cleft, ready for reuptake into the presynaptic nerve, or for further receptor interaction (**1**). Some is then retransported into the presynaptic nerve terminal by the plasma membrane transporter (PLM-TR) (**2**).

3. Once entering the presynaptic nerve terminal, about 30% of the neurotransmitters are metabolized by specific catabolic enzymes. Monoamine oxidase type A (MAO_A) is the main enzyme responsible for metabolizing serotonin, norepinephrine and epinephrine. Monoamine oxidase type B (MAO_B) metabolizes dopamine, and histamine-N-methyltransferase along with MAO_A metabolize histamine. Acetylcholine undergoes an extracellular catabolic process by acetylcholine esterase.

4,5. About 70% of the neurotransmitters uptaken by the PLM-TR are re-stored in intracellular vesicles located in the presynaptic nerve terminal (**4**). Each of these vesicles contains only specific biogenic amine: norepinephrine is accumulated and stored in specific vesicles in adrenergic nerves, serotonin in specific vesicles in serotonergic nerves, etc. All monoamine neurotransmitters are transported from the cytoplasm into their corresponding vesicle by a non-specific transporter termed the vesicular monoamine transporter (VMAT). There are two main isoforms involved in such processes: VMAT1 and VMAT2. VMAT1 has, to date, been located exclusively in adrenal tissue while the VMAT2 is found in brain tissue (**5**), as well as in peripheral and enteric neurons. VMAT2 is located on the membrane of the intracellular storing vesicle, and it transports all biogenic amines (e.g. serotonin, norepinephrine, dopamine, acetylcholine, histamine) with practically equivalent affinity. Regional localization of VMAT2 is consistent with the known monoamine nerve terminal density; highest in the striatum, lateral septum, substantia nigra pars compacta, raphe nuclei and the locus ceruleus. Lower density is evident in the cerebral cortex and in the cerebellum. The VMAT transporter is a protein with 12 transmembrane segments and both of its extremities are located in the cytoplasmatic side.

6,7. The mechanism of VMAT2 action is complex and only partially understood. It is thought that the transport of the biogenic amines is dependent on the pH gradient between the cytoplasm and the intravesicular space. The cytoplasm is a relative high-pH region (**6**) compared with the intravesicular space (low-pH region; pH = 4–5) (**7**). This pH gradient provides an essential driving force for the transport of the biogenic amine from the cytoplasm into the vesicle in exchange for a proton, which is transported in the opposite direction. Some data suggest that a serine residue in the third transmembrane domain of VMAT2 is the most important factor for recognizing the transported biogenic amine by the VMAT2, and that hydroxyl groups on the different biogenic amines serve as substrates that are recognized by the serine residues. Other factors are also likely to be important.

8. The most studied substances that affect the VMAT2 are **reserpine** and **tetrabenazine**. Both inhibit VMAT2 activity with a consequent decrease in biogenic amine transport into storing vesicles. This results in a reduced amount of biogenic amine available for release into the synaptic cleft. **Reserpine** and **tetrabenazine** have different binding sites on the VMAT2 and they are presumed to exert their inhibitory effects on biogenic amine transport via different mechanisms. There is some evidence for the existence of two conformations of VMAT2, binding either **reserpine** or **tetrabenazine**. This means that when **reserpine** (or **tetrabenazine**) binds VMAT2, it inhibits its capacity to uptake monoamines but at the same time prevents the binding of the other antagonist (**tetrabenazine** or **reserpine** respectively). Chronic use of these drugs leads to a relative depletion of amine stores which is why they can cause depressions.

9. Other possible inhibitors of VMAT2 activity are cytotoxic compounds such as **ethidium**, **isometamidium**, **tetraphenyl-phosphonium** and **rhodamine**, as well as agents such as **tacrine**, **verapamil** and the hormones **estrogen** and **progesterone**. The way in which **estrogen** and **progesterone** affect the VMAT2 is unclear, and might be via an indirect action (e.g. reduced VMAT2 gene expression for example).

1.12 Receptor/transporter-mediated reactions
Assumed side-effects

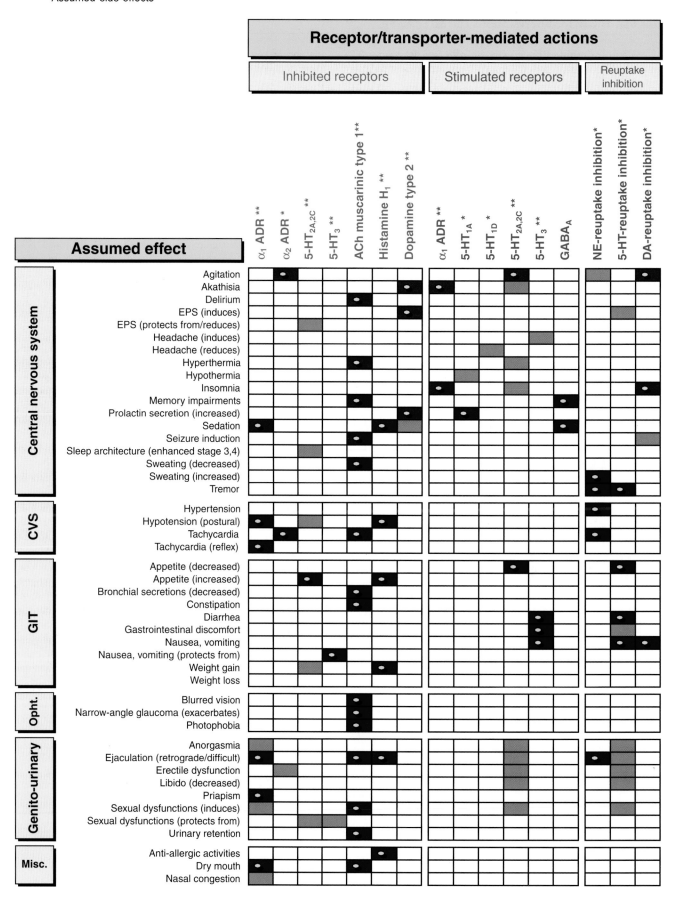

1.13 Receptor-mediated psychiatric symptoms

Assumed roles of specific receptors in major psychiatric syndromes

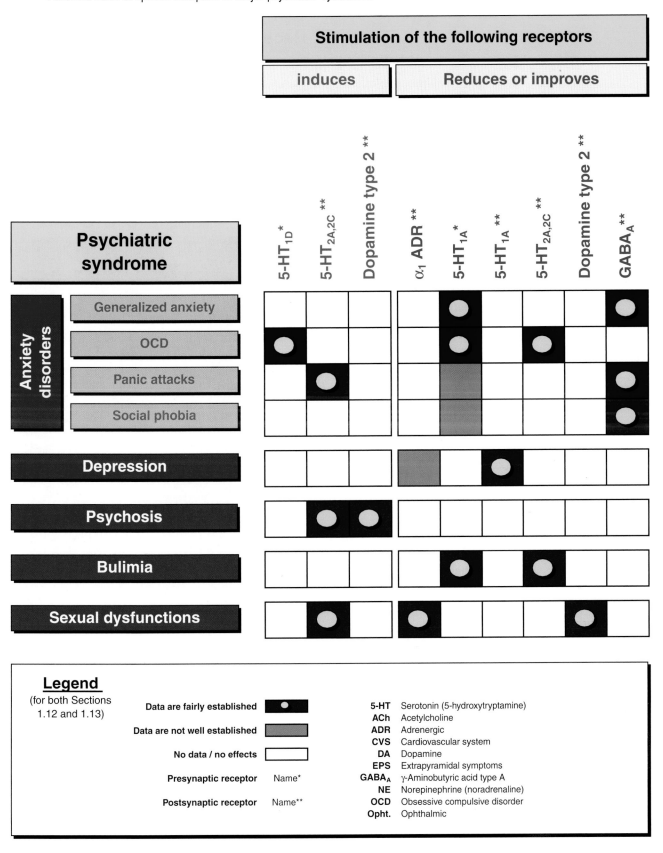

Psychiatric syndrome		Stimulation of the following receptors								
		induces			Reduces or improves					
		5-HT$_{1D}$*	5-HT$_{2A,2C}$**	Dopamine type 2**	α_1 ADR**	5-HT$_{1A}$*	5-HT$_{1A}$**	5-HT$_{2A,2C}$**	Dopamine type 2**	GABA$_A$**
Anxiety disorders	Generalized anxiety					●				●
	OCD	●				●		●		
	Panic attacks		●			▨				●
	Social phobia					▨				●
Depression					▨		●			
Psychosis			●	●						
Bulimia						●		●		
Sexual dysfunctions			●		●				●	

Legend
(for both Sections 1.12 and 1.13)

Data are fairly established	⬛●	5-HT	Serotonin (5-hydroxytryptamine)
		ACh	Acetylcholine
Data are not well established	▨	ADR	Adrenergic
		CVS	Cardiovascular system
No data / no effects	☐	DA	Dopamine
		EPS	Extrapyramidal symptoms
Presynaptic receptor	Name*	GABA$_A$	γ-Aminobutyric acid type A
		NE	Norepinephrine (noradrenaline)
Postsynaptic receptor	Name**	OCD	Obsessive compulsive disorder
		Opht.	Ophthalmic

1.14 Various receptor subtypes

Comparative distribution in different brain regions

Receptor subtype

Brain region

	5-HT 1A	5-HT 1D	5-HT 2A	5-HT 2C	Acetylcholine M₁	Acetylcholine nicotinic	α₁ adrenergic	α₂ adrenergic	AMPA	β adrenergic	Dopamine type 1	Dopamine type 2	Dopamine type 4	GABA A / BDZ type 1	GABA A / BDZ type 2	GABA B	KAINATE	NMDA
Amygdala																		
Caudate																		
Cerebellum																		
Cortex																		
Globus pallidus: lateral																		
Globus pallidus: medial																		
Hippoccampus																		
Hypothalamus																		
Locus ceruleus																		
Nucleus accumbens																		
Putamen																		
Raphe nuclei																		
Red nucleus																		
Substantia nigra - pars compacta																		
Substantia nigra - pars reticulata																		
Subthalamic nucleus																		
Thalamus																		

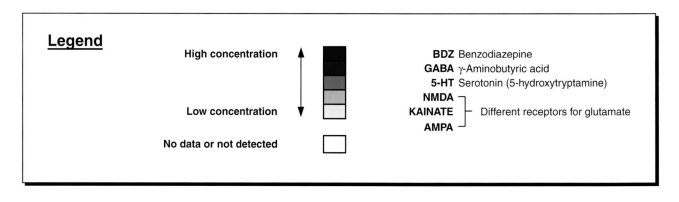

Legend

High concentration ↑

Low concentration ↓

No data or not detected

BDZ Benzodiazepine
GABA γ-Aminobutyric acid
5-HT Serotonin (5-hydroxytryptamine)
NMDA
KAINATE ⎤ Different receptors for glutamate
AMPA

1.15 Specific ligands for various receptor subtypes

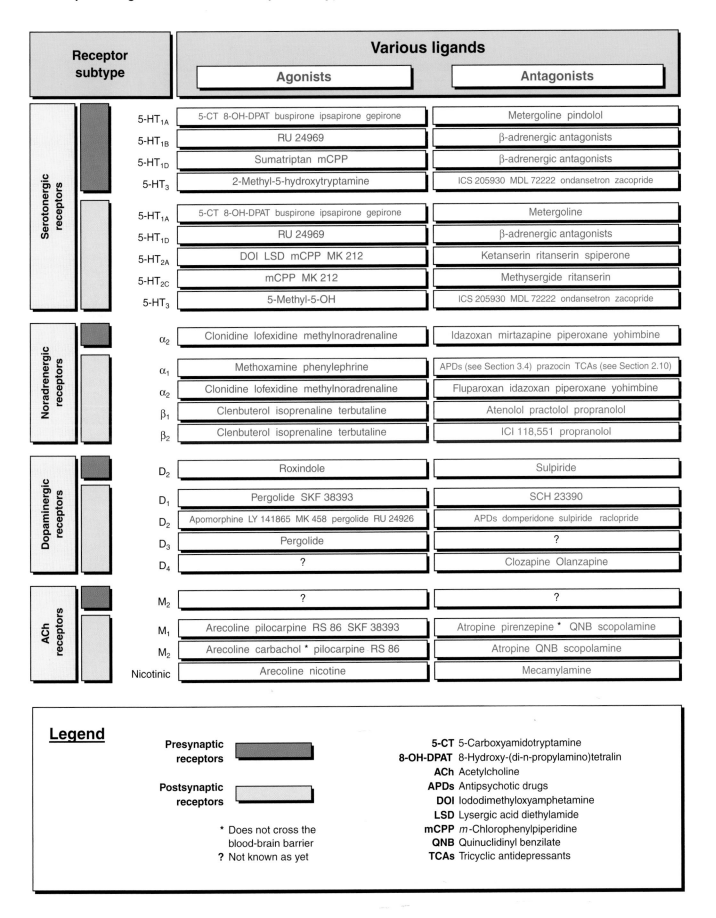

Receptor subtype		Agonists	Antagonists
Serotonergic receptors	5-HT$_{1A}$	5-CT 8-OH-DPAT buspirone ipsapirone gepirone	Metergoline pindolol
	5-HT$_{1B}$	RU 24969	β-adrenergic antagonists
	5-HT$_{1D}$	Sumatriptan mCPP	β-adrenergic antagonists
	5-HT$_3$	2-Methyl-5-hydroxytryptamine	ICS 205930 MDL 72222 ondansetron zacopride
	5-HT$_{1A}$	5-CT 8-OH-DPAT buspirone ipsapirone gepirone	Metergoline
	5-HT$_{1D}$	RU 24969	β-adrenergic antagonists
	5-HT$_{2A}$	DOI LSD mCPP MK 212	Ketanserin ritanserin spiperone
	5-HT$_{2C}$	mCPP MK 212	Methysergide ritanserin
	5-HT$_3$	5-Methyl-5-OH	ICS 205930 MDL 72222 ondansetron zacopride
Noradrenergic receptors	α$_2$	Clonidine lofexidine methylnoradrenaline	Idazoxan mirtazapine piperoxane yohimbine
	α$_1$	Methoxamine phenylephrine	APDs (see Section 3.4) prazocin TCAs (see Section 2.10)
	α$_2$	Clonidine lofexidine methylnoradrenaline	Fluparoxan idazoxan piperoxane yohimbine
	β$_1$	Clenbuterol isoprenaline terbutaline	Atenolol practolol propranolol
	β$_2$	Clenbuterol isoprenaline terbutaline	ICI 118,551 propranolol
Dopaminergic receptors	D$_2$	Roxindole	Sulpiride
	D$_1$	Pergolide SKF 38393	SCH 23390
	D$_2$	Apomorphine LY 141865 MK 458 pergolide RU 24926	APDs domperidone sulpiride raclopride
	D$_3$	Pergolide	?
	D$_4$	?	Clozapine Olanzapine
ACh receptors	M$_2$	?	?
	M$_1$	Arecoline pilocarpine RS 86 SKF 38393	Atropine pirenzepine * QNB scopolamine
	M$_2$	Arecoline carbachol * pilocarpine RS 86	Atropine QNB scopolamine
	Nicotinic	Arecoline nicotine	Mecamylamine

Legend

Presynaptic receptors

Postsynaptic receptors

* Does not cross the blood-brain barrier
? Not known as yet

5-CT 5-Carboxyamidotryptamine
8-OH-DPAT 8-Hydroxy-(di-n-propylamino)tetralin
ACh Acetylcholine
APDs Antipsychotic drugs
DOI Iododimethyloxyamphetamine
LSD Lysergic acid diethylamide
mCPP *m*-Chlorophenylpiperidine
QNB Quinuclidinyl benzilate
TCAs Tricyclic antidepressants

1.16 Drug pharmacokinetics
Principles and major agents affecting the hepatic microsomal enzymes

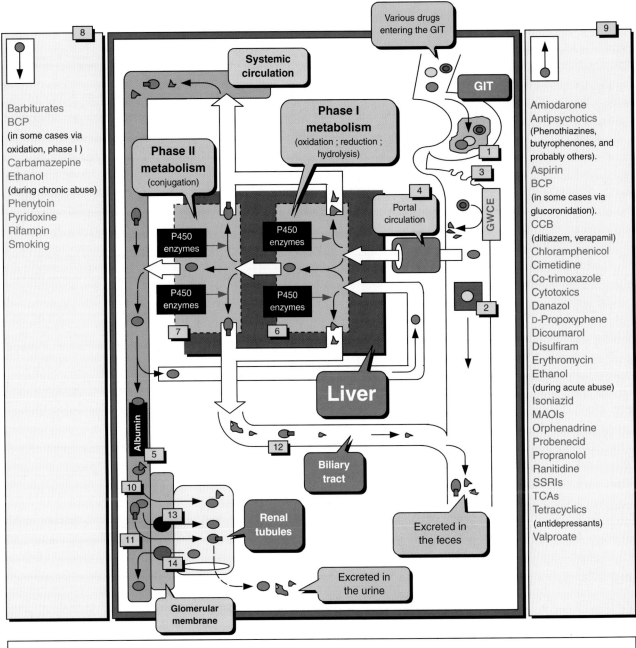

Notes about the numbered items in the scheme

Pharmacokinetic interactions are subdivided into **absorption, distribution, metabolism** and **excretion**.

A. Absorption. Orally administered drugs can undergo a number of interactions or processing while passing through the gastrointestinal tract. Most of these interactions interfere with absorption, mainly affecting the rate and total amount of drug absorbed. The rate of absorption is important if a rapid response is needed. It has little importance if the drug is given chronically or in multiple daily doses. In the case of a drug given in a single dose, with a need for an immediate response, altered absorption might prevent the expected therapeutic response, mainly due to inability to reach appropriate serum level. The most relevant factors governing its absorption are as follows:

a. Gastrointestinal pH (1). Absorption from the gastrointestinal tract (mostly from the proximal parts of the ileum) depends on the solubility of the agent (the more lipid-soluble, the better is the diffusion through the intestinal membrane) and on the electrical charge of the agent (the non-ionized form usually diffuses well through the mucus membrane). The gastrointestinal pH may alter these parameters, with a consequent impairment in the rate of absorption or the total amount of drug absorbed.

b. Adsorption – precipitation. Many agents may form a larger complex - precipitates (**2**) with other particles such as metallic ions (aluminum, bismuth, calcium, iron) while passing via the gastrointestinal tract. These complexes are sometimes poorly absorbed.

c. Gut motility. Some agents can alter gut motility (**3**), which can have opposite effects. Decreased gut motility, or delayed emptying of the stomach, causes the drug to spend more time in the gastrointestinal tract and can either enhance absorption (with drugs for which prolonged time enables better dissolution) or impair it (with drugs that are metabolized by gut wall catabolic enzymes).

B. Distribution. Once absorbed from the gastrointestinal tract, drugs pass through the liver via the portal circulation (**4**) and are metabolized to various extents (the first-pass effect). Following passage through the liver, the drugs are distributed to the tissues by the systemic circulation. The major parameters relevant to alterations in distribution are as follows:

a. The extent of perfusion to a target organ or tissue. Initially, highly perfused tissues (central nervous system, heart, kidneys, liver) exhibit a rapid blood–tissue equilibration of drugs. Then, the drug may be redistributed to less perfused tissues (muscle, adipose). This redistribution can mean that a drug with long elimination half-life might exert a shorter therapeutic effect than a second drug with a shorter elimination half-life due to the former drug's greater affinity for adipose tissue (or a larger volume of distribution).

b. Protein-binding properties. Most drugs are bound to plasma proteins, particularly to albumin (**5**). The bound fraction depends on the concentration of albumin and the number of binding sites for the drug. The bound fraction is pharmacologically inactive. Once some of the free drug has been metabolized, a portion of the bound drug becomes unbound and can exert its pharmacological activities and, at the same time, is subjected to metabolic processing and excretion. Significant drug–drug interactions are associated with drugs that are more than 90% bound to plasma proteins. Although potentially important, protein binding interactions exert minimal effects on clinical response.

C. Metabolism. Metabolism is the biotransformation of a drug to another chemical and a less lipid-soluble form that is more easily excreted by the kidneys. The vast majority of metabolic processing is done by a group of enzymes located in microsomes of the endoplasmatic reticulum of hepatic cells. There are four main types of metabolic reactions: oxidation, reduction, hydrolysis [termed phase I (**6**)] and conjugation [termed phase II (**7**)]. Phase I reactions change the parent compound into a more-polar form, which may be still pharmacologically active, partially active or inactive. Phase I oxidation requires the presence of NADPH and the heme-containing protein cytochrome P450. When a drug is metabolized by phase I reactions it can further be metabolized by phase II, or it can be hydrophilic enough to be eliminated without further metabolism (phase II). Phase II reactions involve the conjugation (coupling) of a drug with a polar substrate such as glucuronic, acetic, sulfuric or an amino acid, which generally leads to total inactivation of the parent compound. Many drugs alter the activities of these metabolic processes by either stimulating some of the catabolic enzymes (**8**) or inhibiting them (**9**), and many drug–drug interactions are due to this.

D. Excretion. Most drugs are excreted via the bile to be finally eliminated in the feces or the urine. Renal excretion is composed of three major steps, each of which can be a target for drug interactions:

a. Glomerular filtration. Small compounds (water, salts, a few drugs, metabolites) diffuse relatively freely through the glomerular membrane into the lumen of the renal tubules (**10**). Larger compounds such as protein-bound drugs (**5**) are not filtered and are retained in the systemic circulation until they become unbound. Conjugated drugs are eliminated either by renal (**11**) or biliary (**12**) excretion.

b. Active tubular secretion. Some drugs are actively excreted (**13**). When two drugs using the same transport mechanism are co-administered, one compound can impair the excretion of the other leading to reduced excretion of one or both of the drugs.

c. Tubular reabsorbption. Following filtration into the renal tubules, some drugs can be actively reabsorbed into the systemic circulation, [especially lipid soluble compounds, (**14**)]. Increased urinary pH enhances the excretion of weak acids and decreases excretion of weak bases, while the opposite happens if the urinary pH is reduced.

1.17 The P450 microsomal enzymes (I)

Various psychotropic substrates of the P450 enzymes

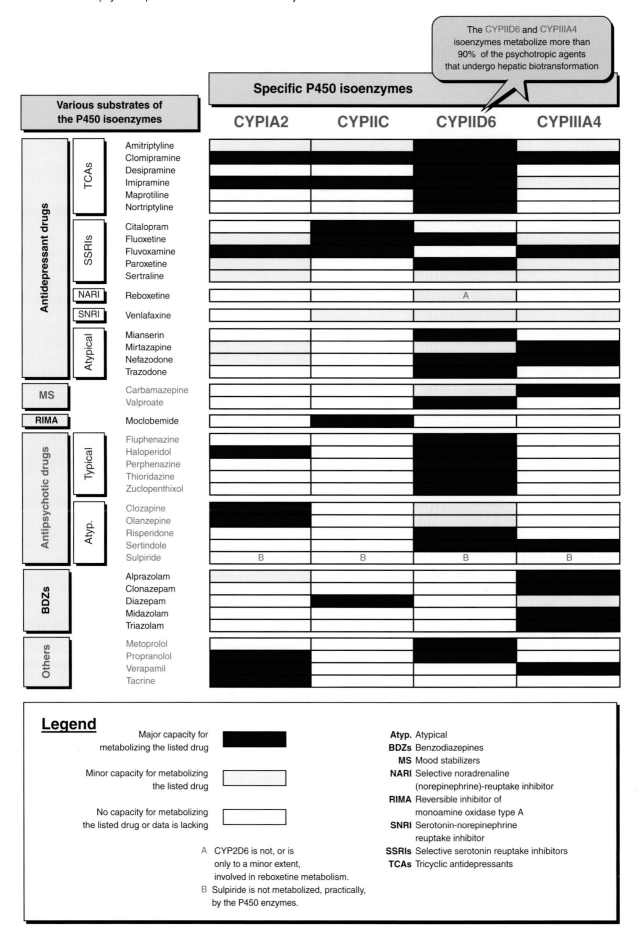

The CYPIID6 and CYPIIIA4 isoenzymes metabolize more than 90% of the psychotropic agents that undergo hepatic biotransformation

Legend

Major capacity for metabolizing the listed drug ▮ (black)

Minor capacity for metabolizing the listed drug ▯ (gray)

No capacity for metabolizing the listed drug or data is lacking ▯ (white)

Atyp. Atypical
BDZs Benzodiazepines
MS Mood stabilizers
NARI Selective noradrenaline (norepinephrine)-reuptake inhibitor
RIMA Reversible inhibitor of monoamine oxidase type A
SNRI Serotonin-norepinephrine reuptake inhibitor
SSRIs Selective serotonin reuptake inhibitors
TCAs Tricyclic antidepressants

A CYP2D6 is not, or is only to a minor extent, involved in reboxetine metabolism.

B Sulpiride is not metabolized, practically, by the P450 enzymes.

1.18 The P450 microsomal enzymes (II)

Psychotropic drugs or compounds known to inhibit or stimulate specific P450 isoenzymes

> The CYPIIIA4 isoenzyme is the most abundant metabolizing isoenzyme in the intestinal mucosa. It usually refered to as 'gut wall metabolism'.

Affected P450 isoenzymes

Various inhibitors of the P450 isoenzymes

		CYPIA2	CYPIIC	CYPIID6	CYPIIIA4
Antidepressant drugs — TCAs	Amitriptyline			black	
	Clomipramine			black	
	Desipramine			black	
SSRIs	Fluoxetine		dark gray		dark gray
	Fluvoxamine	black	light gray	black	light gray
	Paroxetine			black	
	Sertraline		dark gray	dark gray	dark gray
Misc.	Nefazodone				black
	Reboxetine	A	A	A	A
	Venlafaxine	light gray	light gray	light gray	light gray
RIMA	Moclobemide			black	
Typical APDs	Fluphenazine			black	
	Haloperidol			black	
	Perphenazine			black	
	Thioridazine			black	
Others	Diltiazem				black
	Verapamil				black

Various stimulators of the P450 isoenzymes

		CYPIA2	CYPIIC	CYPIID6	CYPIIIA4
Misc.	Carbamazepine				black
	Cigarette smoking *	black			
	Phenobarbital				black

Legend

black	Most potent inhibitor/inducer of a specific CYP isoenzyme
dark gray	Less potent inhibitor of a specific CYP isoenzyme
light gray	Minor inhibitor of a specific CYP isoenzyme
white	No capacity for inhibiting the specific CYP isoenzyme or data is lacking

APDs Antipsychotic drugs
Misc. Miscellaneous
RIMA Reversible inhibitor of monoamine oxidase type A
SSRIs Selective serotonin reuptake inhibitors
TCAs Tricyclic antidepressants

* Through the action of polyaromatic hydrocarbons

A Reboxetine appears to be devoid of any inducing / inhibitory effects on the major hepatic metabolism enzymes

2.1 Antidepressant drugs – supposed mechanism of action (I)

Euthymic state; no treatment

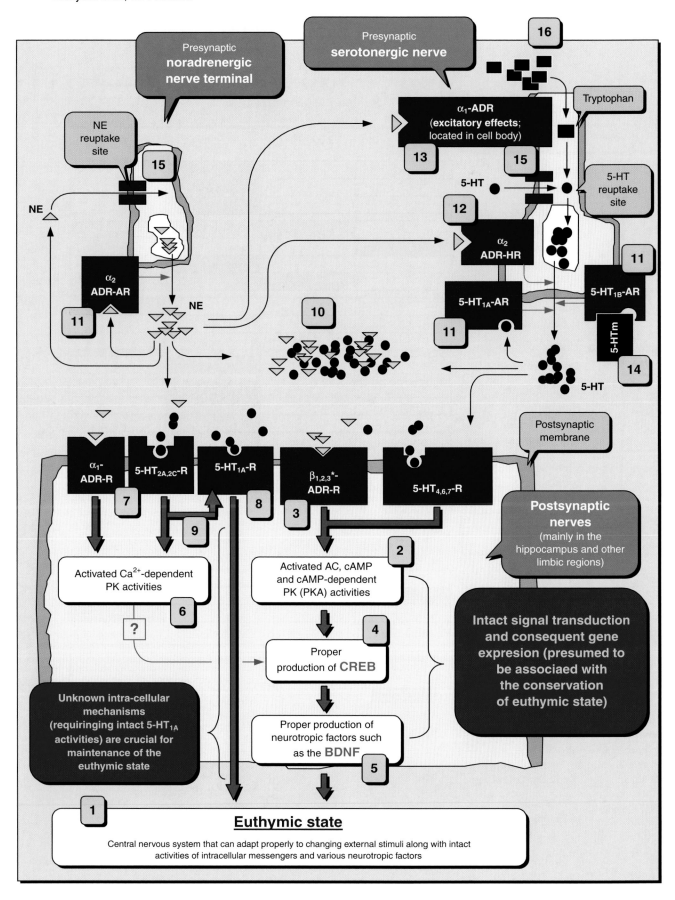

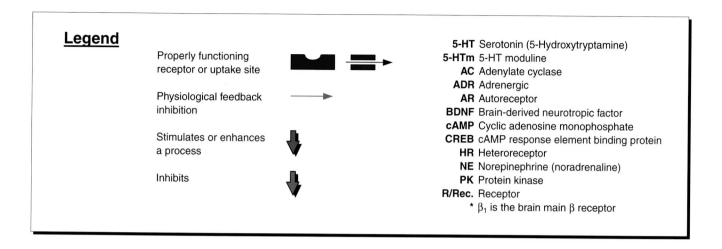

Legend

Properly functioning receptor or uptake site

Physiological feedback inhibition

Stimulates or enhances a process

Inhibits

5-HT Serotonin (5-Hydroxytryptamine)
5-HTm 5-HT moduline
AC Adenylate cyclase
ADR Adrenergic
AR Autoreceptor
BDNF Brain-derived neurotropic factor
cAMP Cyclic adenosine monophosphate
CREB cAMP response element binding protein
HR Heteroreceptor
NE Norepinephrine (noradrenaline)
PK Protein kinase
R/Rec. Receptor
* β_1 is the brain main β receptor

Present knowledge about the biological mechanisms of euthymic mood is limited. Recent advances in understanding signal transduction and consequent cellular processes including gene expression have enriched our insight and pointed the way to new pharmacological agents.

Notes about the numbered items in the scheme

1. Most current data on the biological mechanisms of mood are based on the well-established efficacy of agents that manipulate the adrenergic and serotonergic systems to improve or reduce mood (antidepressants, stimulants and reserpine respectively). Further data show receptor and/or transporter modifications that follow administration of antidepressive drugs and correspond chronologically to the resolution of depression. Practically all antidepressant drugs increase the availability of norepinephrine (NE) and/or serotonin (5-HT) in the synaptic cleft. In many cases (although not in all) this is evident immediately following antidepressant administration, but the initial resolution of the depressive features takes between 10–20 days to develop. This phenomenon made it clear that other mechanisms, presumably gradual and intracellular, are involved in the resolution of depression.

Recent research has emphasized the role of secondary intracellular mechanisms in supporting euthymic state. It is assumed that to maintain normal mood the central nervous system must be able to adapt itself to changing external stimuli through appropriate gene expression and the capacity to modify or maintain certain synaptic connections. This capacity relies, among other things, on the availability of NE and 5-HT for synaptic transmission, on subsequent intact signal transduction and on the succeeding production of certain neurotropic factors. There are many factors under examination, and the best known are brain-derived neurotropic factor (**BDNF**), neurotrophin 3/4/5 (**NT-3/4/5**), nerve growth factor (**NGF**) and clinically neurotropic factor (**CNTF**).

2–7. The production of most neurotropic factors, especially of **BDNF**, is under the control of the adenylate cyclase (AC), cyclic adenosine monophosphate (cAMP) and cAMP-dependent protein kinases (PKs) system (**2**). It is well established that the postsynaptic $\beta_{1,2,3}$ **adrenergic (ADR)** and the **5-HT$_{4,6,7}$ serotonergic** receptors activate the AC–cAMP cascade (**3**). One of the products resulting from this activation of the AC–cAMP cascade is the cAMP response element-binding protein (**CREB**) (**4**) which in turn induces the expression of **BDNF** (**5**). CREB is also presumed to be stimulated by Ca^{2+}-dependent protein kinases (**6**) which are under the control of postsynaptic α_1 ADR and **5-HT$_{2A,2C}$** receptors (**7**).

8,9. There is accumulated evidence (mostly indirect) about the important role of postsynaptic **5-HT$_{1A}$** receptors in modulating mood (**8**). It is presumed that most antidepressant agents that antagonize the postsynaptic **5-HT$_{2A,2C}$** receptors (**trazodone, nefazodone, mianserin, mirtazapine**) exert at least some of their action by enhancing the activities of **5-HT$_{1A}$** receptors (stimulated **5-HT$_{2A,2C}$** receptors are presumed to suppress the **5-HT$_{1A}$** receptors indirectly) (**9**). It is also reported that postsynaptic **5-HT$_{1A}$** agonists (**buspirone** in high doses) have beneficial antidepressive effects.

10–16. All other components of the presynaptic nerve must properly regulate the release and synaptic concentrations of NE and/or 5-HT (**10**) in order to maintain the euthymic state. All the inhibitory auto- or heteroreceptors (**11,12**), the excitatory α_1 ADR receptors located in the presynaptic cell soma or dendrite (**13**), the 5-HT moduline system (**14**; see Section 2.2), and the reuptake mechanisms (**15**) must be intact, along with the availability of important components such as tryptophan (**16**; the precursor of serotonin; see Section 2.2).

2.2 Antidepressant drugs – supposed mechanism of action (II)

Depressive state; no treatment

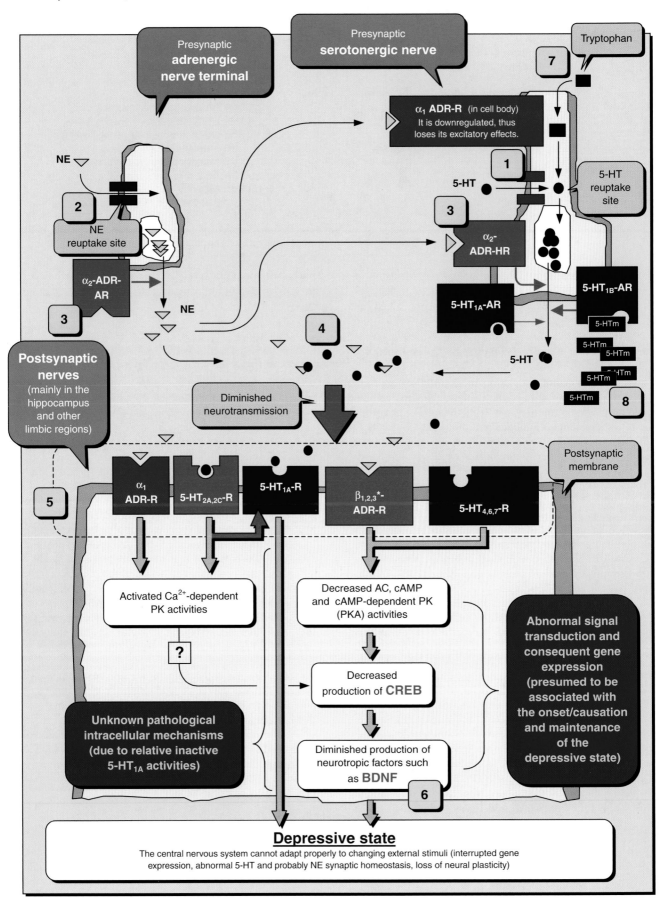

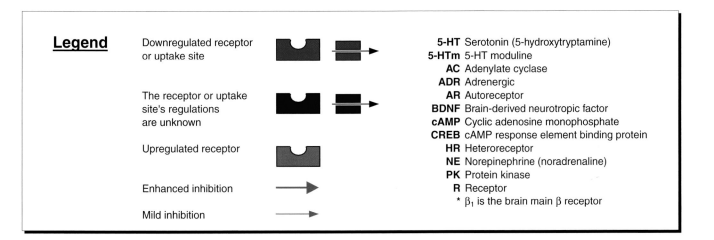

Legend

Downregulated receptor or uptake site		
The receptor or uptake site's regulations are unknown		
Upregulated receptor		
Enhanced inhibition		
Mild inhibition		

5-HT Serotonin (5-hydroxytryptamine)
5-HTm 5-HT moduline
AC Adenylate cyclase
ADR Adrenergic
AR Autoreceptor
BDNF Brain-derived neurotropic factor
cAMP Cyclic adenosine monophosphate
CREB cAMP response element binding protein
HR Heteroreceptor
NE Norepinephrine (noradrenaline)
PK Protein kinase
R Receptor
* β_1 is the brain main β receptor

The primary abnormalities that induce a major depressive episode are unclear, and most of our present knowledge about depression and the effects of antidepressive agents is focused on apparent receptor changes (pre- and post-synaptic) and consequent impairments in signal transduction associated with the administration of antidepressive treatment.

Notes about the numbered items in the scheme

1,2. Dysregulation of the adrenergic and serotonergic systems is thought to be a key factor in the causation or maintenance of an acute depressive state. Some reports demonstrate downregulation of the 5-HT reuptake site (transporter) in untreated depressive episodes (**1**), while the activities of the NE reuptake site (**2**) during acute depression is uncertain.

3,4. Stimulated α_2-**adrenergic** (ADR) receptors suppress the release of NE and 5-HT from presynaptic adrenergic and serotonergic neurons (**3**). α_2-**ADR** receptors may be upregulated during depression, leading to a relative shortage of synaptic NE and 5-HT (**4**).

5. The postsynaptic receptor configurations related to an acute depressive episode are unclear. The $\beta_{1,2,3}$ and **5-HT**$_{2A,2C}$ receptors might be upregulated and the α_1-**ADR** receptors might be downregulated. There are no data about the configuration of the **5-HT**$_{4,6,7}$ or **5-HT**$_{1A}$ receptors. Under normal circumstances the **5-HT**$_{4,6,7}$ and the $\beta_{1,2,3}$-**ADR** receptors stimulate adenylate cyclase (AC) and the production of cyclic adenosine monophosphate (cAMP). The presumed decreased availability of both NE and 5-HT in the synaptic cleft in depressive episodes leads to decreased activities of AC and cAMP. Also under normal conditions, the **5-HT**$_{2A,2C}$ and the α_1-**ADR** receptors indirectly stimulate the Ca^{2+}-dependent protein kinases (PKs). Thus, in untreated depression the Ca^{2+}-dependent PKs are likewise repressed. The important role of intact AC, cAMP, cAMP and Ca^{2+}-dependent PKs along with the postsynaptic **5-HT**$_{1A}$ activities in maintaining a euthymic state is discussed further in Section 2.1.

6. Our understanding of the secondary intracellular changes and global brain abnormalities related to depression is minimal. Some current research efforts are focused on target genes such as brain-derived neurotropic factors (**BDNF**). These factors influence the differentiation and growth of immature neurons and have a major role in the maintenance and vitality of mature nerves along with the possible strengthening of certain synaptic connections in the central nervous system (see Section 2.1). A possible link between **BDNF** and depression is that **BDNF** deficiency is found in the hippocampus of stressed rats, and chronic antidepressant treatment prevents this. Furthermore, the time course for the resolution of a treated depressive episode (about 10–20 days) conforms well with the induction of **CREB** and **BDNF** (unlike the downregulation of β adrenergic and serotonergic receptors, which usually occurs more rapidly). Also, chronic administration of most antidepressive treatments (**tricyclics, selective serotonin reuptake inhibitors, monoamine oxidase inhibitors, electroconvulsive therapy**) is also associated with increased expression of **BDNF** in the hippocampus.

7. Tryptophan is the dietary precursor of serotonin. Depletion of this causes relapse in depressed patients recently made well by antidepressant medication. **Tryptophan** depletion may induce depressive symptoms in both drug-free and in patients on serotonergic treatment.

8. Recent findings in animals have demonstrated the existence of an endogenous ligand termed **5-HT moduline** that is predominantly selective for the presynaptic inhibitory **5-HT**$_{1B}$ autoreceptors, and may be associated with stress-related conditions. An over-active **5-HT moduline** system could inhibit serotonin release from presynaptic nerve terminals, thus leading to depression.

2.3 Antidepressant drugs – supposed mechanism of action (III)

Resolving depressive state; TCA, TeCA and SSRI treatment

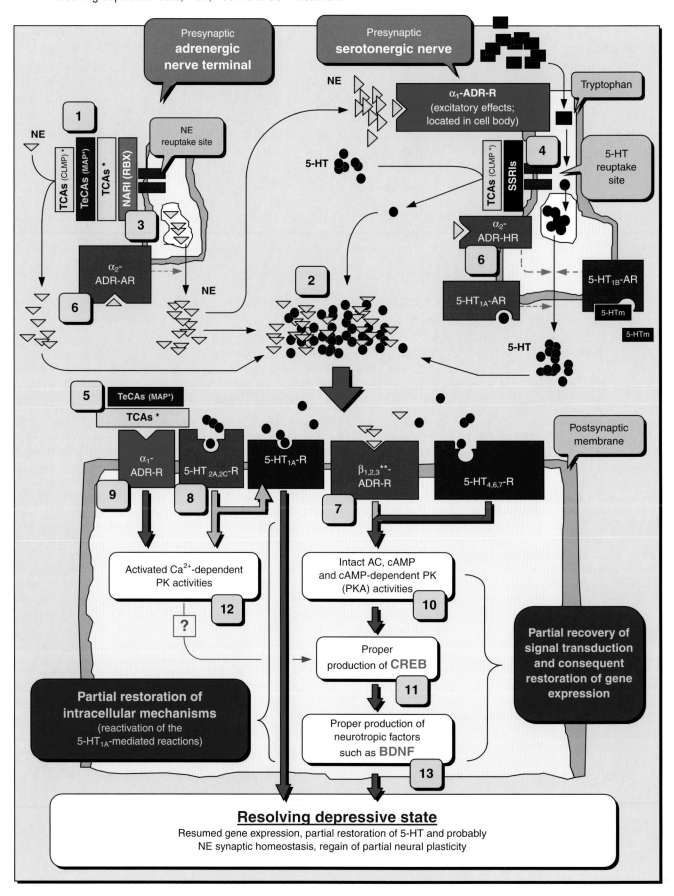

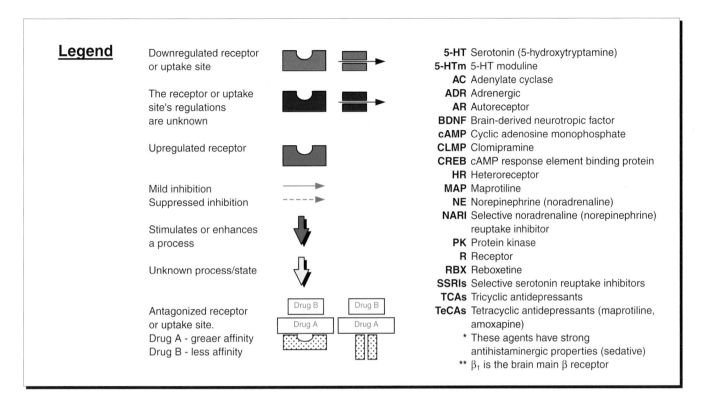

Legend

Downregulated receptor or uptake site

The receptor or uptake site's regulations are unknown

Upregulated receptor

Mild inhibition
Suppressed inhibition

Stimulates or enhances a process

Unknown process/state

Antagonized receptor or uptake site.
Drug A - greaer affinity
Drug B - less affinity

Drug B   Drug B
Drug A   Drug A

5-HT	Serotonin (5-hydroxytryptamine)
5-HTm	5-HT moduline
AC	Adenylate cyclase
ADR	Adrenergic
AR	Autoreceptor
BDNF	Brain-derived neurotropic factor
cAMP	Cyclic adenosine monophosphate
CLMP	Clomipramine
CREB	cAMP response element binding protein
HR	Heteroreceptor
MAP	Maprotiline
NE	Norepinephrine (noradrenaline)
NARI	Selective noradrenaline (norepinephrine) reuptake inhibitor
PK	Protein kinase
R	Receptor
RBX	Reboxetine
SSRIs	Selective serotonin reuptake inhibitors
TCAs	Tricyclic antidepressants
TeCAs	Tetracyclic antidepressants (maprotiline, amoxapine)
*	These agents have strong antihistaminergic properties (sedative)
**	β_1 is the brain main β receptor

The resolution of depression is thought to be due to one or more changes in a complex of secondary intra- and intercellular interactions.

Notes about the numbered items in the scheme

1,2. Tricyclic (**TCAs**) and tetracyclic antidepressants (**TeCAs**) block the reuptake of norepinephrine (NE) into presynaptic nerve terminals (**1**), increasing the amount of NE in the synaptic cleft (**2**).

3. Reboxetine is a new selective noradrenaline-reuptake inhibitor (**NARI**) that shows a high affinity for the norepinephrine transporter and very low affinity for other transporters/receptors.

4. Selective serotonin reuptake inhibitors (**SSRIs**) and some **TCAs** (usually to a much lesser extent) block the reuptake of serotonin (5-HT) into presynaptic nerve terminals (**4**) and thus increase the 5-HT concentration in the synaptic cleft (**2**).

5. Some of the **TCAs** and **TeCAs** can antagonize the postsynaptic α_1-**adrenergic** receptors (**5**). The **SSRIs** are usually the least potent at this activity and their antagonizing effects are clinically insignificant. **Mianserin**, a **TeCA** that many consider to be an atypical agent, antagonizes the postsynaptic **5-HT**$_{2A}$ and **5-HT**$_{2C}$ receptors, thus enhancing the postsynaptic **5-HT**$_{1A}$ receptors. It also blocks the α_2–autoreceptors (see Section 2.4 for further details).

6-9. Several receptor modifications are evident following *chronic* treatment with these antidepressive agents. These correlate, although not exactly, with the time course for the therapeutic effects of the antidepressants. The main ones are the downregulation of presynaptic α_2-**adrenergic** receptors (**6**)

and postsynaptic β_1-**adrenergic** (**7**), and **5-HT**$_{2A.2C}$ (**8**) receptors and the upregulation of postsynaptic α_1-**adrenergic** receptors (**9**).

10–13. These receptor effects of the antidepressants lead to various secondary reactions that terminate the depressive episode. The latest research emphasizes the important antidepressive effects of a cascade of reactions initiated by the stimulation of postsynaptic adrenergic and serotonergic receptors (via the increased availability of NE and 5-HT in the synaptic cleft). Stimulated **5-HT**$_{4.6.7}$ and $\beta_{1.2.3}$-**adrenergic** receptors enhance the activities of adenylate cyclase (AC) and cyclic adenosine monophosphate (cAMP), cAMP-dependent protein kinases (**10**) and cAMP response element binding protein (**CREB**) (**11**). **CREB** is also presumed to be stimulated by Ca^{2+}-dependent protein kinases (**12**), which are indirectly activated by **5-HT**$_{2A.2C}$ and α_1 adrenergic receptors. All these stimulatory effects induce the production of **BDNF** (**13**). The potential role of neurotropic factors and especially **BDNF** in the pathogenesis of depression is discussed in detail in Section 2.1. It is assumed that the final common pathway of antidepressive-agent action is the enhanced activities of factors such as **BDNF** and the subsequent resolution of the depressive state. The possible link between **BDNF** and depression is discussed in an earlier section.

2.4   Antidepressant drugs – supposed mechanism of action (IV)

Resolving depressive state; SNRI and atypical antidepressants treatment

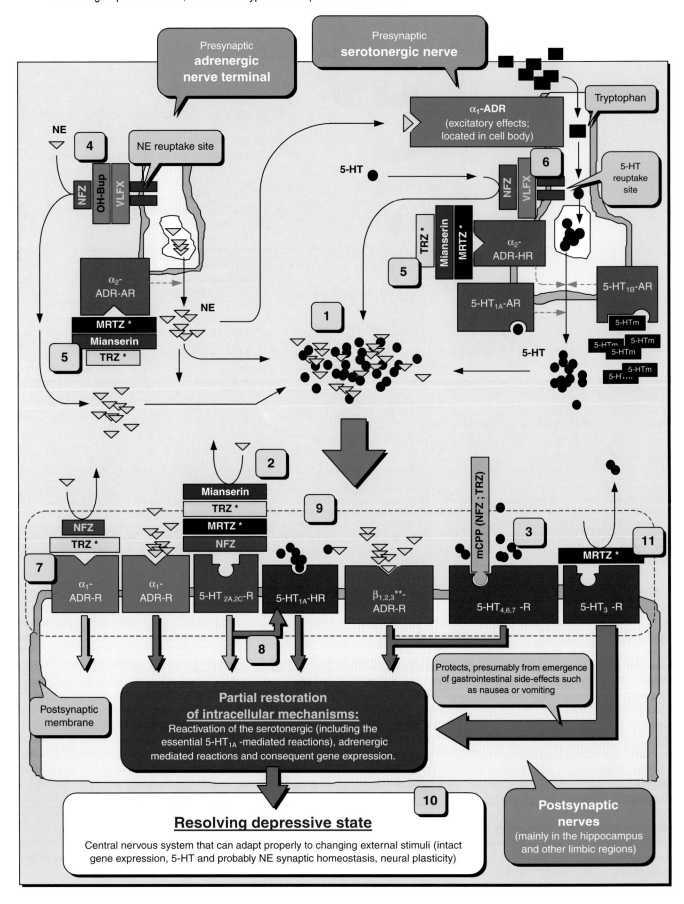

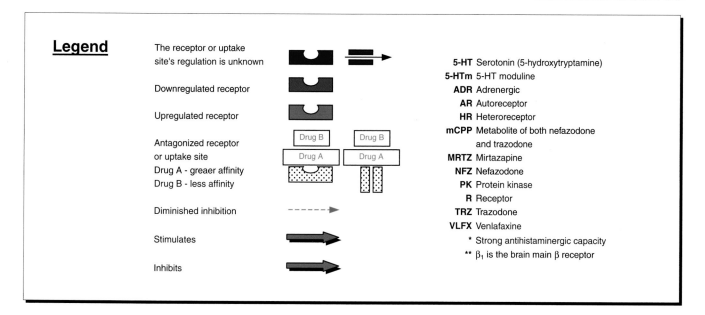

Legend

The receptor or uptake site's regulation is unknown

Downregulated receptor

Upregulated receptor

Antagonized receptor or uptake site
Drug A - greaer affinity
Drug B - less affinity

Diminished inhibition

Stimulates

Inhibits

5-HT Serotonin (5-hydroxytryptamine)
5-HTm 5-HT moduline
ADR Adrenergic
AR Autoreceptor
HR Heteroreceptor
mCPP Metabolite of both nefazodone and trazodone
MRTZ Mirtazapine
NFZ Nefazodone
PK Protein kinase
R Receptor
TRZ Trazodone
VLFX Venlafaxine
  * Strong antihistaminergic capacity
 ** β_1 is the brain main β receptor

All antidepressant drugs manipulate the serotonergic and/or adrenergic systems in a way that enhances the neuronal transmission of serotonin (5-HT) and/or norepinephrine (NE). Tricyclic antidepressants (**TCAs**), tetracyclic antidepressants (**TeCAs**) and selective serotonin reuptake inhibitors (**SSRIs**) exert their effects via reuptake inhibition of either NE or 5-HT. These are direct effects, and it is well established that there are also cross and indirect effects between the NE and the 5-HT systems. For example, the α_2 adrenergic receptor serves as an heteroreceptor that regulates the release of serotonin from presynaptic vesicles, and stimulation of the α_1 adrenergic receptor (located in the soma or dendrites of serotonergic nerves) serves as an excitatory modulator that enhances the firing rate of the serotonergic nerve. Serotonin–norepinephrine reuptake inhibitors (**SNRIs–venlafaxine**) and atypical antidepressant drugs (**AtypADs**) such as **bupropion**, **mianserin**, **mirtazapine**, **nefazodone** and **trazodone**, differ from the other subclasses in two major aspects: firstly, their direct mode of action is not aimed solely at inhibiting the reuptake of NE or 5-HT. The **SNRIs** do exert their effects via reuptake inhibition but they manipulate both the 5-HT and NE systems. The **AtypADs** might have NE or 5-HT reuptake inhibition properties, but they also enhance NE transmission by effecting the presynaptic α_2 adrenergic receptors. Secondly, the **SNRIs** and the **AtypAD** have a unique receptor binding affinity profile that might account for their specific beneficial effects such as **mirtazapine's** relative lack of gastrointestinal adverse effects such as nausea or vomiting (presumably due to its 5-HT$_3$ antagonistic properties) and the relative lack of sexual adverse effects (related mostly to their 5-HT$_{2A,2C}$ antagonistic actions).

Notes about the numbered items in the scheme

1–7. Both **SNRIs** and **AtypADs** manipulate the 5-HT and/or NE systems via presynaptic mechanisms, and the initial result of these actions is the increased availability of 5-HT and NE in the synaptic cleft (**1**). Some of the **AtypADs** also exert postsynaptic effects (mainly 5-HT$_{2A,2C}$ antagonistic actions) which are presumed to influence their therapeutic effects and at the same time, reduce sexual adverse effects (**2**). **Nefazodone** and **trazodone** stimulate, at the same time and via their metabolite mCPP, some serotonergic receptors (**3**). **Bupropion** has some dopamine-reuptake inhibition properties but their clinical significance is probably much less prominent than its NE-reuptake inhibition capacity (via its metabolite **OH-bupropion**) (**4**). There are two main presynaptic actions of **SNRIs** and the **AtypAD**. **Mirtazapine**, **mianserin** and (to a lesser extent) **trazodone** antagonize the presynaptic α_2-adrenergic receptors (**5**), and thus prevent its inhibitory effects on the release of 5-HT and NE into the synaptic cleft. **Venlafaxine** inhibits the reuptake of both NE and 5-HT (**4,6**) as its sole major direct effect. **Nefazodone** has a somewhat different and wider antagonistic profile and it blocks both the postsynaptic 5-HT$_{2A,2C}$ receptors (**2**) and the reuptake of 5-HT and NE into the presynaptic nerve terminals (**4,6**). **Trazodone** also inhibits the α_1-adrenergic receptors (**7**) and this effect probably accounts for

some of its adverse side-effects (postural hypotension, reflex tachycardia, sedation, ejaculatory difficulties and priapism). **Nefazodone** has also some antagonistic effects on the α_1-adrenergic receptor (**7**) but its clinical significance is unclear.
8. The therapeutic role of antagonizing the postsynaptic 5-HT$_{2A,2C}$ receptors is discussed in detail elsewhere (Section 2.1) but it seems that blocking these receptors enhances the activity of the postsynaptic 5-HT$_{1A}$ receptors, which in turn are assumed to play a major role in the antidepressive action.
9. Pre- and postsynaptic receptor modifications (up- or down-regulation) are observed following the chronic administration of both **SNRIs** and **AtypADs**. Their significance is unclear.
10. The final common pathway of the described antidepressant interactions are just beginning to be revealed. They involve and probably necessitate the stimulation of the adenylate cyclase and cyclic adenosine monophsphate (cAMP) systems (via stimulation of postsynaptic 5-HT$_{4,6,7}$ receptors) with a consequent production of certain neurotropic factors (see Section 2.1). It also requires the activation of the serotonergic transmission via postsynaptic 5-HT$_{1A}$ receptors.
11. Mirtazapine antagonizes the postsynaptic 5-HT$_3$ receptors and it seems that this action reduces its capacity to induce gastrointestinal side-effects such as nausea or vomiting.

2.5 Antidepressant drugs – supposed mechanism of action (V)

Resolving depressive state; MAOIs and RIMAs treatment

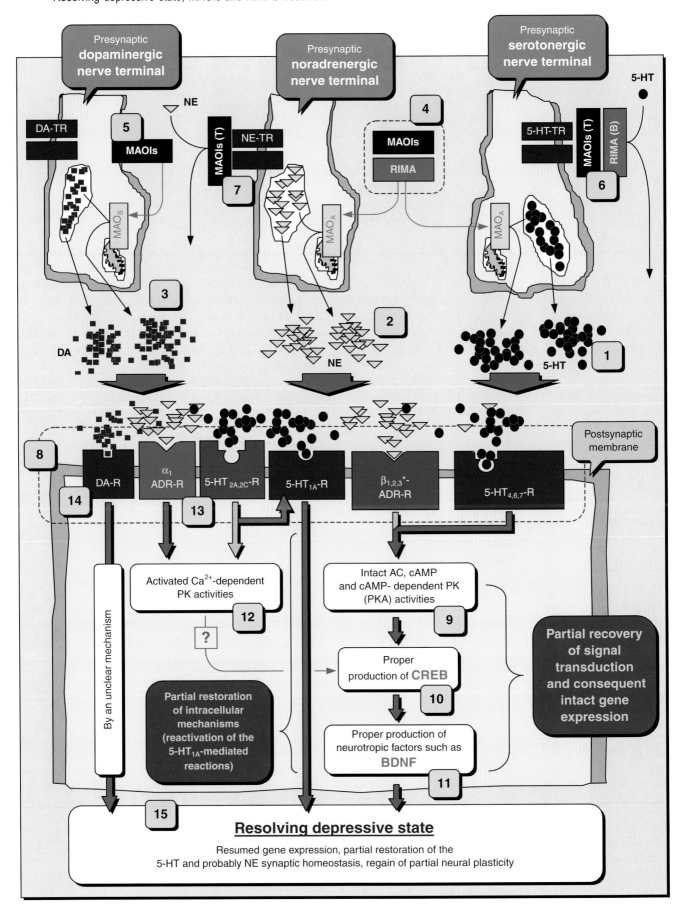

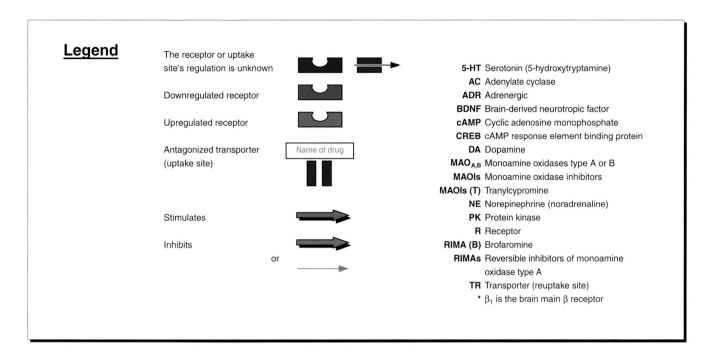

Legend

The receptor or uptake site's regulation is unknown

Downregulated receptor

Upregulated receptor

Antagonized transporter (uptake site)

Name of drug

Stimulates

Inhibits

or

5-HT	Serotonin (5-hydroxytryptamine)
AC	Adenylate cyclase
ADR	Adrenergic
BDNF	Brain-derived neurotropic factor
cAMP	Cyclic adenosine monophosphate
CREB	cAMP response element binding protein
DA	Dopamine
MAO$_{A,B}$	Monoamine oxidases type A or B
MAOIs	Monoamine oxidase inhibitors
MAOIs (T)	Tranylcypromine
NE	Norepinephrine (noradrenaline)
PK	Protein kinase
R	Receptor
RIMA (B)	Brofaromine
RIMAs	Reversible inhibitors of monoamine oxidase type A
TR	Transporter (reuptake site)
*	β_1 is the brain main β receptor

Notes about the numbered items in the scheme

1–3. The monoamine oxidase inhibitors (**MAOIs**) and the reversible inhibitors of monoamine oxidase type A (**RIMAs**) effect both the serotonergic and adrenergic systems, although in a different way than the other antidepressants such as the tricyclics, selective serotonin reuptake inhibitors, etc. The **MAOIs** (**isocarboxazid, phenelzine, tranylcypromine**) are non-reversible inhibitors of the monoamine oxidases (MAOs) type A and B, which are the main metabolizing enzymes of norepinephrine (NE), serotonin (5-HT) and dopamine (DA) respectively. The **RIMAs** (**moclobemide, brofaromine**) are reversible inhibitors, which in clinical doses affect only the MAO type A. Under normal conditions, the MAOs metabolize about 30% of the neurotransmitters uptaken by the plasma transporter into the cytoplasm (the other 70% are stored in vesicles to be released again when needed). When these enzymes are inhibited, the fraction of the neurotransmitters that are stored and available for future release is higher. Therefore, the concentration of 5-HT (**1**), NE (**2**) and DA (**3**) in the synaptic cleft increases.

4–7. All **MAOIs** are relative non-selective and they inhibit the activities of both MAO type A (MAO$_A$) (**4**) and MAO type B (MAO$_B$) (**5**). **Tranylcypromine** has a weak action to block the reuptake of serotonin (**6**) and norepinephrine (**7**) into the presynaptic nerve terminals. **Brofaromine** also blocks the reuptake of serotonin (**6**).

8-13. Pre- and postsynaptic receptor modifications (up- or downregulation) are observed following chronic administration of **MAOIs** and **RIMAs**. The most consistant are the down-

regulation of the 5-HT$_{2A,2C}$ and the $\beta_{1,2,3}$-adrenergic receptors along with the upregulation of the α_1-adrenergic receptors (**8**). The exact role of these modifications is unclear but they presumably influence the initiation of a cascade of reactions, starting with the stimulation of the adenylate cyclase (AC) and cyclic adenosine monophsphate (cAMP) systems (**9**). One of the products resulting from this activation of the AC–cAMP cascade is the cAMP response element binding protein (**CREB**) (**10**), which in turn induces the expression of certain protective neurotropic factors such as **BDNF** (**11**). **CREB** is also presumed to be stimulated by Ca^{2+}-dependent protein kinases (**12**), which are under the control of postsynaptic α_1-**ADR** and **5-HT$_{2A,2C}$** receptors (**13**) (see Section 2.1 for further details).

14. The inhibition of MAO$_B$ increases the availability of DA for synaptic transmission. The antidepressive effects of the increased dopaminergic transmission are unclear and there are mainly indirect data that links the dopaminergic system and depression. One of these is the increased incidence of depression in Parkinson's disease which is a good example of a state of decreased dopaminergic activity. Some research suggests that the antidepressant effects of some antidepressant drugs are due to their enhancement of dopaminergic transmission in limbic structures (nucleus accumbens for example). This effect might be secondary to increased serotonergic transmission; as stimulation of 5-HT serotonergic receptors can enhance dopaminergic activity.

15. The final common pathway of the mentioned processes is the re-establishment of a euthymic state (see Section 2.1).

2.6 Mood stabilizers – lithium

Supposed mechanism of action

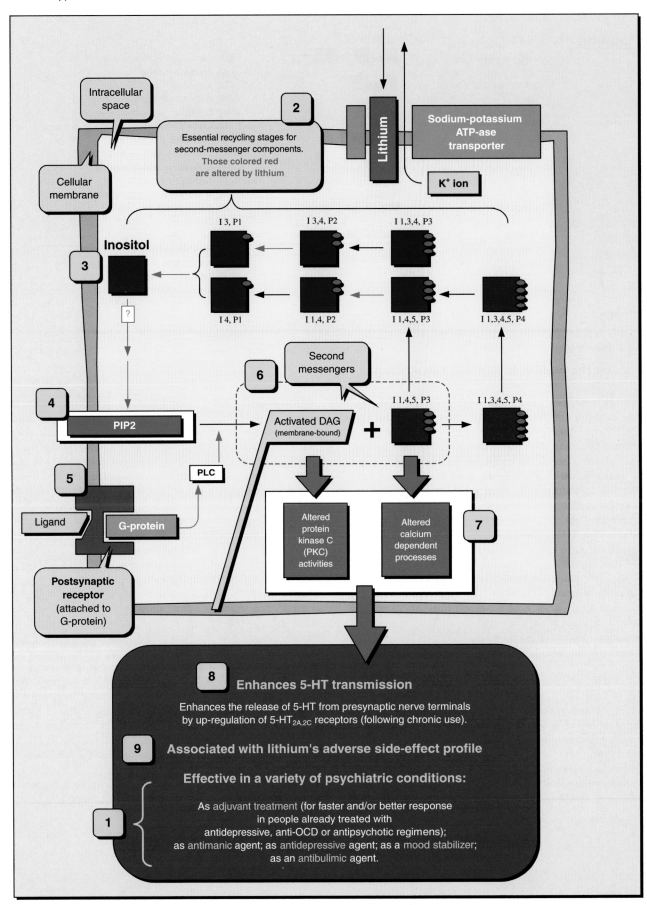

Legend

Induces	⟹	
Stimulates	⟶	
Intracellular reactions or transformations inhibited by lithium	⟶	

5-HT Serotonin (5-hydroxytryptamine)
DAG Diacylglycerol
K⁺ Potassium ion
OCD Obsessive-compulsive disorder
P1,2,3,4 Number of phosphate residues attached to inositol
PIP2 Phosphatidil inositol biphosphate
PLC Phospholipase C

Lithium (Li ; atomic number 3) is one of the group IA alkali metals (like potassium and sodium) and is not normally present in the body. **Lithium** acts predominantly through the PI second-messenger causing alterations in calcium- and protein kinase C-mediated processes. Lithium can also alter the adenylate cyclase (AC) system and this action is probably related to toxic effects. Many enzyme or other calcium-dependent systems may be affected by **lithium**. Calcium-mediated regulation of receptor sensitivity, parathyroid hormone release and proper functioning of the intracelluar microtubule structures are examples of some processes altered by **lithium**.

Notes about the numbered items in the scheme

1. Lithium is one of the most widely used drugs in psychiatry since it exerts beneficial effects in many disorders both as an adjuvant to another treatment modality and as a first-line drug. Interestingly, **lithium's** beneficial effects as an adjuvant drug are apparent only if it is administered to an already pharmacologically treated patient. For example, in cases of unresponsive major depressive disorder, the co-administration of **lithium** to an ongoing antidepressant treatment increases the response rate by up to 50% and, at the same time, it shortens the time for achieving beneficial effects to about 10–14 days. In most cases the response to **lithium** augmentation is either considerable or not at all ('all-or-none' phenomenon). **Lithium** is most efficacious in the treatment of acute manic episodes (beneficial in up to 80% of cases) but good results have been reported in 20–50% of other psychiatric entities, such as maintenance treatment of bipolar I disorder (mood stabilizer), major depression and bulimia. **Lithium** also exerts antiaggressive effects independent of any mood disorder, and can reduce behavioral dyscontrol and self-mutilation in mentally retarded patients.

2–8. Lithium's specific mode of action is not fully established. These are two main theories:

a. Lithium has been found to alter intracellular building stages (**2**) essential for the proper production of inositol (**3**) and consequently phophatidyl inositol biphosphate (PIP2) (**4**). PIP2 itself serves as a substrate for the G-protein-activated phospholipase C (PLC) (**5**), which, when activated, stimulates the production of both diacylglycerol (DAG) and inositol-1,4,5-triphosphate (I 1,4,5 P3) from PIP2. Both DAG and I 1,4,5 P3 are second messengers (**6**) and under normal conditions they regulate the activities of protein kinases and intracellular calcium balance respectively (**7**).

b. Lithium also enhances serotonergic transmission (**8**). It may enhance the uptake of tryptophan (the precursor of 5-HT) into serotonergic nerves, it increases the presynaptic release of serotonin (5-HT) and also upregulates postsynaptic 5-HT_{2A} and 5-HT_{2C} receptors following chronic use. These effects of **lithium** might explain its efficacy in several psychiatric disorders that respond favorably to serotonergic agents (depression, obsessive–compulsive disorder, bulimia, aggression).

9. The most commonly observed adverse side-effects of **lithium** are gastrointestinal (weight gain, nausea, diarrhea), polyuria and polydipsia, fine tremor and hypothyroidism. **Lithium's** side-effect profile is presented in detail in Section 2.14.

2.7 Mood stabilizers – carbamazepine

Supposed mechanism of action

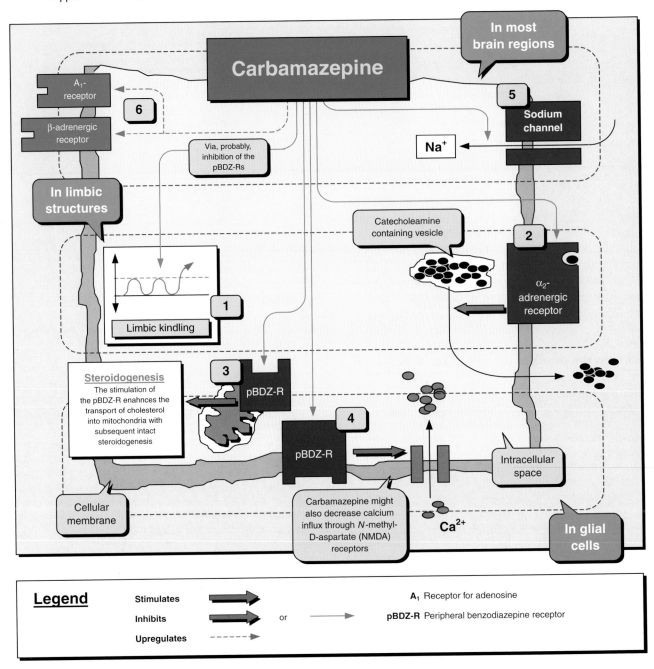

Carbamazepine's mode of action in psychiatric disorders is not totally understood; figure shows some of the more likely explanations.

Notes about the numbered items in the scheme

1. Limbic kindling is the repeated subthreshold stimulation of limbic neurons that over time grow in response, and subsequent action potentials are generated with behavioural changes following. Carbamazepine supresses these activities via, probably, inhibition of peripheral benzodiazepine receptors (pBDZ-R).

2. There is some evidence that carbamazepine may inhibit the α_2-adrenergic receptors. This so causing an increased release of catecholamines into the synaptic cleft.

3. Carbamazepine interferes with glial cell steroidogenesis via inhibition of cholesterol transport into the mitochondria, presumably by carbamazepine's antagonism of the pBDZ-R.

4. Carbamazepine reduces calcium influx into glial cells, by an antagonism of the pBDZ-R.

5. Carbamazepine blocks sodium channels in most brain regions.

6. Carbamazepine has consistantly shown to upregulate β adrenergic and the A_1 receptor for adenosine.

2.8 Mood stabilizers – valproate
Supposed mechanism of action

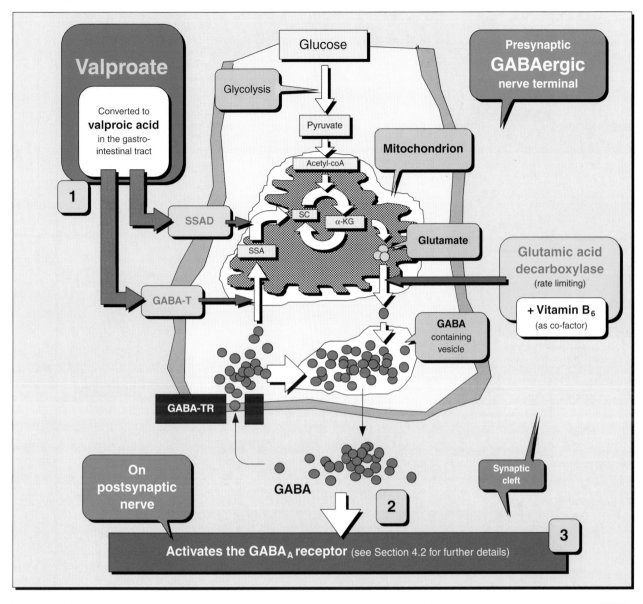

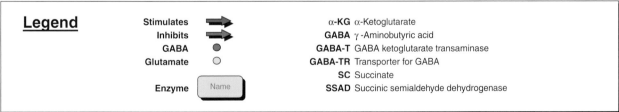

Legend

Stimulates	⟹	**α-KG** α-Ketoglutarate
Inhibits	⟹	**GABA** γ-Aminobutyric acid
GABA	●	**GABA-T** GABA ketoglutarate transaminase
Glutamate	○	**GABA-TR** Transporter for GABA
		SC Succinate
Enzyme	Name	**SSAD** Succinic semialdehyde dehydrogenase

Notes about the numbered items in the scheme

1. Valproic acid inhibits the activities of key catabolic enzymes of GABA (GABA-T and SSAD).
2. Consequently, intracellular GABA concentrations are increased and more GABA is released to the synaptic cleft.

3. When activated, the GABA$_A$ receptor induces a configurational change in an adjunct chloride channel that makes it more permeable for chloride ions. The increased intracellular chloride concentrations hyperpolarize the neuronal membrane, with a concomitant decrease in neuronal excitability.

2.9 Antimanic treatments
Supposed mechanism of action

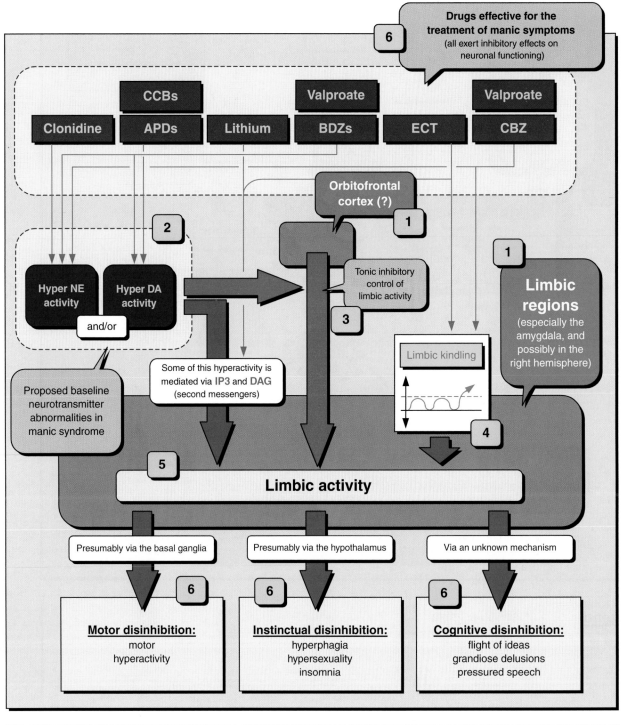

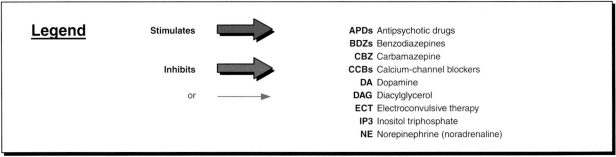

The most common manic symptoms are euphoria, inflated self-esteem, decreased need for sleep, talkativeness, hyperactivity, irritability, low frustration tolerance, emotional lability, pressured speech, flight of ideas, decreased concentration, mood-congruent (e.g. grandiose) delusions, impaired impulse control, excessive involvement in pleasurable activities and impaired judgment. Manic symptoms can be either **primary** (as part of bipolar I disorder), or **secondary** (post-stroke, post-traumatic brain injury, post-electroconvulsive therapy, or induced by drugs such as **antidepressants, amphetamines, cocaine, bromocriptine, cimetidine, corticosteroids** and **disulfiram**.

Notes about the numbered items in the scheme

1,2. The limbic system is presumed to be a major region involved in mania (**1**), since secondary mania is almost always the consequence of lesions involving the orbitofrontal or basotemporal cortex, or subcortical regions of the limbic system. Some of the drugs ameliorating manic symptoms (**antipsychotics, clonidine, calcium channel blockers**) suppress the adrenergic and dopaminergic systems, so hyperactivity of these systems is also implicated in the pathophysiology of manic symptoms (**2**).

3. The orbitofrontal and basotemporal cortex tonically inhibit limbic activity. Hyperadrenergic or hyperdopaminergic states could suppress this tonic inhibitory effect or be related to its failure.

4. Limbic kindling is the process where repeated subthreshold stimulations of limbic neurons lead eventually to generation of an action potential. The theory is based mainly on the effectiveness of **carbamazepine** and **valproic acid** in ameliorating manic symptoms.

5,6. The consequence of the above lead to disinhibition of limbic activity (**5**), and thus the emergence of most typical manic symptoms (**6**).

Treatment effective for manic symptoms

Lithium. An estimated 60–80% of patients with euphoric mania respond well to **lithium** therapy. The enhanced stimulation of adrenergic and dopaminergic receptors in manic states initiates a cascade of intracellular reactions, among them the activation of the second messengers diacylglycerol (DAG) and inositol triphosphate (IP3). **Lithium** exerts its therapeutic effects presumably via inhibiting the intracellular buildup and activities of these second messengers (see Section 2.6), thus opposing the presumed hyperadrenergic and/or hyperdopaminergic activities.

Antipsychotic drugs (APDs). These suppress dopaminergic overactivity. The use of **APDs** for manic symptoms should be restricted to severe cases of agitation, aggressiveness or purely delusional states, since other treatment modalities (e.g. **lithium, carbamazepine, valproate**) are as effective and much safer.

Calcium channel blockers (CCBs). Beneficial effects of **CCBs** are reported in a few case reports. **CCBs** presumably act by decreasing the release of biogenic amines from intracellular vesicles into the synaptic cleft (these are calcium-dependent processes). **CCBs** also have inhibitory effects on tyrosine hydroxylase, the rate limiting enzyme for the synthesis of dopamine, thus decreasing the availability of dopamine for neuronal transmission.

Clonidine. This stimulates the presynaptic α_2 adrenergic autoreceptor (in adrenergic neurons) or heteroreceptor (in serotonergic neurons), and so decreases the release of these neurotransmitters into the synaptic cleft.

Benzodiazepines. These enhance GABAergic activity in many brain regions, thus generating an inhibitory effect on neuronal activity (including on adrenergic and dopaminergic neurons).

Valproate. This enhances GABAergic activity, and thus, like **benzodiazepines**, generates an inhibitory effect on neuronal activities. It may also ameliorate limbic kindling, which might be associated with the induction of manic symptoms.

Carbamazepine. This can reduce manic symptoms via, presumably, a couple of mechanisms:

 a. It might have suppressing effects on limbic kindling.

 b. Carbamazepine has some agonist activity on the presynaptic α_2 receptors, which decreases the release of biogenic amines, especially norepinephrine, into the synaptic cleft. However, this capacity of **carbamazepine** is presumed to have only a negligible effect in clinically used doses.

 c. Carbamazepine decreases sodium influx via a specific action on sodium channels. This leads to an increase in the neuronal threshold for developing an action potential, with a consequent inhibitory effects on neuronal activities in many brain regions.

 d. Carbamazepine decreases calcium influx and alters steroidogenesis via its inhibitory effects on the peripheral benzodiazepine receptors. The role of these actions in suppressing manic symptoms is as yet unclear.

Electroconvulsive therapy (ECT). This is used mainly for severe or life-threatening mania. Its various intra- and intercellular activities are described in detail in Section 8.1. Its inhibitory effects on limbic kindling and on the coupling of various neurotransmitters to their corresponding G-proteins, may explain its suppressing, antimanic properties.

2.10 Antidepressant drugs

Comparative affinity for different receptors/transporters

Receptor or transporter interaction

Class	Generic name	NE reuptake inhibition	5-HT reuptake inhibition	Dopamine reuptake inhibition	H_1 blockade	ACh muscarinic blockade	Dopamine 2 blockade	α_1-ADR blockade	α_2-ADR blockade	$5\text{-}HT_{2A}$ blockade	Approximate NE/5-HT blocking ratio	Approximate 5-HT/NE blocking ratio
TCAs - Tertiary amines	Amitriptyline										4	
	Clomipramine											5
	Doxepin										15	
	Imipramine										2	
TCAs - Secondary amines	Desipramine										85	
	Nortriptyline										35	
	Protriptyline										25	
TeCAs	Amoxapine										25	
	Maprotiline										450	
SSRIs	Citalopram											>400
	Fluoxetine											15
	Fluvoxamine											150
	Paroxetine											>200
	Sertraline											150
NARI	Reboxetine										>150	
SNRI	Venlafaxine											5
Atypical	Bupropion										7	
	Mianserin										**	**
	Mirtazapine										2.5	
	Nefazodone											4
	Trazodone											25

Legend

5-HT Serotonin (5-hydroxytryptamine)
ACh Acetylcholine
ADR Adrenergic receptor
H1 Histamine type 1 receptor
NARI Selective noradrenaline (norepinephrine)-reuptake inhibitor
NE Norepinephrine (noradrenaline)
SNRI Serotonin-norepinephrine reuptake inhibitor
SSRIs Selective serotonin reuptake inhibitors
TCAs Tricyclic antidepressants
TeCAs Tetracyclic antidepressants

Approximate IC_{50} values (nM)*

Lowest (0.1-1)

Highest (>100 000)

* IC_{50} is the concentration of a drug required to occupy
50% of the available receptors. Most data are based on animal studies.
Lower values correspond to higher affinity of the compound to the receptor/transporter.

** Mianserin does not significantly inhibit, in clinically used doses, the uptake of either serotonin or norepinephrine.

2.11 Antidepressant drugs

Subclasses according to presumed mode of therapeutic action

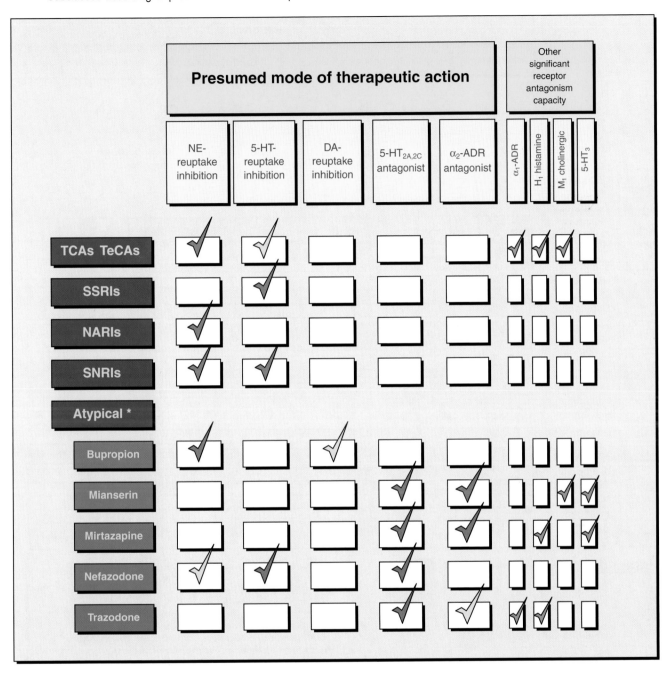

	Presumed mode of therapeutic action					Other significant receptor antagonism capacity			
	NE-reuptake inhibition	5-HT-reuptake inhibition	DA-reuptake inhibition	5-HT$_{2A,2C}$ antagonist	α_2-ADR antagonist	α_1-ADR	H$_1$ histamine	M$_1$ cholinergic	5-HT$_3$
TCAs TeCAs	✓	✓				✓	✓	✓	
SSRIs		✓							
NARIs	✓								
SNRIs	✓	✓							
Atypical *									
Bupropion	✓		✓						
Mianserin				✓	✓			✓	✓
Mirtazapine				✓	✓		✓		✓
Nefazodone	✓	✓		✓					
Trazodone				✓	✓	✓	✓		

Legend

Main mode of action (related to therapeutic action)		**5-HT**	Serotonin (5-hydroxytryptamine)
		ADR	Adrenergic
Minor mode of action (related to therapeutic action)		**Atypical ***	Agents whose main mode of action is not solely via NE- or 5-HT-reuptake inhibition
		DA	Dopamine
		H$_1$	Histamine type 1 receptor
Other clinical significant receptor antagonism capacities (related mainly to side-effect profile)		**M$_1$**	Acetylcholine muscarinic receptor type 1
		NARI	Selective noradrenaline (norepinephrine)-reuptake inhibitor (reboxetine)
		NE	Norepinephrine (noradrenaline)
		SNRI	Serotonin-norepinephrine (noradrenaline)-reuptake inhibitors (venlafaxine)
		SSRIs	Selective serotonin reuptake inhibitors
		TCAs	Tricyclic antidepressants
		TeCAs	Tetracyclic antidepressants

2.12 Antidepressant drugs

Comparative side-effect profile

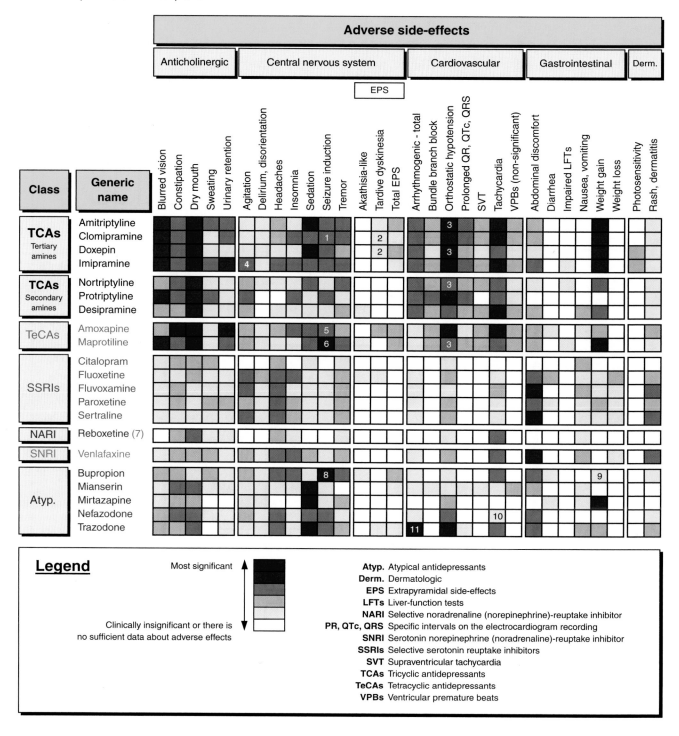

Notes about the numbered items in the scheme

1. Higher incidence if doses > 250 mg / day.

2. Tardive dyskinesia is very rare. It is usually seen when TCAs are given with a combined antipsychotic regimen, so it is difficult to differentiate the exact etiological cause.

3. Can also cause hypertension.

4. Agitation, in the case of imipramine (mainly in panic disorder), could reflect the overstimulation that appears, usually, during the first few days or weeks of treatment.

5. Higher incidence if doses > 300 mg / day.

6. Higher incidence if doses > 225 mg / day.

7. Reboxetine has no anticholinergic properties. Its anticholinergic-like adverse effects may be related to its ability to block the reuptake of norepinephrine in preganglionic neurons (in salivary nucleus for example) and thus to inhibit the parasympathetic output.

8. Higher incidence if doses > 450 mg / day.

9. It could also cause weight loss (rarely).

10. Also decreases heart rate (relatively rare).

11. If the patient suffers from a pre-existing cardiac disorder the frequency of ventricular premature beats could exceed 10%.

2.13 Monoamine oxidase inhibitors

Comparative side-effect profile

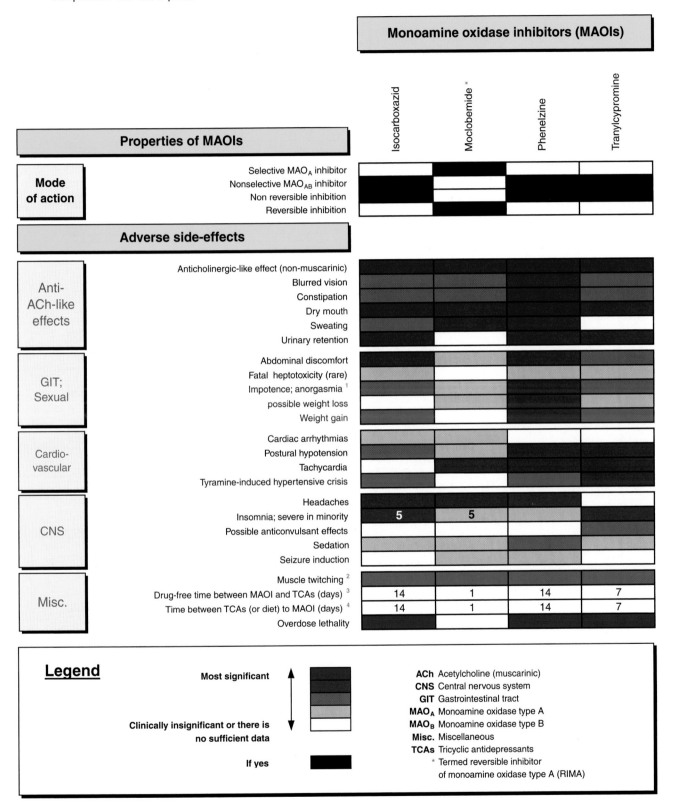

Monoamine oxidase inhibitors (MAOIs)

Properties of MAOIs	Isocarboxazid	Moclobemide *	Phenelzine	Tranylcypromine
Mode of action				
Selective MAO$_A$ inhibitor		■		
Nonselective MAO$_{AB}$ inhibitor	■		■	■
Non reversible inhibition	■		■	■
Reversible inhibition		■		

Adverse side-effects

	Isocarboxazid	Moclobemide	Phenelzine	Tranylcypromine
Anti-ACh-like effects				
Anticholinergic-like effect (non-muscarinic)				
Blurred vision				
Constipation				
Dry mouth				
Sweating				
Urinary retention				
GIT; Sexual				
Abdominal discomfort				
Fatal heptotoxicity (rare)				
Impotence; anorgasmia [1]				
possible weight loss				
Weight gain				
Cardio-vascular				
Cardiac arrhythmias				
Postural hypotension				
Tachycardia				
Tyramine-induced hypertensive crisis				
CNS				
Headaches				
Insomnia; severe in minority	5	5		
Possible anticonvulsant effects				
Sedation				
Seizure induction				
Misc.				
Muscle twitching [2]				
Drug-free time between MAOI and TCAs (days) [3]	14	1	14	7
Time between TCAs (or diet) to MAOI (days) [4]	14	1	14	7
Overdose lethality				

Legend

Most significant ↕ Clinically insignificant or there is no sufficient data

If yes ■

- **ACh** Acetylcholine (muscarinic)
- **CNS** Central nervous system
- **GIT** Gastrointestinal tract
- **MAO$_A$** Monoamine oxidase type A
- **MAO$_B$** Monoamine oxidase type B
- **Misc.** Miscellaneous
- **TCAs** Tricyclic antidepressants
- * Termed reversible inhibitor of monoamine oxidase type A (RIMA)

Notes about the numbered items in the scheme:

1. Sometimes reversible with cyproheptadine.
2. May respond to supplementation of pyridoxine (vitamin B$_6$).
3. Following stopage of MAOIs and before starting tricyclic antidepressants.

4. Following stopage of tricyclic antidepressant regimen, or time needed to elapse before starting MAOIs following consumption of tyramine-rich diet.
5. Especially when given in the evening.

2.14 Mood stabilizers

Comparative side-effect profile

Side effects	CBZ	Lithium	Valproate
Neurologic			
Ataxia	■	1	■
Cognitive impairments (non-specific)	■		
Diplopia	■		
Dizziness	■		
Dysarthria		1	
EPS			
Impaired motor functioning	■	■	
Memory impairments	■	■	
Nystagmus	■		
Parkinsonism		1	
Sedation	■		2
Tolerance to drug effect	■	3 ??	
Tremor		4	5
Hematologic			
Agranulocytosis	6		
Aplastic anemia	7		
Leukocytosis		8	
Leukopenia	■		
Other hematological abnormalities	9		
Thrombocytopenia			10
Gastro-intestinal			
Alkaline phosphatase, SGPT, SGOT (elevated)	■		11
Diarrhea		12	
Hepatitis (cholestatic)	13		
Hepatotoxicity	14		15
Nausea or vomiting	■	16	17
Pancreatitis			18
Dermatologic			
Acne, peritibial ulcers		19	
Alopecia		■	20
Dermatitis (exfoliative)	21		
Psoriasis (worsening or new)		22	
Rash (benign)	21		
SLE-like , Steven Johnson syndromes	21		
Teratogenic			
Cranial facial defects (CFD)	23		
Developmental delay (DD)	23		
Ebstein's anomaly		24	
Fingernail hypoplasia (FH)	23		
Spina bifida	25		
CVS			
AV block		26	
Hypokalemic-like syndrome		27	
Miscellaneous			
Excreted in breast milk		28	
Intracranial pressure (increased ; benign)		■	
Kidney damage		29	
Polyuria		30	
Sodium levels: significant hyponatremia	31		
Sodium levels: insignificant hyopnatremia	32		
Thyroid functions (impaired)		33	
Weight gain		34	■

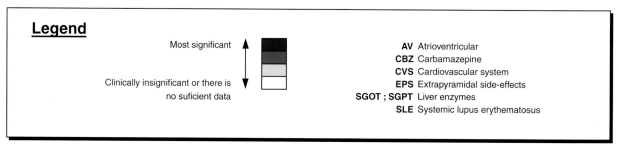

Legend

Most significant ↑ ■

↓ Clinically insignificant or there is no suficient data

AV Atrioventricular
CBZ Carbamazepine
CVS Cardiovascular system
EPS Extrapyramidal side-effects
SGOT ; SGPT Liver enzymes
SLE Systemic lupus erythematosus

Notes about the numbered items in the scheme

1. Ataxia and dysarthria are usually due to intoxication.

2. About 50% suffer from some degree initially.

3. Tolerance is controversial, but stoppage of lithium can cause 'discontinuation refractoriness', which means that the patients become unresponsive to other treatments including lithium, following a 'drug holiday'.

4. Responds well to β-adrenergic blockers.

5. Responds well to β-adrenergic blockers.

6. In about 5/10000 treated patients.

7. In about 2/10000 treated patients.

8. It is very common and practically always benign. It almost never exceeds 15000.

9. Transient decrease in polymorphonuclears (PMN) count is found in about 10% of patients. Persistent decrease in PMN count is found in 2% of patients, while 2% suffer from thrombocytopenia, and about 5% from decreased red blood cell count.

10. Could be with a normal count along with dysfunctional platelets.

11. In 5–40%. It is persistent and asymptomatic. It usually resolves following discontinuation of **valproate**.

12. If diarrhea or abdominal discomfort occurs, try to administer **lithium** after the meals. Give smaller doses and more often, try slow-release form or lower dose.

13. It is very rare and idiosyncratic. Can be fatal.

14. Idiosyncratic. Early in treatment. 25% fatal.

15. The hepatotoxicity of **valproate** can be fatal. Is always in the young (2–10 years), on multiple anticonvulsants and with another neurological disorder. It is rare (incidence is about 1/120000).

16. It is usually dose-related and transient. Can be reduced by administering with meals.

17. Nausea is evident in about 25% of treated patients and vomiting in about 5% and it is usually experienced during the first month of treatment (generally transient).

18. It occurs almost always during the first 6 months of treatment. It is rare, but fatal.

19. If acne is treated with tetracycline antibiotics, **lithium** retention may occur (with consequent toxicity).

20. It might occur in about 5–10% of treated patients. It is probably unrelated to genetic predisposition.

21. Benign rashes appear in about 3% of treated patients. Starting with low doses and increasing slowly can minimise the risk.

22. **Lithium** can cause an exacerbation in known psoriatic patients or can provoke psoriatic episodes in people not known to suffer from psoriasis. Psoriasis is usually refractory while on **lithium**, so, if on **lithium**, consider switching to **carbamazepine**.

23. Cranial facial defects (most are minor) are observed in up to 10% of newborns. Fingernail hyperplasia might occur in up to 25% and developmental delay in about 20% of newborns.

24. Early studies suggested an incidence of major congenital malformation in about 10% of **lithium** treated mothers. The present data suggests a much lower incidence.

25. Occurs in up to 1% of newborns.

26. **Lithium** depresses the endogenous pacemaker activity, causing, possibly, sinus arrhythmias and syncope. **Lithium** is contraindicated in Sick Sinus Syndrome.

27. **Lithium** displaces intracellular potassium, causing T-wave inversion or flattening.

28. The concentration in the milk is about 50% of its plasma level.

29. Pathological, nonspecific renal interstitial fibrosis is observed in some chronic **lithium** users. The clinical significance of this finding is considered negligible.

30. **Lithium** reduces the ability to concentrate urine due to antagonism of the antidiuretic hormone (ADH). Polyuria occurs in about 25–35% of patients and is not always reversible when **lithum** is discontinued.

31. About 20% of patients develop hyponatremia, which is practically always mild. In these cases the plasma levels of sodium do not decrease beyond 130 mEq/l.

32. Most of the patients suffer from a minimal (average 2 mEq/l) and transient decrease in plasma sodium levels (relative to their baseline).

33. **Lithium** causes clinical and/or laboratory hypothyroidism in 7–9% of treated patients. The plasma levels of thyroid stimulating hormone (TSH) are increased in up to 30% of treated patients. There is also an abnormal thyroid releasing hormone (TRH) response in about 50% of patients on **lithium** therapy.

34. It is due to a poorly understood effect on carbohydrate metabolism and/or due to increased edema. Appetite is sometimes reduced on **lithium**.

3.1 Antipsychotic drugs – supposed mechanism of action (I)

Schizophreniform psychosis; no treatment

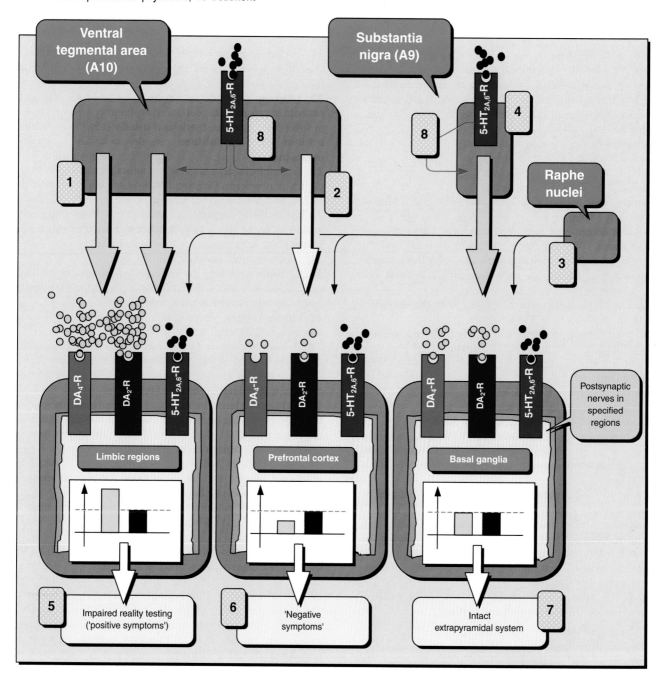

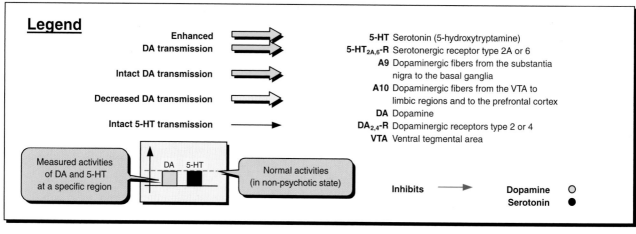

The term 'schizophreniform psychosis' refers to the clinical symptoms observed during the chronic course or as part of the psychotic exacerbation of schizophrenia. There are many possible etiological factors in schizophrenia including genetic components, infectious origins, environmental factors, abnormal autoimmune responses, socio-economic status, seasonal modifications and neurotransmitter abnormalities. Among these, some of the hypothesized neurotransmitter abnormalities (especially the overactive dopamine hypothesis) are widely accepted as directly inducing or at least mediating certain symptoms. There are four major empirical observations concerning the role of abnormal neurotransmitter functioning in schizophrenia:

1. Evidence of dopaminergic (DA) overactivity

The most widely accepted and consistant abnormality relies mainly on the following findings:

a. Psychotic symptoms, indistinguishable from the characteristic symptoms found in schizophrenia, can be induced by the use of dopaminergic agents such as **amphetamines**, **bromocriptine**, **cocaine**, **L-dopa** and **phencyclidine (PCP)**.

b. The efficacy of almost all antipsychotic drugs (**APDs**) has been found to be correlated with their ability to antagonize dopamine receptors.

c. The plasma levels of homovanillic acid (HVA), a metabolite of dopamine, are correlated with the severity of the psychotic symptoms, and with the consequent response to **APD** treatment.

2. Possible serotonergic (5-HT) overactivity

5-HT involvement in schizophrenia and other psychotic disorders is based on the following:

a. Psychotic symptoms (mainly hallucinations) can be induced by the administration of the partial 5-HT agonist lysergic acid diethylamide (LSD).

b. The beneficial role of the **atypical APDs** in ameliorating psychotic symptoms. These agents and especially **clozapine**, have been proved superior to typical antipsychotic drugs in treatment-resistant schizophrenic patients. Many possible factors might explain **clozapine's** enhanced efficacy but its serotonergic antagonism (along with its dopamine inhibition properties) is one of the most widely accepted.

3. α_1-adrenergic overactivity

This is based on few studies that suggested that the therapeutic effects of several **APDs** are associated with their antagonistic activities at adrenergic receptors, and with findings of increased cerebral spinal fluid norepinephrine levels during an acute relapse of psychotic episodes.

This possibility is further supported by several studies that found that a chronic use of **APDs** can decrease the norepinephrine firing rate from the locus ceruleus.

4. γ-Aminobutyric acid (GABA) hypoactivity

GABAergic neurons are inhibitory and a loss of these inhibitory effects can produce, at least in part, the overactivity seen with other neurotransmitter systems (dopaminergic, serotonergic, and adrenergic). Some findings, mainly the loss of GABAergic neurons in the hippocampus of schizophrenic patients, are consistent with such a notion. Furthermore, addition of benzodiazepines to **APDs** may augment their therapeutic activity.

Notes about the numbered items in the scheme

1–3. The presumed neurotransmitter abnormalities are: enhanced dopaminergic transmission in the mesolimbic pathway (from the VTA to limbic regions) (**1**) and the decreased dopaminergic transmission in the mesocortical pathway (from the VTA to the prefrontal cortex) (**2**). At the same time, the serotonergic transmission from the raphe nuclei to these regions is unaltered (**3**).

4. The dopaminergic transmission in the nigro-striatal pathway (from the substantia nigra to the basal ganglia) is unaffected. Extrapyramidal side-effects (EPS) are a consequence of inhibited dopaminergic transmission in these regions.

5. The clinical consequences of increased dopaminergic activity in limbic areas are positive psychotic symptoms (delusions, hallucinations, bizarre behavior, thought disorder).

6. The decreased dopaminergic activity in the prefrontal cortex is thought to induce the characteristic negative symptoms (affective flattening, anhedonia, avolition, alogia, asociality).

7. The extrapyramidal system is unaltered by the primary pathological mechanisms that induce the typical schizophreniform psychosis and there are no evident EPS.

8. Postsynaptic 5-HT_{2A} and 5-HT_6 receptors are also located on the soma and dendrites of the dopaminergic pathways originating from the VTA (**1,2**) or the substantia nigra (**4**). Under normal circumstances when these receptors are stimulated by serotonin they exert inhibitory effects on the firing rate of these dopaminergic neurons.

3.2 Antipsychotic drugs – supposed mechanism of action (II)
Schizophreniform psychosis; treatment with typical antipsychotic drugs

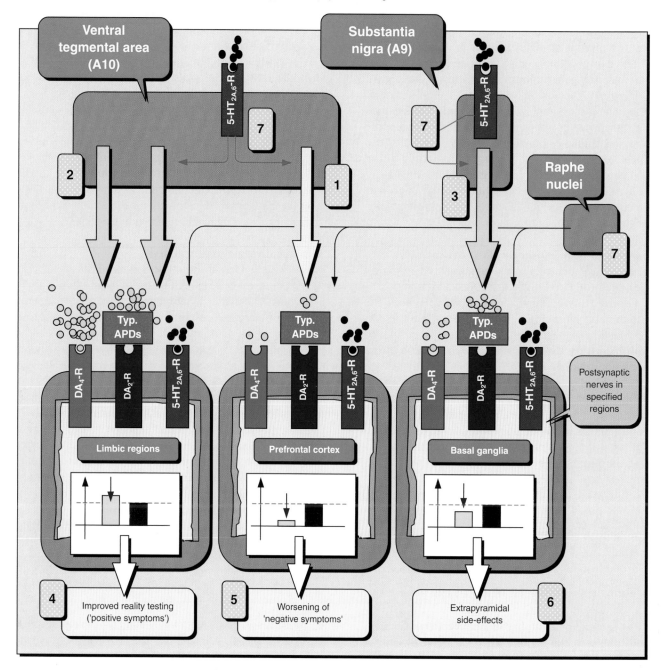

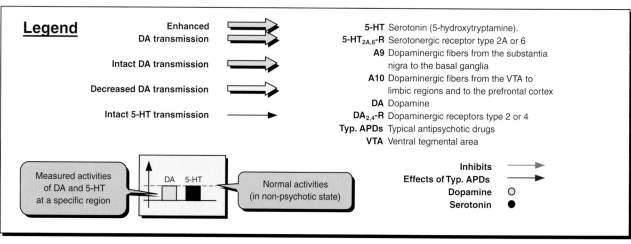

Typical antipsychotic drugs (**APDs**) are believed to work via antagonizing dopamine receptors. The clinical potency is closely related with the drugs' affinity for D_2 dopamine receptors. Although the antagonism of the D_2 receptors takes place almost immediately, it takes a few weeks for the amelioration of the psychotic symptoms to occur, implying a secondary mechanism. **APDs** are usually divided into 'typical agents' (also termed neuroleptics) and 'atypical agents'. Virtually all **APDs** are non-selective. They possess a wide range of receptor-antagonizing capacities, particularly dopaminergic, adrenergic, serotonergic, cholinergic and histaminergic. Most of the neurological and endocrinological adverse side-effects associated with the use of **APDs** can usually be related to their antagonistic effects at these receptors.

Many different **typical APDs** are in use (see the following sections); and practically all have a high affinity for D_2 dopamine receptors. PET scan studies have shown that therapeutic effects are evident if more than 70% of D_2 receptors are bound with an **APD**. Many **APDs** have some affinity for serotonergic (5-HT), α_1-adrenergic, cholinergic and/or histaminergic receptors. All typical **APDs** are equally efficacious, although they exert their maximal antipsychotic effects in various doses (different potency). Hence, **APDs** are further divided as to their potency – high, intermediate and low-potency agents and – for convenience, they are usually related to a **chlorpromazine** equivalence of 100 mg.

Notes about the numbered items in the scheme

1–3. All typical **APDs** block (at least to some extent) all dopamine receptors except **sulpiride** which is relatively selective for D_2. All typical **APDs** affect all major dopaminergic pathways. The major dopaminergic pathways which are most relevant to schizophrenia and **APDs** treatment are as follows:

A. Mesolimbic and mesocortical. These are dopaminergic neurons that project from the VTA to frontal and other cortical areas (**1**) and to limbic structures such as the nucleus accumbens, amygdala, and the olfactory tubercle (**2**).

B. Nigrostriatal. These are dopaminergic neurons that project from the substantia nigra (pars compacta ; A9) to the basal ganglia (caudate nucleus, putamen and globus pallidus) (**3**). Extrapyramidal side-effects are mostly related to the antagonistic effects of **APDs** on this dopaminergic pathway.

C. Tuberoinfundibular (not illustrated in the scheme). These are dopaminergic projections from the posterior hypothalamus to the median eminence and the posterior and intermediate lobes of the pituitary. Prolactin secretion is enhanced following this blockade, since dopamine inhibits prolactin secretion.

4. At the mesolimbic pathway, typical **APDs** block mainly the D_2 component, whereas atypical **APDs** like **clozapine** block other dopamine receptors (D_4 for example) so perhaps yielding better efficacy (in treatment-resistant populations; see next section). The D_2 blockade induces a subsequent improvement, of 'positive' psychotic symptoms (delusions, hallucinations, bizarre behavior, thought disorder).

5. Decreased dopaminergic transmission in the mesocortical pathway might induce 'negative' symptoms (affective flattening, anhedonia, avolition, alogia, asociality). Typical **APDs** further decrease these dopaminergic activities and so potentially worsen these symptoms.

6. Typical **APDs** decrease dopaminergic transmission in the nigro-striatal pathway. Normal functioning of the extrapyramidal system relies on intact dopaminergic and associated cholinergic (see section 6.1) activities in this pathway. Hence, extrapyramidal side-effects (EPS) are induced especially by high-potency agents (significant D_2 blockade without concomitant anticholinergic capacity). The main EPS are as follows:

A. Dystonia. This occurs usually during the first few hours or days of treatment to about 10% of patients. Risk factors associated with dystonia are: men; age < 40 years; high-potency antipsychotic agents and intramuscular administration. Dystonic reactions are presumed to be the consequence of dopaminergic hyperactivity in the basal ganglia, which occurs when central nervous system levels of the antipsychotic agent begins to fall between doses (see Section 6.1).

B. Parkinsonism. This usually occurs during the first 3 months of treatment, and affects up to 10% of treated patients. It is characterized by muscle stiffness (lead pipe or cogwheel rigidity), shuffling gait, stooped posture, drooling, regular and coarse tremor, bradykinesia, and masked face. The associated risk factors are: women (twice as common as in men) ; age > 40 years; and high-potency antipsychotic agents (without significant anticholinergic properties).

C. Akathisia. This is a subjective feeling of muscular discomfort which leads to restless pacing, agitation and dysphoria. It reflects a possible imbalance between the noradrenergic, serotonergic and the dopaminergic systems. It occurs in up to 90% of patients during the first 10 weeks of treatment.

7. The activities of the serotonergic system seem to be unaltered by the use of typical **APDs**.

3.3 Antipsychotic drugs – supposed mechanism of action (III)

Schizophreniform psychosis; treatment with atypical antipsychotic drugs

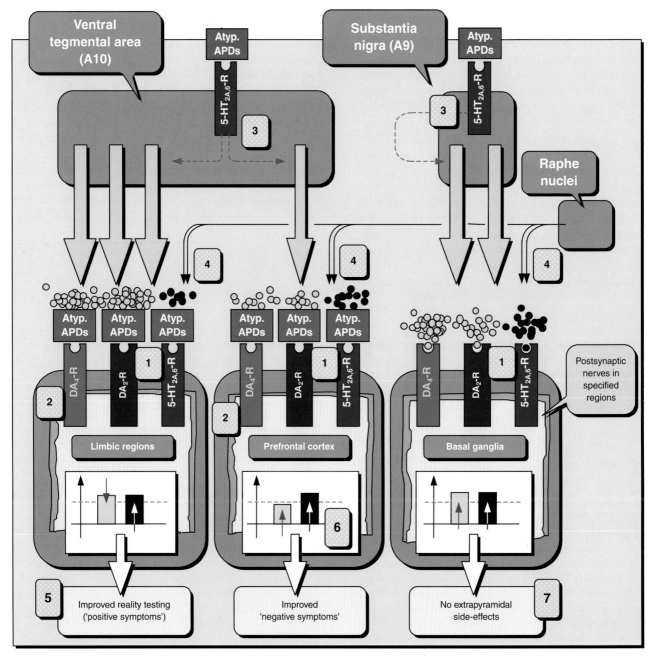

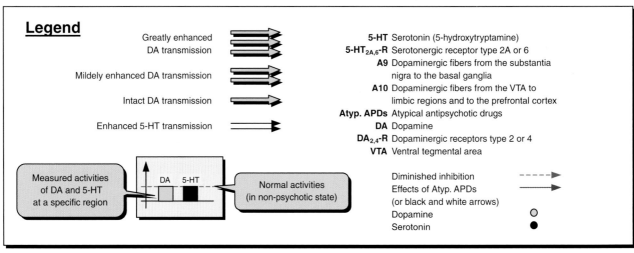

The 'atypical' antipsychotic drugs (**atyp. APDs**) are a class of new antipsychotic agents that share a diminished capacity to cause extrapyramidal side effects (including tardive dyskinesia) and a minimal effect on serum prolactin levels. Some researchers believe that having some efficacy on 'negative' symptoms is a necessary criterion for an 'atypical' drug. This criterion is controversial because only **clozapine** and **risperidone** have been shown to improve negative symptoms in some large and well-established studies.

Clozapine, olanzapine, quetiapine, risperidone, sertindole, amisulpiride and **ziprasidone** are new-generation antipsychotic drugs designated as atypical, and are either marketed or just on the verge of being marketed. All these agents possess at least some of the listed atypical features.

There is no one specific receptor interaction responsible for atypical propensities, but a few have been postulated.

The first is a high affinity for antagonizing the postsynaptic 5-HT$_{2A}$ serotonergic receptors. Secondly, there is a high ratio of serotonin (5-HT) compared with dopamine (DA) blockade. There is no well-accepted ratio, but all **APDs** claimed to be atypical have a 5-HT/DA blocking ratio larger than 1. **Atyp. APDs** vary greatly with respect to how big this ratio is. **Quetiapine**, the atypical agent with the smallest ratio, exhibits a 5-HT/DA blocking ratio of about 2 to 1 while **sertindole**, at the other extreme, has a 110 to 1 ratio. 5-HT blockade is not a specific enough criterion as **chlorpromazine**, for example, has a 5-HT/DA blocking ratio of about 15 and still exerts many 'typical' effects [induces tardive dyskinesia, elevates serum prolactin and can cause extrapyramidal side effects (EPS)]. Thirdly, there is a high affinity for blocking other subclasses of receptors, particularly the D$_4$ dopaminergic and/or the newly cloned 5-HT$_6$ serotonergic receptors, and the noradrenergic α_2-adrenoceptors.

Notes about the numbered items in the scheme

1–4. Most **atyp. APDs** (**sertindole, clozapine, olanzapine** and **ziprasidone**) are potent blockers of both 5-HT$_{2A}$ and 5-HT$_6$ receptors (besides their mild–moderate capacity to antagonize the D$_2$ receptors)(**1**). **Clozapine**, and to a lesser extent **olanzapine** are also potent D$_4$ dopaminergic blockers (**2**). 5-HT$_{2A}$ antagonism increases dopaminergic (**3**) and serotonergic (**4**) transmission in limbic regions, and it is hypothesized to happen in prefrontal and other brain regions as well. It does so, presumably, by decreasing the inhibitory potential of these serotonergic receptors on the firing rate of these neurons. Following treatment with **atyp. APDs,** serotonergic activity is increased, counterbalancing, perhaps, the increased dopaminergic activity observed in schizophrenic patients. This may explain a superior efficacy in improving positive symptoms in some cases (treatment-resistant psychosis for example).

5. Atyp. APDs antagonize the D$_2$ receptors in the mesolimbic regions; this explains their equal efficacy in ameliorating positive psychotic symptoms compared with typical agents.

6. The increased dopaminergic firing rate in the mesocortical pathway (following treatment with **atyp. APDs**) converts the relatively deficient dopaminergic state presumed to exist in baseline psychotic patients into a more or less intact transmission. This might explain the possible improvement in negative symptoms seen mostly with **clozapine**. Accumulating data suggest that other **atyp. APDs** likewise have at least some capacity to improve negative symptoms. Another possible explanation for this action is that some **atyp. APDs** (**clozapine, risperidone, quetiapine**) block α_2 adrenoreceptors and so increase norepinephrine levels in prefrontal cortex.

7. Atyp. APDs are relatively selective for the mesolimbic and mesocortical compared with the tuberoinfudibular and/or nigro-striatal dopaminergic pathways. This helps explain especially their diminished potential to increase serum prolactin levels or to cause EPS.

3.4 Antipsychotic drugs

Comparative affinity for different receptors

Affinity for receptors

Class		Generic name	D_1 blockade	D_2 blockade	D_3 blockade	D_4 blockade	ACh Mus. blockade	H_1 blockade	α_1-ADR blockade	α_2-ADR blockade	$5\text{-}HT_{2A}$ blockade	$5\text{-}HT_{2A}$ / D_2 affinity ratio	D_2 / $5\text{-}HT_{2A}$ affinity ratio
Typical antipsychotic drugs	Phenothiazines	Chlorpromazine										10:1	
		Fluphenazine											2:1
		Levomepromazine										5:1	
		Perphenazine										2:1	
		Thioridazine										5:1	
		Trifluoperazine										2:1	
	Thio-xanthenes	Chlorprothixene										30:1	
		Thiothixene											40:1
		Zuclopenthixol											3:1
	Miscelaneous APDs	Clothiapine										15:1	
		Haloperidol											25:1
		Loxapine										7:1	
		Molindone											8:1
		Pimozide											5:1
Atypical APDs		Clozapine										30:1	
		Olanzapine										50:1	
		Quetiapine										1:1	
		Risperidone										8:1	
		Sertindole										100:1	
		Sulpiride											50:1
		Ziprasidone										3:1	

Legend

* IC_{50} = the concentration of the drug required to occupy 50% of the available receptors. Most data are based on animal studies. Lower values correspond to higher affinity of the compound to the receptor

5-HT$_2$ Serotonergic receptor type 2
ACh Mus. Acetylcholine muscarinic
ADR Adrenergic
APDs Antipsychotic drugs
D_1 - D_4 Different dopaminergic receptor subtypes
H_1 Histaminergic receptor type 1

Approximate IC_{50} values (nM)*

Lowest (0.1-1)

Highest (>100 000)

No conclusive data

3.5 Antipsychotic drugs

Subclasses according to presumed mode of therapeutic action

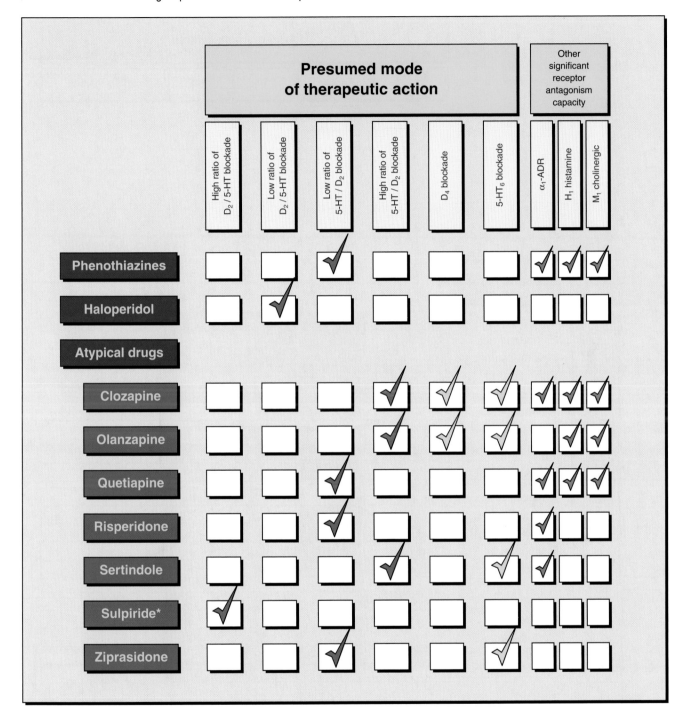

	Presumed mode of therapeutic action						Other significant receptor antagonism capacity		
	High ratio of D_2 / 5-HT blockade	Low ratio of D_2 / 5-HT blockade	Low ratio of 5-HT / D_2 blockade	High ratio of 5-HT / D_2 blockade	D_4 blockade	$5\text{-}HT_6$ blockade	α_1-ADR	H_1 histamine	M_1 cholinergic
Phenothiazines			✓				✓	✓	✓
Haloperidol		✓							
Atypical drugs									
Clozapine				✓	✓	✓	✓	✓	✓
Olanzapine				✓	✓	✓		✓	✓
Quetiapine			✓				✓	✓	✓
Risperidone			✓				✓	✓	
Sertindole						✓	✓	✓	
Sulpiride*	✓								
Ziprasidone			✓			✓			

Legend

Main mode of action (related to therapeutic action)	✓	
Minor mode of action (might be related to therapeutic action)	✓	
Other clinical significant receptor antagonism capacities (related, mainly, to side-effect profile)	✓	

5-HT Serotonin (5-hydroxytryptamine)
ADR Adrenergic
DA Dopamine
H_1 Histamine type 1 receptor
M_1 Acetylcholine muscarinic receptor type 1
* Sulpiride is claimed by many to be an atypical agent because its low propensity to cause extrapyramidal side-effects or tardive dyskinesia

3.6 Antipsychotic drugs
Comparative side effect profile

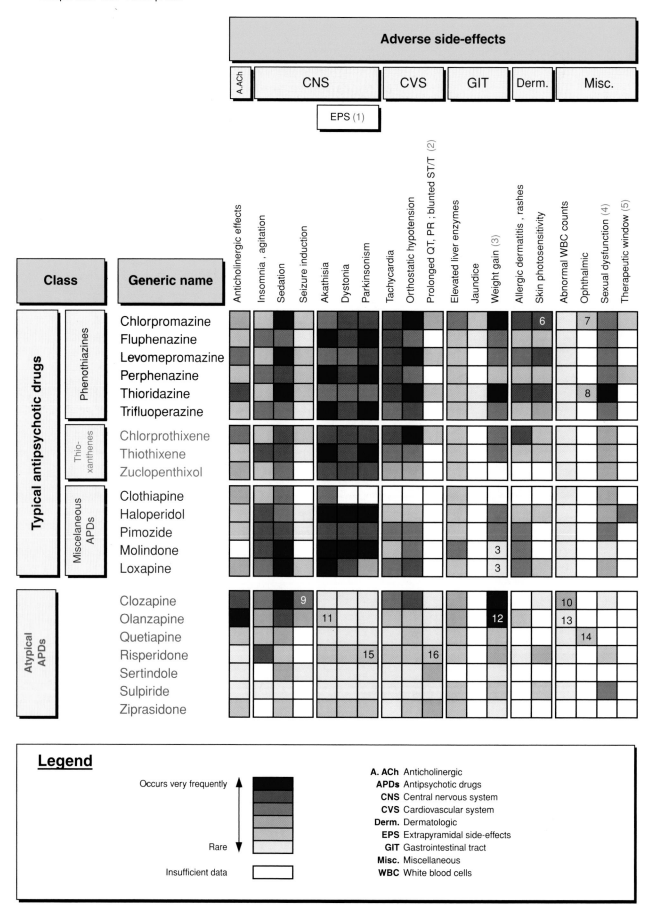

Legend

Occurs very frequently ↑

Rare ↓

Insufficient data

A. ACh	Anticholinergic
APDs	Antipsychotic drugs
CNS	Central nervous system
CVS	Cardiovascular system
Derm.	Dermatologic
EPS	Extrapyramidal side-effects
GIT	Gastrointestinal tract
Misc.	Miscellaneous
WBC	White blood cells

Notes about the numbered items in the scheme

1. Extrapyramidal side effects (EPS) (see Section 6.1): these are mainly due to D_2 blockade and are more common with the use of high and intermediate-potency antipsychotic drugs. The main EPS encountered while using antipsychotic agents are dystonia, parkinsonism and akathisia (see Section 3.2 for details).

2. QT, PR, ST/T are specific intervals of the ECG.

3. The mechanism of weight gain on antipsychotics is unclear, although H_1 antagonism in the hypothalamus is likely to be relevant. **Clozapine** and low-potency **phenothiazines** usually cause a greater weight gain than other agents. **Amantadine** is sometimes used successfully to reverse the weight gain. **Molindone** and **loxapine** have the least weight-gaining properties, perhaps none at all.

4. See Section 7.7 for further details.

5. The term therapeutic window refers to an n-shaped plasma concentration–efficient relationship. Monitoring of plasma levels of such drugs can be beneficial in enhancing the responsiveness of fast metabolizers or reduce the risk of toxicity in slow metabolizers. The most studied agent associated with therapeutic window is **haloperidol**, and data (albiet inconsistent) suggest a therapeutic window around 30–100 ng/ml. **Chlorpromazine** and **perphenazine** are also well studied, and **perphenazine** might have a therapeutic window between 0.8–2.4 ng/ml (data are less well established than with **haloperidol**).

6. The phenomena resembles severe sunburn tan. Patients treated with **phenothiazines**, and especially with **chlorpromazine**, should be advised to use protective sunscreens and to limit their exposure to direct sunlight to periods not longer than 30–60 minutes per day.

7. This is a benign and reversible whitish-brown pigmentation which appears as granular deposits mainly in the anterior lens and posterior cornea. The lesions are visible only by slit-lens. Vision is almost never impaired. The occurrence of these lesions is almost entirely in chronic users of **chlorpromazine** with a lifetime user of 1–3 kilograms (about 6–18 years of treatment with daily doses of about 500 mg.

8. Irreversible pigmentation of the retina can occur in high doses (800–1600 mg/d). Impaired or lost night vision along with nocturnal confusion is often a first sign of the up-coming retinal damage. The damage resembles retinitis pigmentosa and often causes blindness. Cessation of **thioridazine** administration does not reverse the damage, which can even progress.

9. Seizure disorder is evident in 1–2% of patients on **clozapine** if doses up to 300 mg/d are used. Above 600 mg/d the frequency increases to about 3–5%. Lowering the dose to a previous tolerable one is generally effective.

10. Clozapine causes agranulocytosis in about 1–2% of treated patients, which can often be fatal. Female gender and increased age are possible risk factors. The incidence is much higher than in patients treated with **typical antipsychotics** (estimated to be 0.05–0.5%). About 75% of cases emerge during the first 18 weeks of treatment, and up to 90% during the first 26 weeks of treatment. When the white blood cell count is monitored, the percentage of fatal cases is reduced to about 0.06%. The adverse reaction is not dose-related. The incidence of agranulocytosis with other atypical antipsychotic drugs is not known. Available data suggests that the use of **quetiapine**, **risperidone** or **sulpiride** does not increase the risk of developing agranulocytosis (compared with placebo) while there is no sufficient information for **olanzapine**, **sertindole** or **ziprasidone**.

11. Olanzapine induces akathisia in doses equal to or higher than 10 mg/day. Other EPS are rare, and usually occur for doses higher than 15 mg/day.

12. Weight gain is reported in 6–29% of patients. The average weight gain is about 3 kg in 6 weeks. There are no well-established data about the more chronic effects of **olanzapine** on weight.

13. Benign eosinophilia occurs in less than 0.3% of patients treated with **olanzapine**. Thrombocytopenia and leukocytosis have been reported to occur, but they are very rare.

14. Quetiapine has been shown to induce cataracts in dogs at high doses, possibly as a result of inhibited cholesterol synthesis in the dogs lens.

15. The incidence of parkinsonism is rare for therapeutic doses (2–4 mg/d) but it might significantly rise for higher doses.

16. Prolongation of the QT interval is observed, infrequently and seems to be clinically insignificant.

4.1 Drugs effective in anxiety disorders

Potential mechanisms involved in anxiolytic effects; empirical findings

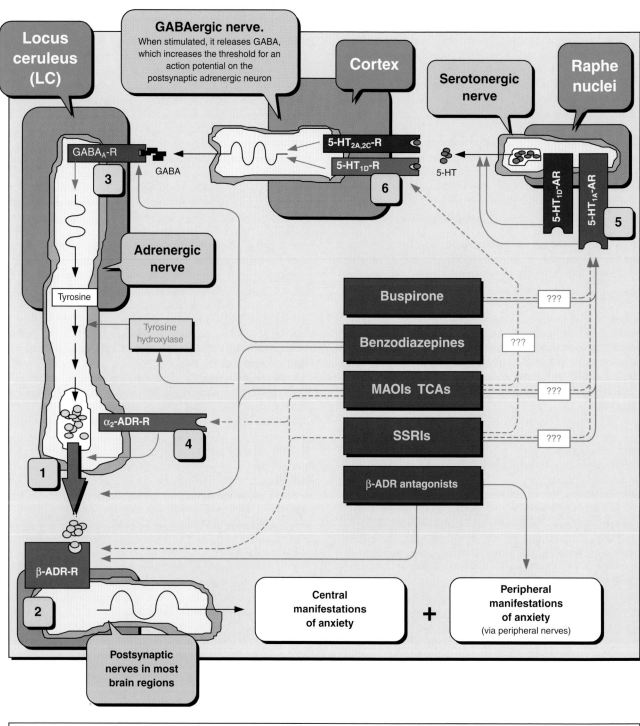

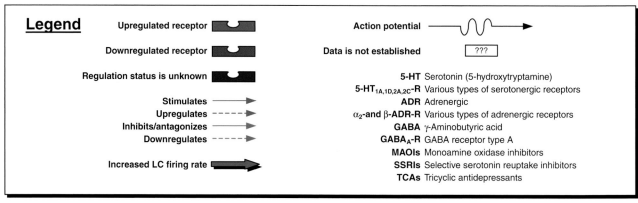

The pathophysiology of anxiety probably differs between the various anxiety disorders. Therefore, pharmacological agents that suppress one sort of anxiety do not necessarily exert the same anxiolytic effects in other anxiety disorders. Anxiety related to panic attacks is the most studied and presented here as a general model. No definitive pathophysiological or etiological mechanisms of anxiety disorders have been firmly established, but the adrenergic, GABAergic, and serotonergic systems are widely accepted as the major determinants of anxiety. The following findings are encountered in anxiety disorders (usually when panic attacks are evident) and therefore are assumed to be involved in the pathophysiology of anxiety.

Notes about the numbered items in the scheme

1. Increased locus ceruleous (LC) firing rate. This is seen in most of the anxiety disorders, and agents that do not suppress the LC firing rate (e.g. **trazodone**) do not suppress panic attacks. **Benzodiazepines** (BDZs) exert agonistic activities at the GABAergic neurons, and consequently decrease the LC firing rate.

2. Hypersensitive β-adrenergic receptors are often found in brain. **Isoproterenol**, a peripheral and selective β-adrenergic agonist can provoke panic attacks in patients suffering from panic disorder, presumably via stimulating the already hypersensitive β receptors. **Tricyclic antidepressants** (TCAs) which downregulate the β-adrenergic receptors, are beneficial in the treatment of panic disorder. They were also found to suppress **isoproterenol**-induced panic attacks, which suggests that the mechanism of panic induction is via the stimulation of hypersensitive β-adrenergic receptors. **Bupropion**, an antidepressant that does not downregulate the β-receptors, is not effective in panic disorder.

3. Subsensitive GABAergic receptors. The data are not conclusive. **Flumazenil**, a benzodiazepine-receptor antagonist, provokes panic attacks in patients suffering from panic disorder. Patients with panic disorder are often found to be less sensitive to **diazepam** administration suggesting a baseline subsensitive GABAergic system.

4. Upregulated α_2 adrenergic receptors. It is possible that, in response to the increased LC firing rates, there is a compensatory upregulation of the presynaptic α_2 receptors in order to counteract the increased norepinephrine (NE) neurotransmission. Up to 70% of panic disorder patients diagnosed as suffering from panic disorder experience **yohimbine**-induced panic attacks. **Yohimbine** is an α_2 antagonist that reduces the inhibitory effects of the presynaptic α_2 receptors on the release of NE so increasing their synaptic concentrations and resulting in panic attacks. Other evidence for dysfunctional α_2 receptors in panic disorder is the blunted growth hormone response to administration of **clonidine** (an α_2 agonist).

5. Alterations in the serotonergic (5-HT) system are evident, and are most apparent in the raphe nucleus and hippocampus.

When **ipsapirone** (a selective 5-HT$_{1A}$ agonist) is administered to patients with panic disorder, a blunted response of ACTH, and cortisol secretion is evident, which suggests a basal downregulation of the 5-HT$_{1A}$ receptors.

6. 5-HT$_{1D}$ receptors. 5-HT stimulates the LC activity and 5-HT agonists **mCPP** and **fenfluramine** (a 5-HT-releasing agent) provoke anxiety in panic disorder patients; thus it seems that in panic disorder there is a hypersensitivity of the inhibitory 5-HT$_{1D}$ receptors. This leads to decreased GABA release and consequent stimulation of the LC.

Specific and relative established effects of anxiolytic agents on different brain systems:

TCAs and MAOIs:	Downregulate postsynaptic β-adrenergic and presynaptic α_2-adrenergic receptors (evidence is inconsistent about the alterations in the α_2-receptors). Decrease LC firing rate. Inhibit tyrosine hydroxylase (in chronic use ; the rate-limiting enzyme for NE synthesis). Decrease the peripheral manifestations of anxiety.
SSRIs:	Downregulate postsynaptic β-adrenergic receptors. Stimulate and upregulate 5-HT$_{1A}$ receptors in the raphe nucleus, which in turn reduces LC firing rates.
BDZs:	Stimulate GABAergic receptors in all major brain regions, and inhibit LC firing rate.
Buspirone:	Stimulates and upregulates (during chronic use) somatodendritic 5-HT$_{1A}$ receptors in the raphe nucleus (see Section 4.4).
Beta blockers:	Antagonize the hypersensitive β-adrenergic receptors. Decrease the peripheral manifestations of anxiety.

4.2 Benzodiazepines and agents that enhance γ-aminobutyric acid type A (GABA_A) activity

Supposed mechanism of action

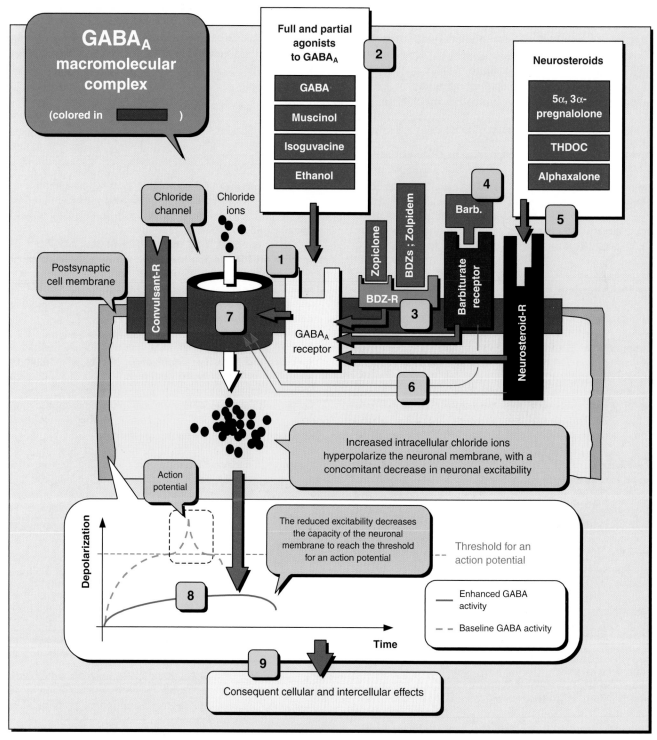

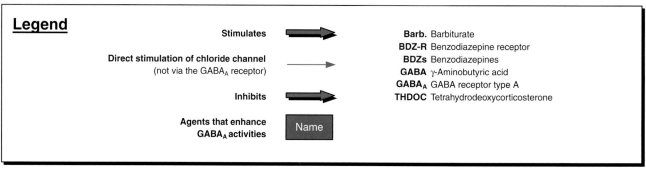

Legend

Stimulates	**Barb.**	Barbiturate
Direct stimulation of chloride channel (not via the GABA_A receptor)	**BDZ-R**	Benzodiazepine receptor
	BDZs	Benzodiazepines
Inhibits	**GABA**	γ-Aminobutyric acid
	GABA_A	GABA receptor type A
Agents that enhance GABA_A activities	**THDOC**	Tetrahydrodeoxycorticosterone

There are two types of γ-aminobutyric acid (GABA) receptors. The $GABA_A$ is a postsynaptic macromolecular complex that includes a chloride channel. These GABAergic receptors are most abundant in limbic regions (amygdala, hippocampus), cerebellum, striatum and cortex. When $GABA_A$ receptor is activated, it increases the chloride influx with a consequent decrease in neuronal excitability (thus exerting an overall inhibitory effect). $GABA_B$ are presynaptic and when stimulated inhibit the release of GABA and several excitatory amino acids, and monoamines. **Baclofen** is the most studied synthetic agonist for the $GABA_B$ receptor. Its antispasticity effects are presumably mediated by inhibiting the release of endogenous excitatory amino acids.

The $GABA_A$ receptor is composed of five different subunits out of a potential pool of 16 different units each coded by a separate gene. The different subunits are further divided into classes according to similarities in their amino-acid sequences (α, β, γ, and ε). Most

benzodiazepines bind to the benzodiazepine receptor, which is located on the α subunits of the $GABA_A$ receptor, though recently developed benzodiazepines (**quazepam, zolpidem**) show a high affinity only to $α_1$ subunits. Even so, for exerting GABA enhancing effects, all **benzodiazepines** are dependent on the co-existence of an intact γ subunit as well. There are two types of benzodiazepine receptors (type 1 and 2). Type 1 receptors are located mainly in the cerebellum and are mostly related to induction and maintenance of sleep. Type 2 receptors are abundant in limbic regions and are more associated with anxiolytic and anticonvulsant effects of **benzodiazepines.** The large number of different $GABA_A$ subunits, and especially a recent finding that some of these subunits are selectively located in distinct brain regions, may lead to the development of new anxiolytics or sedative agents with diminished or significantly reduced adverse side-effect profile.

Notes about the numbered items in the scheme

1–5. Most anxiolytics or sedatives directly enhance $GABA_A$ activity (**1**). The $GABA_A$ receptor serves an intermediate component that governs the permeability of a chloride channel. Some are agents that directly bind to the $GABA_A$ receptor (**GABA, muscinol, isoguavacine** and **ethanol**, which is probably selective to distinct γ subunits) (**2**). Others, indirectly enhance the $GABA_A$ receptor, by binding to various sites on the complex and enhance the function of the $GABA_A$ receptor. None of these agents can exert anxiolytic or sedative effects if the $GABA_A$ receptor is substantially impaired, or if there is not enough GABA available for neuronal transmission. Among the indirect enhancers of $GABA_A$ receptor are the **benzodiazepines, zolpidem** and the cyclopyrolone **zopiclone**. The former two bind to the benzodiazepine site while **zopiclone** binds to another distinct site on the benzodiazepine receptor (**3**). **Zolpidem** is a hypnotic agent without a significant anxiolytic, anticonvulsant or muscle relaxant effects. This is due presumably to its relative selectivity to the benzodiazepine type 1 receptor. The **barbiturates** (**4**) and various **neurosteroids** (**5**) also have distinct receptors. **Neurosteroids** are derivates of progesterone and cortisol, and some of them exert enhancing effects on the $GABA_A$ receptor [**5-α-3-α-pregnalolone, tetrahydro-deoxy-corticosterone (THDOC)** and **alphaxalone**], while other derivatives (**pregnalolone sulfate**) exert the opposite effect. The existence of these neurosteroid modulators can potentially explain at least some psychiatric clinical manifestations related to pregnancy or to the menstrual cycle.

6. Some agents e.g., **barbiturates** and **alcohol** in high doses and **neurosteroids** are capable of directly stimulating the chloride channel, independent of the presence of $GABA_A$. This explains their toxicity in overdose as excessive inhibition of respiratory neurones leads to respiratory arrest.

7,8. All the GABAergic agents share a common final pathway in which they increase the permeability of cross-membrane chloride channels (**7**). As a result, chloride influx increases and intracellular chloride concentration rises. The increased intracellular chloride hyperpolarizes the neuronal membrane, with a subsequent increase in the threshold for reaching an action potential (**8**).

9. The effects of enhancing GABA activities can meet either physiological or clinical needs. The physiological availability and an intact functioning of GABA has major roles in almost all normal brain functions. These include limiting and directing sensory inputs, governing motor outputs, modulating memory and possibly regulating anxious attitudes. The role of GABAergic transmission is most evident either in modulating anxiety (**benzodiazepines** are potent anxiolytic agents) and in memory. Enhanced GABA activity (as with the use of **benzodiazepines**) induces amnesia, and it is speculated that memory acquisition may require, at least in part, the loss of certain GABAergic inhibitions.

The physiological role of the GABA receptors is not fully understood since no endogenous ligand has yet been found to modulate their activities in humans. Even so, **benzodiazepine**-like susbstances are naturally present in various plants, and it could be that they have a natural role in humans.

The most prominent therapeutic and adverse side-effects of **benzodiazepines** are:

Hypnotic. They facilitate onset and maintenance of sleep.
Sedative. They decrease daytime anxiety and excitement along with a concomitant calming effect.
Adverse effects. Cognition and attention impairments, Drowsiness: 10%. Ataxia: < 2%. Enhance effects of alcohol.

4.3 Agents that suppress γ-aminobutyric acid type A (GABA_A) activity

Supposed mechanism of action

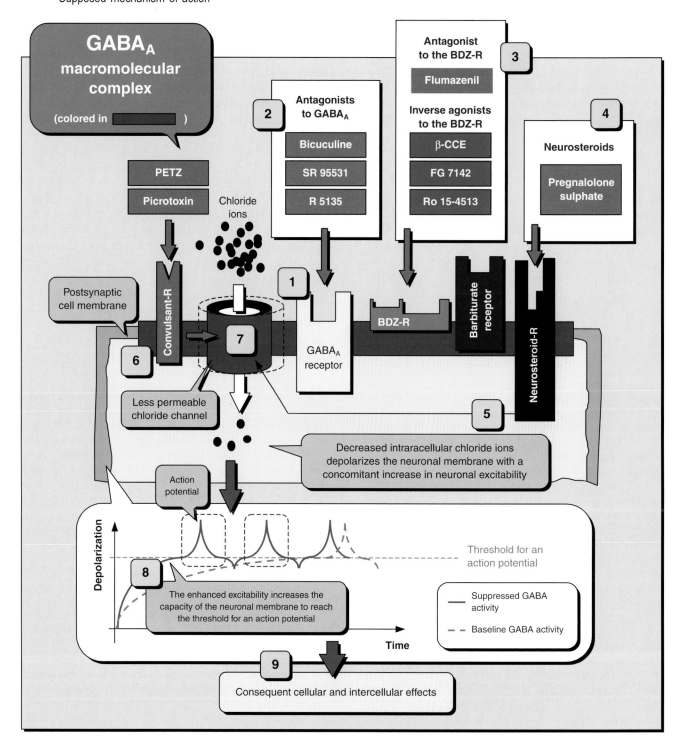

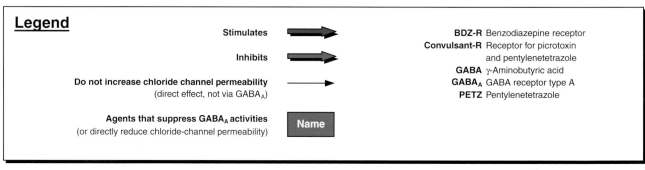

Legend

Stimulates

Inhibits

Do not increase chloride channel permeability
(direct effect, not via GABA_A)

Agents that suppress GABA_A activities
(or directly reduce chloride-channel permeability) — Name

BDZ-R Benzodiazepine receptor
Convulsant-R Receptor for picrotoxin
and pentylenetetrazole
GABA γ-Aminobutyric acid
GABA_A GABA receptor type A
PETZ Pentylenetetrazole

There are several classes of compounds, which either suppress GABA$_A$ activity or act directly on the chloride channel to decrease its permeability to chloride ions (see Section 4.2 for further details on the GABA macromolecular complex).

Notes about the numbered items in the scheme

1–4. There are several types of GABA$_A$ receptor inhibitors: GABA$_A$-receptor antagonists (**2**), benzodiazepine-receptor antagonists and inverse agonists (**3**) and neurosteroids (**4**). The GABA$_A$ receptor antagonists act by directly suppressing the activity of GABA$_A$ (e.g. **bicuculine**, **SR 95531** and **R 5135**). The most well known and clinically used benzodiazepine-receptor antagonist is **flumazenil**. It inhibits the binding of both **benzodiazepines** and **cyclopyrolones** to their corresponding binding sites on the benzodiazepine receptor, as well as possible compounds that have not yet been identified. The latter effect can be demonstrated as **flumazenil** can partially reverse endogenous symptoms of hepatic encephalopathy. **Flumazenil** has two major clinical applications: it shortens the postoperative anesthetic adverse effects of **benzodiazepines** (mainly sedation and recall) and for diagnosing and treating **benzodiazepine** overdose. In **benzodiazepine**-intoxicated patients **flumazenil** is commonly administered intravenously (due to predominant first-pass metabolism), and full beneficial effects are seen in a few seconds to minutes. **Flumazenil** is also widely known for its panic-attack-provoking capacities in untreated patients suffering from panic disorder (70–90% will exhibit a panic attack). These effects are not observed when it is administered to healthy subjects implying that in normal physiological functioning there is no apparent activity associated with the benzodiazepine receptors. **Flumazenil** has no significant adverse effects except for occasional nausea and vomiting. More infrequent though serious side-effects of **flumazenil** are seizure induction including status epilepticus, and induction of acute psychosis if it is given to benzodiazepine-dependent individuals.

Inverse agonists are substances that produce effects at a specific receptor that are opposite to those produced by the usual agonist to the same receptor. The most studied of the benzodiazepine-receptor inverse agonists is the β-carboline-3-carboxylic acid ethyl ester (**β-CCE**). **β-Carboline's** effects are evident both in animals (it increases serum cortisol levels and causes tachycardia in monkeys) and in humans, where they induce anxiety resembling panic attacks.

Pregnalolone sulfate is a neurosteroid (Section 4.2), but, unlike the other neurosteroids, it exhibits antagonistic effects on the receptor for neurosteroids thus decreasing chloride influx (**4**). **5–7. Pregnalolone sulfate** (**5**) and the two convulsants **picrotoxin** and **pentylenetetrazole** (**6**) can decrease chloride influx via directly blocking the chloride channel (**7**). The receptor for **picrotoxin** and **pentylenetetrazole** is termed the convulsant receptor or the **picrotoxin**-binding site. **Picrotoxin** is a convulsant agent derived from the shrub anamirta cocculus. **Pentylenetetrazol** was used since the late 1940s to produce convulsions in psychiatric patients. Later it was replaced by electroconvulsive therapy due to its profound anxiogenic actions.

8. All the mentioned agents share a common final pathway in which they decrease the permeability of cross-membrane chloride channels. As a result, chloride influx decreases and intracellular ion concentrations are lowered. This decreases the threshold for reaching an action potential.

9. There is insufficient data about the clinical effects on humans of the various agents described. Most of our knowledge comes from animal and human studies with **flumazenil** and some from **picrotoxin** and **pentylenetetrazole. Flumazenil's** effects were described earlier, and the most prominent clinical effects of the latter agents are their anxiogenic and convulsant activities. **Pentylenetetrazole** was used as convulsant for treating depression before electro-convulsive therapy was introduced and its predominant disturbing adverse effect was the provocation of anxiety reactions.

4.4 Buspirone
Supposed mechanism of anxiolytic effect

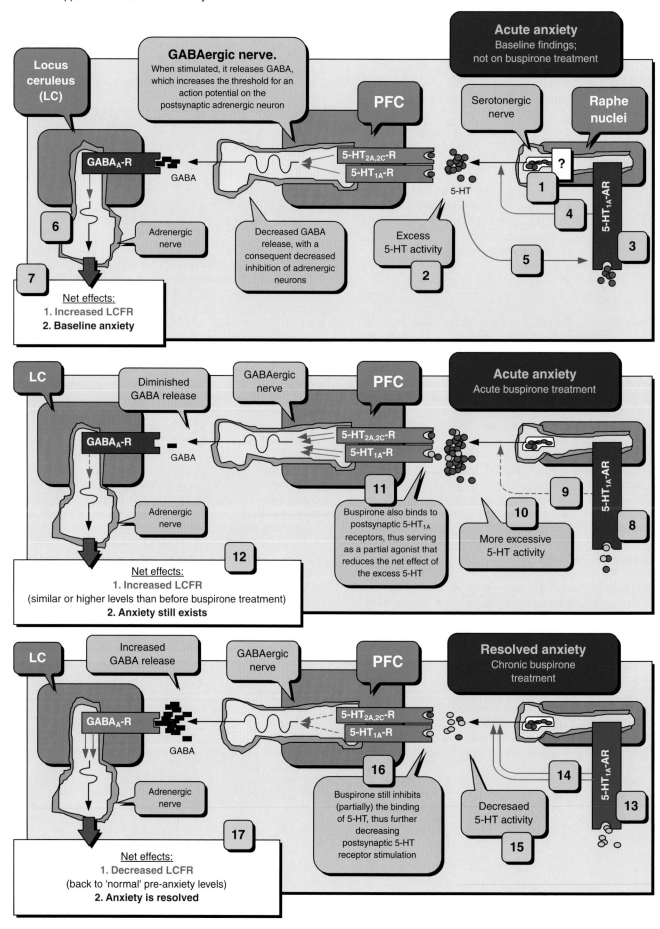

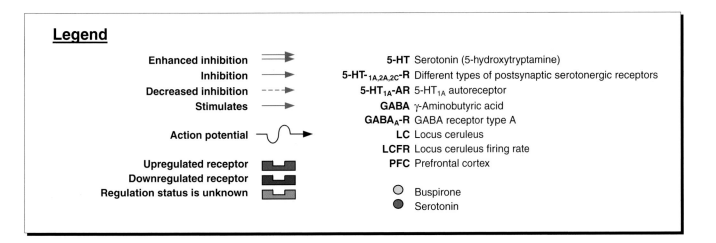

Legend

Enhanced inhibition ⟹	**5-HT** Serotonin (5-hydroxytryptamine)
Inhibition ⟶	**5-HT-$_{1A,2A,2C}$-R** Different types of postsynaptic serotonergic receptors
Decreased inhibition ⇢	**5-HT$_{1A}$-AR** 5-HT$_{1A}$ autoreceptor
Stimulates ⟶	**GABA** γ-Aminobutyric acid
	GABA$_A$-R GABA receptor type A
Action potential	**LC** Locus ceruleus
	LCFR Locus ceruleus firing rate
Upregulated receptor	**PFC** Prefrontal cortex
Downregulated receptor	◯ Buspirone
Regulation status is unknown	● Serotonin

Buspirone is a partial agonist to the 5-HT$_{1A}$ receptor. A partial agonist is an agent that has certain agonistic capacities at a specific receptor, but less efficacy (lower maximal response) than the endogenous ligand that stimulates it. Partial agonists therefore displace or partially inhibit the binding of the endogenous ligand to that receptor. This leads to a decrease in the stimulatory input to the receptor with consequent suppression of its intracellular effects. The 5-HT$_{1A}$ receptors can be either presynaptic (termed somatodendritic autoreceptors, – SDARs) or postsynaptic. The SDARs serve as regulatory receptors that, when stimulated by synaptic 5-HT (serotonin), inhibit the further release of stored 5-HT from intracellular vesicles located in the presynaptic nerve terminal into the synaptic cleft, leading to decreased serotonergic transmission.

Notes about the numbered items in the scheme

A major element in understanding the role of **buspirone** as an anxiolytic agent is the presumed primary excessive serotonergic activity, which affects several brain regions, especially the locus ceruleus (LC), in anxiety. The excessive serotonergic activity increases the LC firing rate, with a consequent increase in adrenergic activities in most major brain regions. The mechanism involved in **buspirone's** anxiolytic effects is presumed to be via the following substeps:

1,2. Unknown intracellular (or extracellular) events (**1**) increase the 5-HT concentrations in the synaptic cleft, leading to excessive serotonergic activity (**2**) in many brain regions.

3,4. The presynaptic 5-HT$_{1A}$-AR is assumed to be downregulated (**3**) in the baseline condition of an acute untreated anxiety. Although downregulated, it still exerts some inhibitory effects on the release of 5-HT from presynaptic nerve terminals into the synaptic cleft (**4**).

5. Synaptic 5-HT serve as feeback mechanism by inhibiting the SDARs but it is not sufficient enough to inhibit the excessive release of 5-HT properly. The net result is an excess of 5-HT.

6,7. This increased serotonergic activity stimulates various postsynaptic 5-HT receptors located in many brain regions (5-HT$_{2A}$, 5-HT$_{2C}$, 5-HT$_3$, 5-HT$_4$ and 5-HT$_{1A}$). Especially relevant to anxiety is the stimulation of serotonergic receptors in the frontal cortex, which in turn suppress GABAergic projections from the cortex to the LC (**6**). This results in increased LCFR (LC firing rate), with a consequent increase in adrenergic activities, which induce the primary symtoms of anxiety (**7**).

8–10. **Buspirone** binds to the presynaptic 5-HT$_{1A}$-AR so inhibits the excessive binding of 5-HT to that receptor, leading to less stimulation of these receptors, and less inhibitory effects on the release of 5-HT into the synaptic cleft (**9**). During the acute phase of **buspirone** treatment (usually less than 2 weeks), the 5-HT-AR are still downregulated and the decreased stimulation of the 5-HT-AR causes a further increase in the release of 5-HT into the synaptic cleft, leading to a further increase in 5-HT availability for synaptic transmission (**10**).

11,12. The increased 5-HT availability in the synaptic cleft is not translated into an increase in postsynaptic 5-HT stimulatory effects since **buspirone** also binds to postsynaptic 5-HT$_{1A}$ receptors with consequent partial inhibition of endogenous 5-HT binding to these receptors (**11**). The net effect of acute **buspirone** treatment is little change in the LCFR, and anxiety does not resolve (**12**).

13–17. Chronic **buspirone** treatment causes upregulation of the 5-HT$_{1A}$-AR (**13**). The postsynaptic 5-HT$_{1A}$-R are not modified by such treatment. The upregulated 5-HT$_{1A}$-AR exert an enhanced inhibition on the release of 5-HT from the presynaptic terminal (**14**), which leads to a significant decrease in 5-HT concentration in the synaptic cleft (**15**). The serotonergic activities are further decreased since **buspirone** binds to the postsynaptic 5-HT$_{1A}$-R (**16**), with a consequent decrease in the already-diminished effects of 5-HT on postsynaptic receptors. The net effects of these reactions decrease the LCFR to 'normal', pre-anxiety levels, which in turn modulates the resolution of the anxiety state.

4.5 Treatments for OCD (obsessive–compulsive disorder)

Supposed mechanism of action

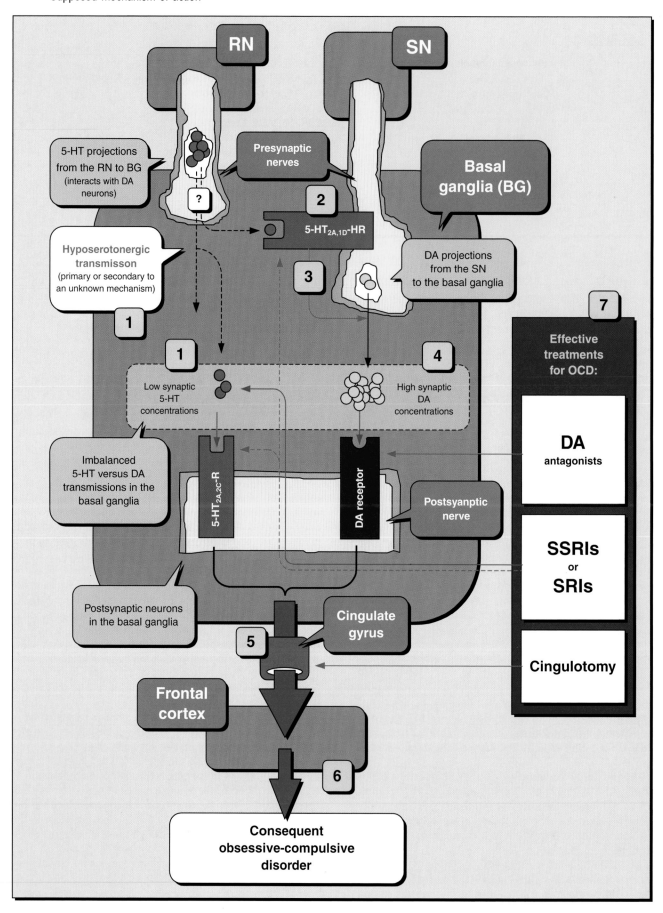

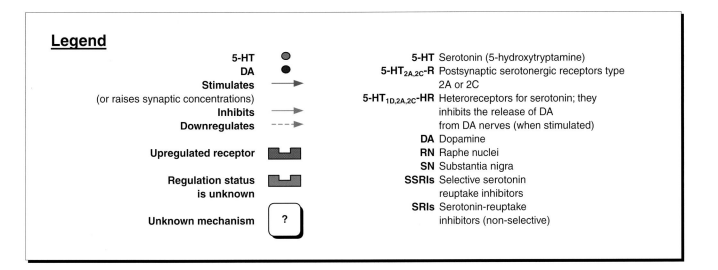

Legend

5-HT	●	5-HT	Serotonin (5-hydroxytryptamine)
DA	●	5-HT$_{2A,2C}$-R	Postsynaptic serotonergic receptors type 2A or 2C
Stimulates (or raises synaptic concentrations)	→	5-HT$_{1D,2A,2C}$-HR	Heteroreceptors for serotonin; they inhibits the release of DA from DA nerves (when stimulated)
Inhibits	→	DA	Dopamine
Downregulates	---→	RN	Raphe nuclei
Upregulated receptor	⊔	SN	Substantia nigra
Regulation status is unknown	⊔	SSRIs	Selective serotonin reuptake inhibitors
Unknown mechanism	?	SRIs	Serotonin-reuptake inhibitors (non-selective)

There are accumulating data indicating that the basal ganglia (BG) and the serotonergic and dopaminergic systems are involved in obsessive–compulsive disorder (OCD). The best evidence for serotonergic involvement is the beneficial effects of non-selective serotonin reuptake inhibitors (**SRIs**). **Clomipramine**, a tricyclic antidepressant drug, was shown early in the 1960s to ameliorate OCD. Double-blind, placebo-controlled studies with selective serotonin reuptake inhibitors (**SSRIs**) such as **fluoxetine**, **fluvoxamine**, **sertraline**, **citalopram** and **paroxetine** have confirmed this. The **SSRIs** and **SRIs** increase the availability of serotonin in the synaptic cleft, with a consequent increase in postsynaptic serotonergic transmission.

The best evidence for DA involvement in OCD is the link between OCD and Gilles de la Tourette Syndrome (GTS). As many as 50–90% of GTS patients have also obsessive behaviors, and many have OCD. Other evidence includes the observation that OCD patients may benefit from the addition of various antidopaminergic agents (**neuroleptics**) to **SRIs**. **Cocaine**, which increases dopaminergic transmission, can aggravate OCD in patients suffering from GTS. Dopamine agonists such as **amphetamines**, **cocaine**, L-dopa, **apomorphine** or **bromocriptine**, have been shown to induce purposeless and repetitive activities, resembling OCD, in previously healthy subjects.

Various structural and functional abnormalities, mostly in BG, have been demonstrated in patients with OCD. Computed tomography (CT) scans have demonstrated reduced caudate volumes, and cavitation of the basal ganglia. Association between OCD and several neurological disorders that involve basal ganglia dysfunction (Sydenham's chorea, postencephalitic parkinsonism) is evident in epidemiological studies. Positron emission tomography (PET) studies have demonstrated increased brain metabolism in the caudate nuclei, cingulate regions, frontal lobe and orbital gyri. Symptomatic improvements in OCD have been found to correlate with restoration of metabolism to normal in the basal ganglia and frontal regions.

Notes about the numbered items in the scheme

1. Decreased serotonergic activity is presumed to be involved with the emergence of OCD. It is unclear if this hyposerotonergic state is primary or secondary.

2–4. Under normal conditions, serotonin stimulates 5-HT$_{1D,2A,2C}$-HR (heteroreceptors for serotonin) located on dopaminergic nerves (**2**), with consequent inhibition of DA release from the presynaptic nerve terminal into the synaptic cleft (**3**). The hyposerotonergic state assumed in OCD decreases the inhibition so increasing DA concentration in the synaptic cleft (**4**). The 5-HT$_{1D,2A,2C}$-HR may also be hypersensitive in OCD which could serve as compensatory mechanism to decrease DA release.

5. The imbalanced 5-HT/DA system in the basal ganglia is reflected in other brain regions, by efferent projection fibers through the cingulate gyrus.

6. Inputs from the basal ganglia to the frontal cortex are assumed to produce the symptoms encountered in syndromes such as OCD and GTS.

7. The most efficacious pharmacological treatments for OCD are the **SRIs** or the **SSRIs** which work in between 30% and 70% of patients but only on chronic administration. There are some preliminary data that this therapeutic effect is associated with the downregulation of postsynaptic 5-HT$_{1D,2A,2C}$-HR. Surgical procedures that interrupt the pathways from the basal ganglia to the frontal cortex are also effective in ameliorating OCD. **Cingulotomy** is the most often used, and long-term remissions are achieved in up to 30% of patients. Adverse side-effects such as seizure disorder might occur so the use of this procedure is limited to the most intractable cases.

4.6 Benzodiazepines and other sedative hypnotics
Comparative clinical and side-effect profiles

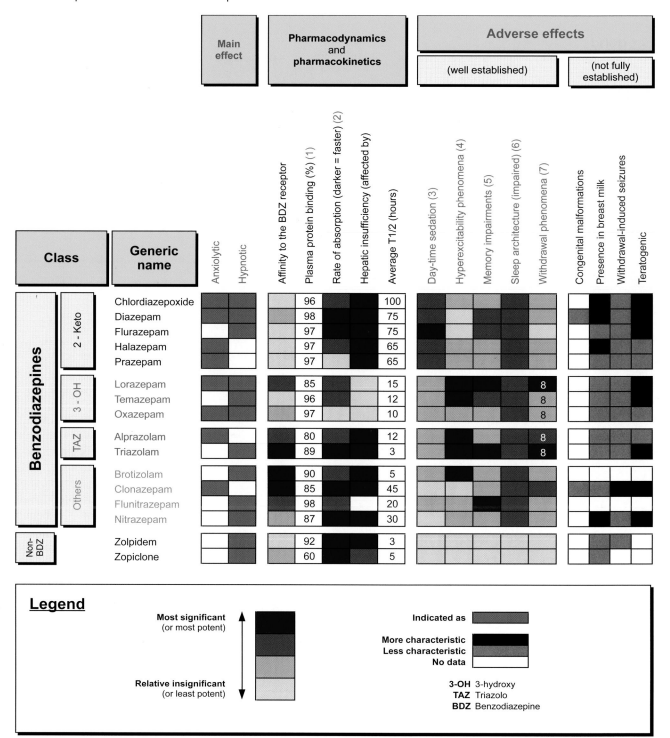

Notes about the numbered items in the scheme

1. The more protein that is bound, the more the agent is affected by pharmacokinetic interactions.

2. Faster rate causes more immediate anxiolytic effect (if given acutely and on a short-term basis).

3. Associated with higher doses and being elderly.

4. Hyperexcitability phenomena: daytime anxiety, early insomnia, tension, panic and development of tolerance (from 1 to 4 weeks).

5. Potent benzodiazepines (**BDZs**) are associated with more memory impairments (mostly anterograde amnesia).

6. All **BDZs** decrease REM and stages 3 and 4 of sleep to various extents. **Zopiclone** and **zolpidem** do not.

7. Mostly rebound insomnia and anxiety. Associated, predominantly, with agents that have short $T_{1/2}$.

8. Only if stopped quickly.

4.7 Benzodiazepines
Metabolism

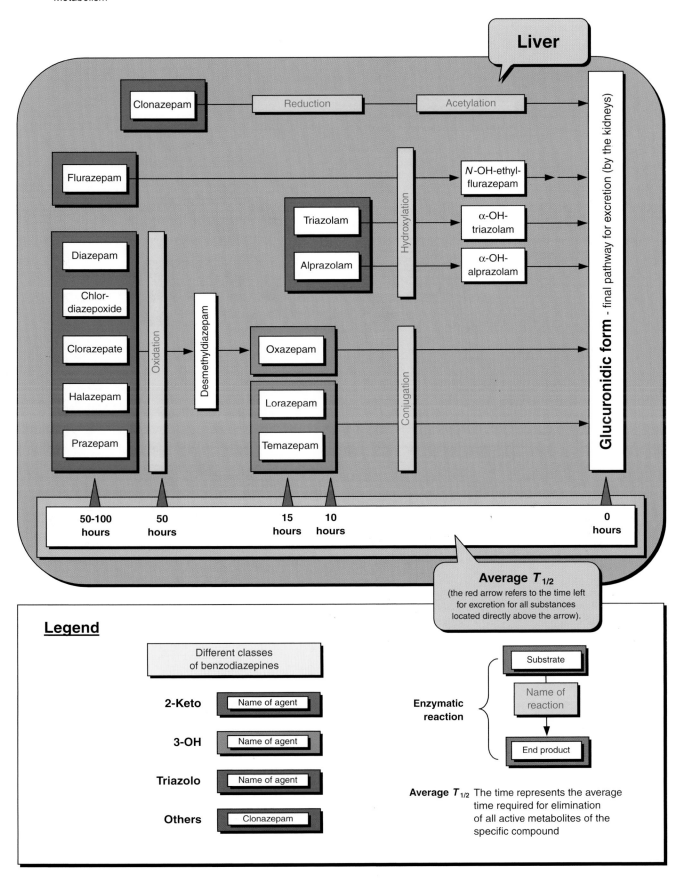

Liver

Clonazepam — Reduction — Acetylation —

Flurazepam — Hydroxylation — *N*-OH-ethyl-flurazepam

Triazolam — α-OH-triazolam

Alprazolam — α-OH-alprazolam

Diazepam
Chlor-diazepoxide
Clorazepate
Halazepam
Prazepam

Oxidation — Desmethyldiazepam — Oxazepam — Conjugation

Lorazepam
Temazepam

Glucuronidic form - final pathway for excretion (by the kidneys)

| 50-100 hours | 50 hours | 15 hours | 10 hours | 0 hours |

Average $T_{1/2}$
(the red arrow refers to the time left for excretion for all substances located directly above the arrow).

Legend

Different classes of benzodiazepines

2-Keto — Name of agent

3-OH — Name of agent

Triazolo — Name of agent

Others — Clonazepam

Enzymatic reaction
Substrate
Name of reaction
End product

Average $T_{1/2}$ The time represents the average time required for elimination of all active metabolites of the specific compound

69

5.1 α₂-adrenergic antagonist – yohimbine

Supposed mechanism of improving erectile dysfunction

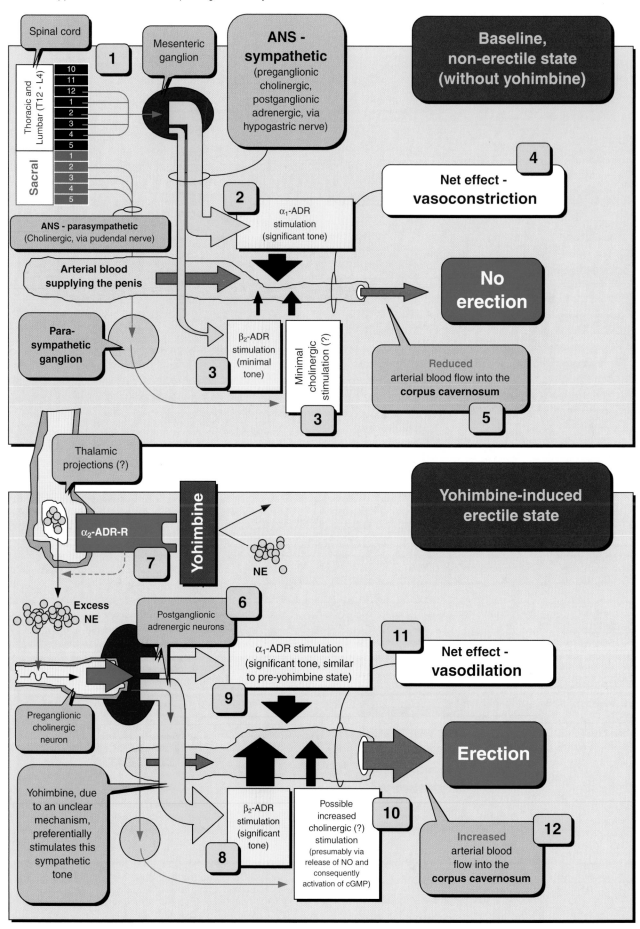

Legend

Stimulates	⟶
Decreased inhibition	----▶
Cholinergic fibers	⟶
Adrenergic fibers	⟹

Effects on vascular masculature

Significant tone	➡
Moderate tone	➡
Mild tone	➡

ADR	Adrenergic
ADR-R	Adrenergic receptor
ANS	Autonomic nervous system
cGMP	Cyclic guanine monophosphate
NE	Norepinephrine
NO	Nitric oxide

Yohimbine has been used for many years as a possible treatment for erectile dysfunction (impotence). Most of the favorable data are case reports or small open-labeled studies. The exact mechanism of action is unclear, but data indicates a major role for the peripheral autonomic nervous system in regulating the **yohimbine**-induced improvements in erectile dysfunction. **Yohimbine** is an α_2-adrenergic receptor antagonist, which causes a net increase in norepinephrine (NE) availability in the synaptic cleft, via the inhibition of the presynaptic α_2-autoreceptor (which regulates and inhibits the release of NE from intracellular vesicles into the synaptic cleft). **Yohimbine** is given in doses of approximately 12–22.5 mg/d for the treatment of impotence (divided into three). At doses above this there are increased frequency of adverse side-effects. The most common side-effects of **yohimbine** are related to stimulation of the adrenergic system: increased blood pressure, tachycardia, tremor, irritability and headaches. Other commonly observed adverse effects are decreased urinary output (which is probably mediated via the release of antidiuretic hormone), impaired renal function, nausea, vomiting, sweating and flushing, as well as emergence of anxiety or panic attacks (especially in predisposed individuals).

Notes about the numbered items in the scheme

1. The erectile mechanism of the male penis is mediated by the autonomic nervous system, both the sympathetic (preganglionic cholinergic fibers from T12 to L4, and postganglionic adrenergic fibers) and parasympathetic (cholinergic fibers from S2 to S4). The corpus cavernosum has to be filled with an appropriate amount of arterial blood via the penile vasculature to achieve penile erection. The blood supply to the corpus cavernosum is regulated by these autonomic fibers.

2. Sympathetic stimulation of the α_1 adrenergic receptors located in the penile vasculature results in vasoconstriction and reduced blood flow into the corpus cavernosum.

3. Parallel sympathetic stimulation of β_2-adrenergic receptors, at the same vascular beds, induces vasodilation. It is also believed that cholinergic (parasympathetic) stimulation induces vasodilatory effects in the penile arterial vasculature.

4,5. At baseline state, when the male is not sexually aroused, and the penis is not erect, the net effect of the adrenergic (both α_1 and β_2) and cholinergic innervations causes significant vasoconstriction, leading to reduced blood flow into the corpus cavernosum. The reduced blood flow is not sufficient to induce erection.

6,7. It is not clear whether or not the major effects of **yohimbine** are via peripheral or central mechanisms, although most data suggests that the peripheral nervous system has the major role in **yohimbine**-induced improvement in erectile dysfunction (**6**). The medial septopreoptic and the medial dorsal nucleus of the thalamus are presumed to be involved in the generation of **yohimbine's** centrally mediated effects (**7**).

8–10. Yohimbine causes a net vasodilatatory effect on the penile vessels. It is assumed that either **yohimbine** causes a preferential increase in the β_2-adrenergic tone (**8**) compared with the α_1 stimulation (**9**), or that it causes a relative increased cholinergic stimulation (**10**). This latter effect might be associated with increased release of nitric oxide (NO) and subsequent activation of cyclic guanine monophosphate (cGMP) which is a potent vasodilator.

11,12. The net effect of **yohimbine** treatment is vasodilation (**11**), which increases the arterial blood flow into the corpus cavernosum, leading eventually to erection (**12**).

5.2 α_2-adrenergic agonists – clonidine/lofexidine
Therapeutic mechanisms in opioid withdrawal. Mechanism of adverse side-effects

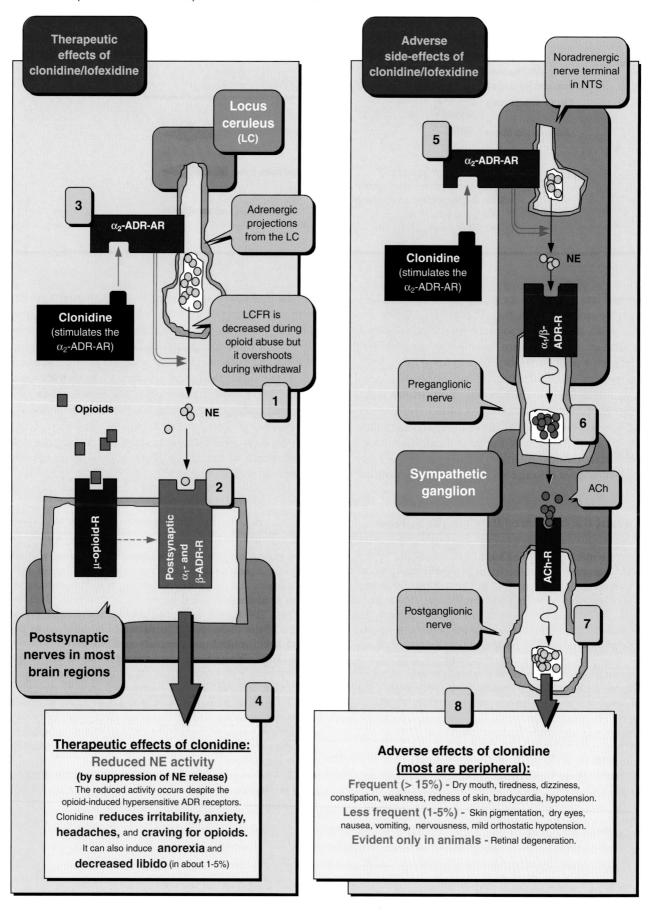

Therapeutic effects of clonidine/lofexidine

Locus ceruleus (LC)

3

α_2-ADR-AR

Adrenergic projections from the LC

Clonidine (stimulates the α_2-ADR-AR)

LCFR is decreased during opioid abuse but it overshoots during withdrawal

1

Opioids

NE

2

μ-opioid-R

Postsynaptic α_1- and β-ADR-R

Postsynaptic nerves in most brain regions

4

Therapeutic effects of clonidine:
Reduced NE activity
(by suppression of NE release)
The reduced activity occurs despite the opioid-induced hypersensitive ADR receptors.
Clonidine **reduces irritability, anxiety, headaches,** and **craving for opioids.**
It can also induce **anorexia** and **decreased libido** (in about 1-5%)

Adverse side-effects of clonidine/lofexidine

Noradrenergic nerve terminal in NTS

5

α_2-ADR-AR

Clonidine (stimulates the α_2-ADR-AR)

NE

α_1/β-ADR-R

Preganglionic nerve

6

Sympathetic ganglion

ACh

ACh-R

Postganglionic nerve

7

8

Adverse effects of clonidine (most are peripheral):
Frequent (> 15%) - Dry mouth, tiredness, dizziness, constipation, weakness, redness of skin, bradycardia, hypotension.
Less frequent (1-5%) - Skin pigmentation, dry eyes, nausea, vomiting, nervousness, mild orthostatic hypotension.
Evident only in animals - Retinal degeneration.

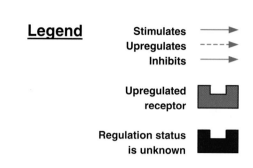

Legend

Stimulates	→
Upregulates	---→
Inhibits	→
Upregulated receiver	
Regulation status is unknown	

ACh Acetylcholine
ACh-R Acetylcholine receptor
ADR-R Adrenergic receptor
ADR-AR Adrenergic autoreceptor
LC Locus ceruleus
LCFR Locus ceruleus firing rate; parameter of adrenergic transmission
NE Norepinephrine (noradrenaline)
μ-opioid-R μ-receptor for opioids
NTS Nucleus tractus solitarius (in the medulla)

Clonidine and **lofexidine** are selective α_2-adrenergic agonists. The α_2 receptor serves as an autoreceptor in presynaptic nerve terminals, where it regulates (via inhibition) the release of norepinephrine (in adrenergic nerves) and serotonin (in serotonergic nerves) into the synaptic cleft. **Clonidine** was initially used as a nasal decongestant, but it is currently and mostly used as an antihypertensive agent, often as an adjuvant to a diuretic. **Clonidine** and **lofexidine's** predominant use in current psychiatric practice is for treating opioid, and to a lesser extent alcohol and nicotine withdrawal symptoms. It is also used as a second-line drug for the treatment of Tourette's disorder and attention-deficit hyperactivity disorder (ADHD) when stimulants are ineffective or contraindicated. It may also be useful in the treatment of stuttering in children, and some reports demonstrate its various efficacy in treating anxiety symptoms related to generalized anxiety or panic disorder. **Clonidine** is also used as a challenge test of the adrenergic system; it stimulates growth hormone release, decreases blood pressure and peripheral 3-methoxy-4-hydroxyphenylglycol (MHPG). Blunted responses in these have been seen in some psychiatric disorders (mainly affective) and it usually indicates favorable response to antidepressant therapy.

Notes about the numbered items in the scheme

Mechanism of action
The following are the main elements in **clonidine** and **lofexidine's** mechanism of action and consequent adverse side-effect profile. The data correspond to those drugs activity in opioid withdrawal, but are assumed to be relevant to withdrawal from other substances as well.
1,2. During chronic use of **opioids**, a decrease in total norepinephrine (NE) activity is found. This is presumably a consequence of suppressed adrenergic transmission originating from the locus ceruleus (LC)(**1**). The α_1- and β-adrenergic receptors located on postsynaptic neurons are upregulated – possibly as a compensatory mechanism (**2**). When a subject withdrawals from **opioids** the adrenergic receptors are still hypersensitive but the adrenergic transmission from the LC is no longer suppressed and usually overshoots as the locus ceruleus firing rate (LCFR) is substantially enhanced. This leads to enhanced adrenergic stimulation which causes the typical withdrawal syndrome which is characterized mainly by autonomic instability, irritability, anxiety, lacrimation, rhinorrhea, and dilated pupils.
3. Clonidine and **lofexidine**, via α_2 agonism, inhibit NE release from presynaptic vesicles into the synaptic cleft, leading to a decrease in NE availability for postsynaptic receptors.

4. These drugs reduce withdrawal symptoms such as irritability, anxiety and headaches. The ability of **clonidine** to reduce craving for **opioids** is also relatively well established. Tolerance develops to the effects of **clonidine,** which is why it is impractical to use this agent for various anxiety disorder (panic disorder, obsessive-compulsive disorder, generalized anxiety disorder) due to the relatively chronic treatment necessary in these cases.

Side effects
5. Clonidine has a troublesome side-effect profile. Most **clonidine**-induced adverse side-effects are mediated via its central agonism at the α_2 receptors in the nucleus tractus solitarius (NTS) in the medulla. **Lofexidine** has less side-effects especially less hypotension.
6. The decreased NE transmission from the NTS results in suppressed preganglionic sympathetic activities (note that acetylcholine serves as a mediator in these nerves).
7,8. As a consequence, diminished sympathetic activity is detected in postganglionic nerves (**7**), resulting in symptoms such as fatigue, dizziness, bradycardia, constipation, hypotension, anorexia, nausea, vomiting and decreased libido (**8**). Skin pigmentation or redness are usually only seen with transdermal preparations.

Dosing strategies for clonidine (oral, for opioid withdrawal syndrome)

A. Day 1: 0.005 mg/kg body weight (about 0.3–0.4 mg/d for a 60–75 kg patient).
B. On days 2–10 (if no adverse side-effects are evident): 0.017 mg/kg body weight (about 1.2 mg/d for a 60-75 kg patient).

C. On days 11, 12, and 13: reduce dose by 50% each day.
D. On day 14: no treatment.
E. Clonidine should be stopped immediately if blood pressure is less than 90/60 mmHg.

5.3 β-adrenergic antagonists (β blockers) – pindolol
Supposed mode of accelerating and augmenting the antidepressant effects of SSRIs

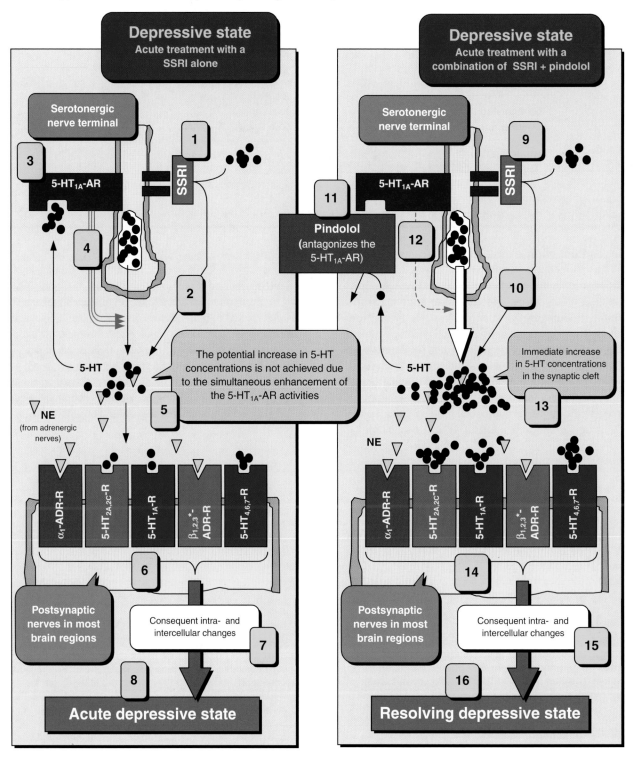

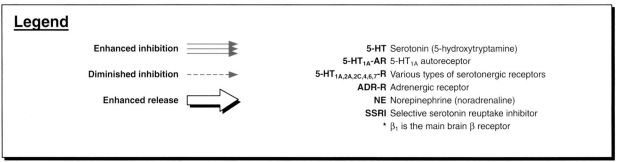

Legend

Enhanced inhibition

Diminished inhibition

Enhanced release

5-HT Serotonin (5-hydroxytryptamine)
5-HT₁ₐ-AR 5-HT₁ₐ autoreceptor
5-HT₁ₐ,₂ₐ,₂C,₄,₆,₇-R Various types of serotonergic receptors
ADR-R Adrenergic receptor
NE Norepinephrine (noradrenaline)
SSRI Selective serotonin reuptake inhibitor
* β₁ is the main brain β receptor

Various β-adrenergic antagonists have a potential use in psychiatric pharmacotherapy. The main agents are **atenolol, metoprolol, nadolol, pindolol** and **propranolol**. There are three distinct β-adrenergic receptors (β_1, β_2, β_3) and two are widely studied: β_1 which is located mainly in the central nervous system and heart, and β_2 which is located predominantly in peripheral tissues such as the liver, pancreas, pulmonary tree, blood vessels and gastrointestinal tract. Some β-adrenergic antagonists (**metoprolol, pindolol** and **propranolol**) are lipid-soluble and cross the blood brain barrier (BBB) with relative ease, while **atenolol** and **nadolol** are more hydrophilic, and so do not cross as easily.

Use of β blockers in psychiatry

Four conditions have been postulated to benefit from β-adrenergic antagonists, namely akathisia, lithium-induced tremor, impulsive or aggressive behaviors, and there is also the recently introduced indication for **pindolol** as an adjunct treatment to a selective serotonin reuptake inhibitor (**SSRI**).

Akathisia. It is believed that a hyperactive noradrenergic activity plays a major role in inducing the disorder. β-adrenergic antagonists (especially **propranolol** and to a lesser extent **nadolol**) are first-line drugs for treating akathisia, via, presumably, reducing adrenergic hyperactivity.

Lithium-induced tremor. A fine tremor is a necessary component of maintaining posture or making a voluntary movement in normal subjects, reflecting unfused motor unit contractions. Agents that increase muscle twitch contractions will exacerbate this physiological tremor. Most of these effects are mediated by increased adrenergic activities, thus β antagonists, via reducing the effects of circulating norepinephrine (NE), are most beneficial in reducing lithium-induced tremor.

Impulsive and aggressive behaviors. Small controlled studies suggest the effectiveness of β-adrenergic antagonists in controlling impulsivity and aggression in patients suffering from organic brain syndromes or schizophrenia (less effective). It could be that these patients suffer from increased adrenergic activities which is blocked by these agents.

Pindolol as an adjuvant to an SSRI for accelerating and augmenting the antidepressant effect. **Pindolol** is a nonselective, lipid-soluble β-adrenergic antagonist with some intrinsic sympathomimetic activity. At the same time, it is also a selective antagonist to the 5-HT$_{1A}$ autoreceptors (it does not interact with the postsynaptic 5-HT$_{1A}$ receptors) – a phenomenon that might explain **pindolol's** unique potential for accelarating and augmenting an antidepressant activity. A few open-label and double-blind studies have been performed to date. In most studies the addition of **pindolol** to an **SSRI** (**fluoxetine, paroxetine**) resulted in a substantial shortening of the time needed to achieve at least 50% reduction in depressive parameters (average 14 days with the combined **pindolol–SSRI** treatment and 26 days with the **SSRI** alone or with placebo). Other studies have demonstrated the capacity of **pindolol** augmentation to an **SSRI** to achieve therapeutic responses both in treatment-resistant patients and in non-resistant patients. In these cases augmentation with **pindolol** has improved the response rate by 25% in the non-resistant group and by about 400% in the treatment-resistant group. Even so, all these data are preliminary and more research is needed to accurately assess **pindolol's** potentials at these indications.

Notes about the numbered items in the scheme

1–5. SSRIs block the reuptake of serotonin (5-HT) into presynaptic nerve terminals (**1**), and thus increase its availability for further synaptic transmission (**2**). However, at the same time, the increased concentration of 5-HT stimulates the 5-HT$_{1A}$ autoreceptors (**3**), which in turn inhibit the release of further 5-HT into the synaptic cleft (**4**). All in all, the concentration of 5-HT available for synaptic transmission is not as high as it could be if the 5-HT$_{1A}$ autoreceptors were not so active (**5**).

6–8. As a result, the postsynaptic modifications (**6**) and the consequent intracellular changes (**7**) that are evident following chronic treatment with **SSRIs** are not evident during the acute treatment and the depressive state is not resolved in these early stages of treatment (**8**).

9–14. When **pindolol** is combined with an **SSRI,** the latter still blocks the uptake of 5-HT (**9**), and thus increases its availability for further transmission (**10**) but at the same time **pindolol** antagonizes the 5-HT$_{1A}$ autoreceptors (**11**), which diminishes their function to suppress 5-HT release from presynaptic terminals (**12**). The net effect of these actions is a prompt and substantial increase in 5-HT concentration in the synaptic cleft (**13**), with a consequent enhanced serotonergic activation of postsynaptic receptors (**14**).

15,16. The exact intra- and intercellular mechanisms involved in the following stages are unclear (**15**), but preliminary evidence suggests that depression resolves more quickly and possibly more effectively with a combined **pindolol–SSRI** regimen than with an **SSRI** alone (**16**).

6.1 Drugs effective for the treatment of extrapyramidal symptoms (EPS)

Suggested mechanisms that induce EPS and relevant drug treatments

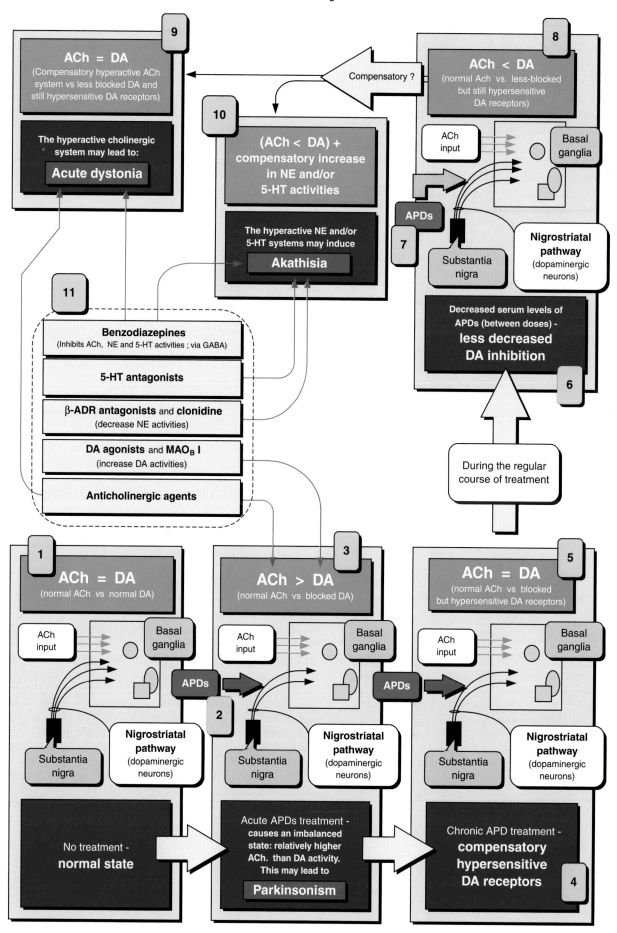

Legend

DA activity	⟶	**5-HT**	Serotonin (5-hydroxytryptamine)
ACh activity	⟶	**ACh**	Acetylcholine
Stimulates activities	⟶	**ADR**	Adrenergic
Inhibits activities	⟶	**APDs**	Antipsychotic drugs
Prominent antagonism by APDs	⟹	**BDZs**	Benzodiazepines
Decreased antagonism by APDs	⟹	**DA**	Dopamine
		GABA	γ-Aminobutyric acid
> ; = ; <	Relative balance	**NE**	Norepinephrine (noradrenaline)
	between different	**MAO$_B$I**	Monoamine oxidase
	neurotransmitter systems		inhibitors (type B)

Notes about the numbered items in the scheme

Antipsychotic Drug Effects

The following cascade of reactions following antipsychotic drug (**APDs**) administration is thought to lead to extrapyramidal side-effects (EPS).

1. Normally and with no **APD** treatment, the basal ganglia, caudate, putamen and globus pallidus (one of the major regions governing motor activity), get a balanced cholinergic versus dopaminergic neural inputs.

2,3. **APDs** antagonize dopaminergic transmission in the nigrostriatal pathway (from the substantia nigra to the basal ganglia) so causing imbalanced dopaminergic-cholinergic neurotransmission. This relative hypercholinergic state (**3**), is believed to be a major factor in drug-induced parkinsonism.

4,5. The dopaminergic receptors, following chronic **APD** treatment (probably as a compensatory mechanism), are up-regulated and become hypersensitive (**4**). This phenomena is partially effective in recovering the baseline balanced cholinergic–dopaminergic activity (**5**).

6–8. Normal administrations of **APDs** is characterized by fluctuating serum drug levels (**6**). When **APD** serum levels are temporarily decreased (**7**) and while the dopaminergic receptors are still hypersensitive (**4**), a relative hyperdopaminergic neurotransmission occurs (**8**).

9. A possible compensatory cholinergic receptor hypersenstitivity occurs, leading to enhanced cholinergic transmission and, in some individuals, to acute dystonic reactions.

10. As a parallel reaction to the relative dopaminergic hypersensitivity, a noradrenergic (which may be serotonergic also) compensatory hyperactivity occurs, leading to akathisia.

11. *Drugs effective for the treatment of EPS:*

Benzodiazepines (BDZs). These, via enhancing GABA$_A$ receptors, have an inhibitory effect on most brain areas, including on the hyperexcitability of the noradrenergic, serotonergic and cholinergic systems.

β-adrenergic (ADR) antagonists. These (**atenolol, metoprolol, nadolol, propranolol**) are beneficial in the treatment of akathisia by blocking the presumed hyperadrenergic activity. They are regarded as first-line agents for this entity, and are considered to be superior to all other anti-akathisia modalities.

Clonidine (see Section 5.2). This is a selective α_2-adrenergic agonist that suppresses the release of norepinephrine from presynaptic vesicles into the synaptic cleft, thus reducing akathisia.

Anticholinergic drugs. These agents block the acetylcholine muscarinic receptors, centrally and peripherally, so decreasing cholinergic activity and, alleviating adverse effects such as acute dystonia and parkinsonism. The main drugs used for such purpose are **benztropine**, **biperidine**, **procyclidine** and **trihexphenidyl**.

Dopaminergic agents. These exert their effects via enhancing dopaminergic transmission.

    MAO$_B$ inhibitors (e.g. **selegiline**). These inhibit the degradation of dopamine, thus increasing its availability for synaptic transmission.

    Amantadine. Exact mechanism is unknown. May act as dopamine-reuptake inhibitor and/or dopamine releaser.

    Bromocriptine. Acts as a postsynaptic dopamine agonist.

Miscellaneous drugs. Various drugs, most with prominent antihistaminergic and/or GABAergic agonistic properties exert some beneficial effects when treating extrapyramidal symptoms (see Section 6.2 for details).

6.2 Drugs effective for the treatment of extrapyramidal symptoms (EPS)
Comparative profile

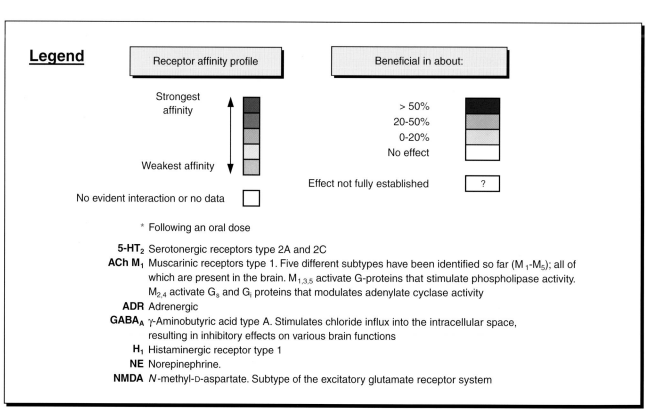

Generic name	5-HT$_2$ antagonism	ACh M$_1$ antagonism	Non-M$_1$ antagonism	α$_2$-ADR antagonism	β-ADR antagonisim	DA releaser	DA-reuptake inhibition	DA agonist (postsynaptic)	GABA$_A$ agonism	H$_1$ antagonism	NE-reuptake inhibition	NMDA antagonism	Akathisia	Akinesia	Dystonia	Rigidity	Tremor	Onset of action (min) *	Duration of action (h)
Amantadine																		up to 48 h	11-15
Benztropine																		60-120	24
Biperiden																		10-30	1-8
Clonazepam																		60-240	18-50
Cyproheptadine													?					up to 48 h	24
Diazepam																		15-60	20-70
Diphenhydramine																		15-180	6-8
Lorazepam																		30-120	10-12
Mianserin																		up to 72 h	24
Orphenadrine																		~ 60	14-25
Procyclidine																		~ 60	~ 4
Propranolol																		60-90	3-5
Trihexphenidyl																		~ 60	6-12

Legend

Receptor affinity profile

Strongest affinity

Weakest affinity

No evident interaction or no data

Beneficial in about:

> 50%
20-50%
0-20%
No effect

Effect not fully established   ?

* Following an oral dose

5-HT$_2$ Serotonergic receptors type 2A and 2C
ACh M$_1$ Muscarinic receptors type 1. Five different subtypes have been identified so far (M$_1$-M$_5$); all of which are present in the brain. M$_{1,3,5}$ activate G-proteins that stimulate phospholipase activity. M$_{2,4}$ activate G$_s$ and G$_i$ proteins that modulates adenylate cyclase activity
ADR Adrenergic
GABA$_A$ γ-Aminobutyric acid type A. Stimulates chloride influx into the intracellular space, resulting in inhibitory effects on various brain functions
H$_1$ Histaminergic receptor type 1
NE Norepinephrine.
NMDA N-methyl-D-aspartate. Subtype of the excitatory glutamate receptor system

6.3 Antihistamines

Comparative profile

Comparative parameters		Cyproheptadine	Diphenhydramine	Hydroxyzine	Promethazine
Antagonizes receptors	Histamine type 1(H$_1$)	Most significant	Most significant	Significant	Most significant
	Acetylcholine muscarinic	Significant	Significant	Significant	
	Serotonin (5-HT) type 2A and 2C	Most significant			
Clinically significant effects	Anorgasmia (reverses)	1			
	Anticough	Weak	2	Weak	Weak
	Anti-motion-sickness	Significant	3	3	
	Anxiolytic	Weak		4	Weak
	Appetite stimulator	5	Weak		
	Dystonic (induces)				
	Dystonic (reduces)		6		
	Glucose serum levels (alters)				Significant
	Hepatotoxic (potentially)				
	Pregnancy test results (alters)				Significant
	Sedative (7)	Significant	Most significant	Significant	Most significant
	Vascular headaches (suppresses)	Most significant			

Legend

Most significant effect	(darkest)
Significant effect	
Weak effect	
Diminished effect / insufficient data	(white)

The role of antihistaminergic drugs in psychiatry is limited. The only well documented indication is the i.v. use of **diphenhydramine** for the treatment of acute dystonic reaction. The use of antihistamines for their sedative effects has diminished since **benzodiazepines** are much better tolerated and have fewer adverse side-effects. As hypnotics, **benzodiazepines** are more effective than antihistaminergic agents in inducing or maintaining sleep. Specific and relative indications for the use of antihistaminergic agents should be limited for patients who are sensitive to or who abuse **benzodiazepines**.

Suggested mechanisms involved in the therapeutic effects of antihistamines

1. Cyproheptadine can reverse anorgasmia caused by selective serotonin reuptake inhibitors (**SSRIs**), by 5-HT$_2$ blockade.

2. Diphenhydramine suppresses the cough reflex more than other antihistamines. The mechanism is unknown.

3. Data are consistent with the role of cholinergic transmission in the induction of motion sickness and vertigo. **Diphenhydramine** and **hydroxyzine** can suppress some of these effects.

4. It is not known how antihistamines, mainly **hydroxyzine**, are anxiolytic. Data suggest a modulating role of the H$_1$ receptor system in anxiety.

5. Cyproheptadine, via its antiserotonergic properties, has a much greater stimulatory effect on appetite since 5-HT (serotonin) might serve as an inhibitory mediator of appetite at the level of the hypothalamus. **Cyproheptadine** may be used for the treatment of anorexia nervosa.

6. Acute dystonia is believed to be a consequence of a hypersensitive cholinergic system. **Diphenhydramine**, by its anticholinergic properties, relieves the dystonic reaction.

7. The sedative effects of all antihistaminergics are believed to be mediated by their antagonistic properties at the postsynaptic central H$_1$ receptor. The exact mechanism is unknown, but it is possible that histamine cause neural depolarization and consequent arousal states.

Peripheral side-effects of antihistamines:

The most common peripheral side effects of antihistamines are: bronchodilation, dried and thickened mucus, tachycardia, hypotension, urinary retention, abdominal distress, diarrhea, constipation, and suppression of allergic reactions.

6.4 Drugs studied for the treatment of dementia of the Alzheimer type (DAT)
Suggested mechanisms involved in DAT and potential drug treatments

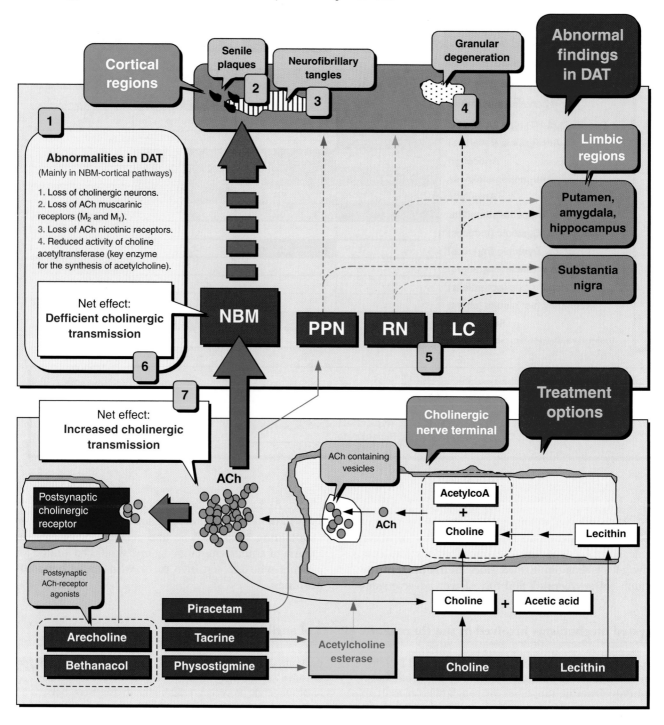

Abnormal findings in DAT

Cortical regions

Senile plaques 2

Neurofibrillary tangles 3

Granular degeneration 4

Limbic regions

1

Abnormalities in DAT
(Mainly in NBM-cortical pathways)

1. Loss of cholinergic neurons.
2. Loss of ACh muscarinic receptors (M_2 and M_1).
3. Loss of ACh nicotinic receptors.
4. Reduced activity of choline acetyltransferase (key enzyme for the synthesis of acetylcholine).

Net effect: **Defficient cholinergic transmission**

6

NBM

PPN **RN** **LC**

5

Putamen, amygdala, hippocampus

Substantia nigra

7

Net effect: **Increased cholinergic transmission**

Treatment options

Cholinergic nerve terminal

ACh

ACh containing vesicles

AcetylcoA + Choline

Lecithin

ACh

Postsynaptic cholinergic receptor

Choline + Acetic acid

Postsynaptic ACh-receptor agonists

Arecoline

Bethanacol

Piracetam

Tacrine

Physostigmine

Acetylcholine esterase

Choline

Lecithin

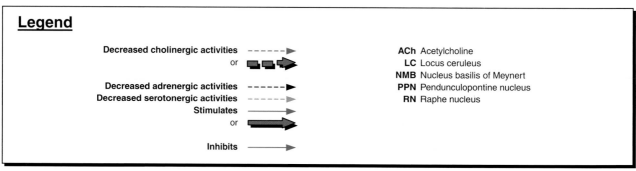

Legend

Decreased cholinergic activities	- - - - ▶
or	▬ ▬ ▶
Decreased adrenergic activities	- - - - ▶
Decreased serotonergic activities	- - - - ▶
Stimulates	──────▶
or	━━━▶
Inhibits	──────▶

ACh Acetylcholine
LC Locus ceruleus
NMB Nucleus basilis of Meynert
PPN Pendunculopontine nucleus
RN Raphe nucleus

Dementia of the Alzheimer type (DAT) is clinically diagnosed by a characteristic decline in multiple cognitive functioning, along with a significant impairment in social, occupational or other major areas of daily activity. Some neurological pathological abnormalities have been identified in DAT, though none are pathognomonic. Some cases of DAT are familial, and genetic analyses suggest non-allelic genetic heterogeneity in both early-onset (age<65) and late-onset (age>65) DAT. Linkage to chromosomes 14 and 21 has been found in early-onset DAT, while late-onset DAT might be linked to chromosome 19 and associated with the gene for apolipoprotein E (APOE). There are 3 major APOE alleles: APOE-e2, APOE-e3 and APOE-e4. The risk of developing late-onset DAT is more than 8 times greater for individuals with two APOE-e4 alleles than that for persons without these alleles and the mean age of onset decreases in these individuals by about 16 years (from 84 to 68 years).

Notes about the numbered items in the scheme:

Pathological lesions in Dementia–Alzheimer Type
1. Major and consistent observations in DAT are the changes seen in the cholinergic system, mainly in projections from the Nucleus Basilis of Meynert (NBM). The main pathological findings are the loss of cholinergic neurons and of acetylcholine muscarinic receptors – both M_1 and M_2, but mainly the M2 type (probably a presynaptic autoreceptor that regulates acetylcholine release into the synaptic cleft). There is also a loss of acetylcholine nicotinic receptors. Note that smoking, which stimulates the nicotinic receptors, has some beneficial effects in DAT. Other findings are the reduced activity of choline acetyl transferase (ChAT), the major and rate-limiting enzyme for the synthesis of acetylcholine. The reduction in ChAT and associated neuronal loss in the basal forebrain, are the most consistent associations with the cognitive impairments seen in DAT patients.
2. Senile plaques (or amyloid bodies) are composed of β A4 deposits (encoded on chromosome 21) and are most prominent in the amygdala, hippocampus and neocortex. They are the most specific findings of DAT (at least in early-onset type), but are also seen in normal aging and in Down's syndrome.
3. Neurofibrillary tangles. These are probably the most specific indicator of neuronal damage, because they are found in neuronal populations that dysfunctions and eventually die. They are formed presumably following modifications in the microtubular associated proteins, mainly Tau.
4. Granular degeneration and pyramidal cell loss, mainly in cortical and hippocampal regions.
5. Some inconsistent findings suggest serotonergic cell loss (projecting from the raphe nucleus) and adrenergic neuronal loss (projecting from the locus ceruleus).
6. The most consistent finding is the deficient cholinergic transmission seen in DAT.
7. Treatment strategies (at present, all are aimed at increasing cholinergic transmission):

Donepezil and tacrine (tetrahydroaminoacridine, THA) are reversible inhibitors of acetylcholine esterase (**donepezil** and **tacrine**), butyrylcholine esterase and cholinesterase (**tacrine**) though **tacrine** also has other effects such as blockade of potassium channels, increasing duration of action potentials, augmenting the release of acetylcholine from presynaptic neurons, inhibition of monoamine oxidase (MAO) type A and type B (less), and inhibiting the reuptake of norepinephrine, serotonin and dopamine into presynaptic neurons. Both drugs have beneficial effects in about 40% of DAT patients both in clinical parameters and by improving scores in several cognitive tests. All these improvements were evident with doses of **tacrine** between 120–160 mg/day and between 5–10 mg/day of **donepezil**. The major adverse side-effects of **tacrine** are elevated serum transaminases (TA) in about 50% of patients, which usually appear during the first 12 weeks of treatment. Twenty-five percent of patients (women are at greater risk) will experience an increase of up to 3 times the normal baseline levels of TA. When TA increases between 3 and 5 times the normal levels, a reduction of 40 mg/day in **tacrine** dosage should be made, until the TA levels return to within the normal range. If TA levels increase by more than 5–10 times, **tacrine** should be stopped. Other relative frequent adverse effects are ataxia, gastrointestinal discomfort, anorexia, nausea, vomiting and diarrhea. **Donepezil** has fewer side effects, the main ones are GI upsets. Monitoring of liver function tests is not required.
Physostigmine. This is an acetylcholinesterase inhibitor which is impractical for clinical use due to its short half-life and significant peripheral adverse side-effects.
Piracetam. This is a γ-aminobutyric acid (GABA) derivative that accelerates the release of acetylcholine from the presynaptic neurons into the synaptic cleft. It has been shown to improve attention and agitation but not cognition in DAT.
Lecithin and **choline**. Both of these are dietary cholinergic supplements. They have not been found, to date, to exert beneficial effects on cognition in DAT patients.
Arecholine. This is a cholinergic agonist. It has shown some inconsistent beneficial effects on cognition in DAT.
Bethanecol. This is a cholinergic agonist. It has not shown any beneficial results in DAT and it also has significant peripheral adverse side-effects, which prevent its clinical use.

7.1 Male sexual behavior

Suggested modulators

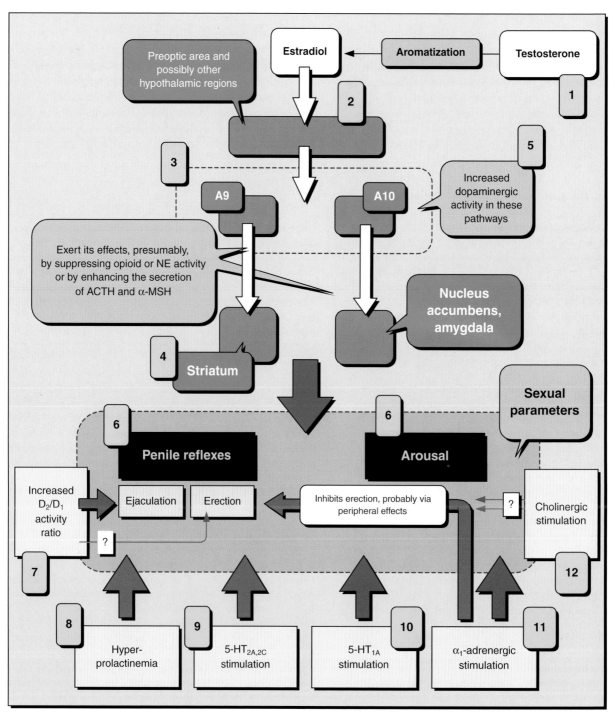

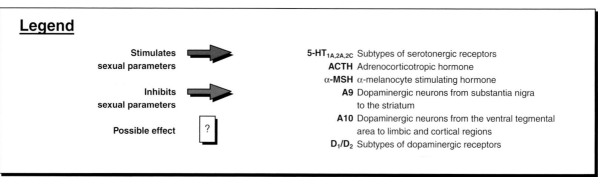

Notes about the numbered items in the scheme

Hormones and sexual functioning

1,2. Testicular steroids are essential to maintain sexual behavior. **Testosterone** is probably the most important hormone modulating male sexual behavior, and it is assumed to exert its effects on the central nervous system following aromatization to **estradiol** (**1**). Note that following castration, a gradual decline in male sexual activity is evident in most mammals. **Testosterone** affects multiple central nervous system sites, particularly the preoptic area in the hypothalamus (**2**). In rodents, **testosterone** has also been shown to interact with both dopaminergic and opioid systems, where it enhances the recognition of various incentive cues emitted by the female. Furthermore, **testosterone** seems to have a role in maintaining normal dopaminergic activity in limbic structures (especially in the nucleus accumbens) since levels of both dopamine and dihydroxyphenylacetic acid (DOPAC, a major metabolite of dopamine) are decreased following castration and increased when testosterone replacement is administered.

Brain mechanisms

3–6. The preoptic area and possibly other hypothalamic regions integrate sensory data from external and internal environments and send impulses to reward centers [mainly to the ventral tegmental area (VTA) and other midbrain structures such as the substantia nigra (**3**)]. These are brain regions containing dopaminergic cell bodies that further project to limbic structures such as the nucleus accumbens and amygdala or pass through the striatum (**4**). The reward system is stimulated by an increase in dopaminergic activity in A9 and especially in A10 which are dopaminergic pathways from the VTA to limbic regions (**5**), with a consequent increased in sexual desire. Dopaminergic agents injected into the nucleus accumbens of rodents stimulate male sexual behavior. These dopaminergic projections project further to the brainstem and spinal cord, where they are presumed to translate sexual desire into motor activity. It is not known if dopamine has a direct sexual role in modulating these sexual parameters or whether it acts via other neurotransmitter systems. The hyperdopaminergic state suppresses opioid and/or noradrenergic activity, and it also stimulates the secretion of several endogenous hormones, such as adrenocorticotropic hormone (ACTH) and α-melanocyte stimulating hormone (α-MSH) which induce penile erection in rats. The net effect of the enhanced dopaminergic activity is an increase in sexual behavior which is evident in two main parameters: desire (sexual arousal) and stimulated penile reflexes (erection and ejaculation) (**6**).

7. In rodents, dopaminergic agonists (e.g. **apomorphine**) or a relative increase in dopamine type 2 receptor transmission versus dopamine type 1 activity (D_2/D_1 ratio) have been shown to reduce ejaculatory latency (thus stimulating ejaculation). This is frequently achieved with a parallel suppression of penile erection. Dopamine's effects on sexual parameters are complex, and although its major effect is estimated to be via central mechanisms, its effect on penile erection might also have a peripheral component, since dopaminergic agonists have been shown to induce penile erection in spinally transected rats.

8. Chronic hyperprolactinemia suppresses all aspects of human sexual behavior. This effect is not due to inhibition of steroid activity, since serum levels of **testosterone** are not altered by chronic hyperprolactinemia. It is also not due to direct alterations in dopaminergic transmission since it does not influence enhanced sexual behavior triggered by dopamine agonists. There is some evidence that it enhances γ-aminobutyric acid (GABA) and opioid activities, which might explain its inhibitory effects on sexual behavior.

9,10. Serotonin (5-HT) has an inhibitory effect on male sexual behavior which is mediated, presumably, via the 5-HT_{2A} and 5-HT_{2C} postsynaptic receptors (**9**). However, stimulation of the serotonergic system can exert different and sometimes opposing effects according to the specific region which is stimulated. Enhanced sexual behavior can be evident following stimulation of presynaptic 5-HT_{1A} autoreceptors in the dorsal or medial raphe of rodents where it apparently decreases the endogenous release of serotonin from presynaptic nerve terminals (**10**). This leads to a consequent decrease in serotonergic inhibition on the striatum (projections from the dorsal raphe) or on the nucleus accumbens, hippocampus and cortex (projections from the medial raphe).

11. Evidence from clinical trials in humans using various adrenergic agents and data based on lesions of adrenergic regions (in animal studies) suggest that norepinephrine increases sexual arousal, probably via stimulating the central postsynaptic α_1-adrenergic receptors located in adrenergic cell bodies of neurons originating from the locus ceruleus. However, it might also have a peripheral and opposing effect where it inhibits penile reflexes (mostly erection; see Section 7.2 for details).

12. Data about the central role of the cholinergic system in male sexual behavior are limited. Some evidence suggests that enhanced muscarinic activity reduces the threshold for ejaculation, but at the same time it exert a parallel reduction in sexual arousal and suppresses penile erection.

7.2 Erection

Supposed mechanism and various agents that can induce erection

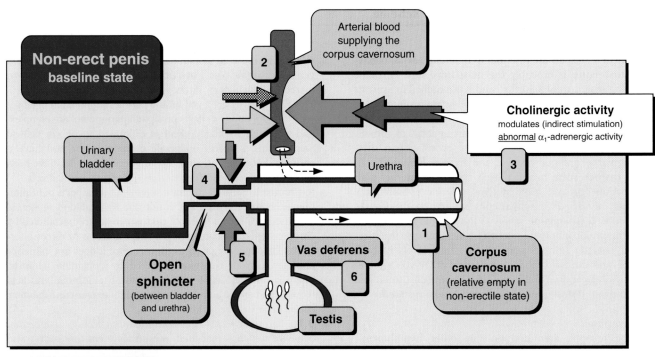

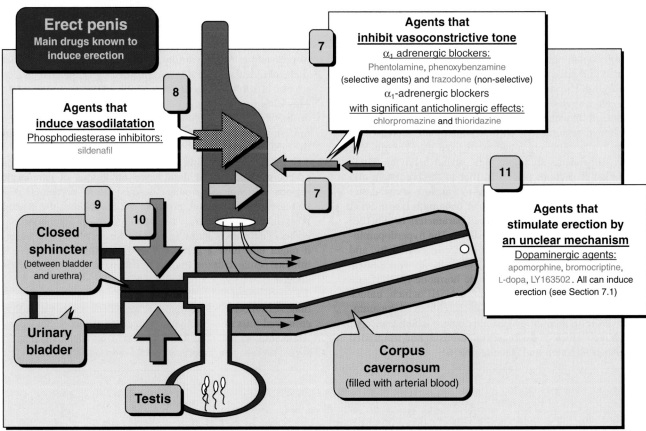

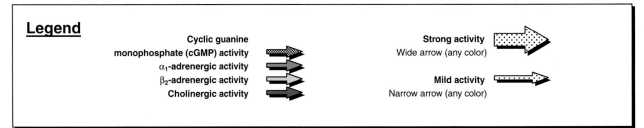

Notes about the numbered items in the scheme

Physiology of penile blood flow

1–3. Penile erection is regulated by both central and peripheral mechanisms. This section discusses mainly the peripheral mechanisms, especially factors controlling the blood supply of the penis. Factors that control the exit of blood from the penis might also be important but current data are insufficient to establish their exact role. For erection to take place, the corpus cavernosum has to be filled with arterial blood (**1**). The arterial vessels supplying the corpus cavernosum are under the predominant innervation and control of the adrenergic system [via α_1-adrenergic (ADR) and β_2-ADR receptors] and cyclic guanine monophosphate (cGMP) activity (**2**). Stimulation of α_1-ADR receptors induces vasoconstriction, and stimulation of the β_2-ADR receptors and/or enhanced cGMP activity brings about vasodilatation. In a baseline, non-erectile state, the arterial vessels supplying the corpus cavernosum are relatively vasoconstricted due to the predominancy of the α_1-ADR tonus over the β_2-ADR activity on these vessels. At the same time, the cGMP activity is not sufficient enough to vasodilate the vessels. The cholinergic system has a modulating role on the α_1-ADR activity. It seems that an enhanced central cholinergic activity stimulates the peripheral α_1-ADR activity, with a consequent increase in vasoconstriction, leading to suppressed erection (**3**). The central cholinergic influence on peripheral α_1-ADR activity is mostly evident when the adrenergic activity is altered and it seems that it has less influence on an intact adrenergic system.

4–6. The tonus of the sphincter between the urinary bladder and the urethra (**4**) is regulated, mainly, by α_1-ADR activity (enhanced α_1-ADR activity contracts the sphincter) (**5**). When the penis is non-erect, the α_1-ADR activity is mild and the tonus on the sphincter is not effective enough to fully constrict it. In such a case, the sphincter between the urinary bladder and the urethra is dilated (e.g. enabling urination). At the same time, and as long as ejaculation is not induced, the vas deferens (**6**), which connects the testis with the urethra and has a role in transporting the ejaculate to the urethra (when it exerts synchronized, directed and rhythmic contractions), is inactive.

Mechanisms of Erection

7,8. For an erection to take place, the β_2-ADR and/or the cGMP activities on the arterial vasculature supplying the penis have to predominate over the α_1-ADR activity. In clinical practice, this effect is achieved, mostly, by the administration of various drugs with a significant α_1-ADR antagonistic effect (**7**). Spontaneous erections can be induced in human males with α_1-ADR blocking agents such as selective α_1-ADR blockers (e.g. **phentolamine, phenoxybenzamine**), or non-selective drugs that have a predominant α_1-ADR blocking effect (e.g. **trazodone**). As mentioned earlier, cholinergic activity has some role in modulating and enhancing α_1-ADR activity. This means that agents that exert a dual action of suppressing both α_1-ADR activity and also decreasing cholinergic transmission (agents with anticholinergic properties) might also induce spontaneous erections, as has been reported for **chlorpromazine** and **thioridazine**.

The role of cGMP in inducing erection is well established following the observed success of the recently introduced selective phosphodiesterase 5 (PDE5) inhibitor **sildenafil** (Viagra) (**8**). PDE5 is probably the most predominant among the phosphodiesterases located in the corpus cavernosum, and inhibition of this enzyme enhances the activity of cGMP, with a consequent decreased smooth muscle tonus and vasodilatation that leads to penile erection. **Sildenafil** is reported to be beneficial in restoring or improving up to 70% of erectile dysfunctions. It induces erection approximately 30 minutes following ingestion and it reaches its peak effect in about 2 hours. **Sildenafil's** most troubling side effects are usually transitory and include: headaches (15%); heatwaves (10%); nasal congestion (4%); and insignificant color blindness (3%). Sudden death is rare and it is invariably associated with the simultaneous use of other vasodilators (e.g. nitrates).

9,10. During erection, the sphincter between the urinary bladder and the urethra is fully constricted (**9**). The constricted sphincter prevents passage of urine into the urethra (from the bladder) and passage of semen (during ejaculation) from the urethra into the bladder. The tonus of the sphincter is enhanced by α_1-ADR activity (**10**). It is confusing how increased α_1-ADR activity suppresses erection and, at the same time, enhances sphincter closure (which is essential for normal ejaculation). It is obvious that there are more parameters involved in this complex mechanism, but current data about other modulators of erection are limited.

11. The effects of dopamine on sexual parameters are complex, and although its major effect is estimated to be via central mechanisms, its effect on penile erection might also have some peripheral component since dopaminergic agonists (e.g. **apomorphine** in low concentrations, **bromocriptine, levodopa, LY163502**) have been shown to induce penile erection in spinally transected rats.

The role of β_2-ADR agonists or antagonists in erection has not been studied well enough, and therefore no conclusions are so far available. There are some data that β_2-ADR agonists (e.g. **clenbuterol**) have a role in regulating arousal and ejaculation but not erection. However, the data are limited and often contradictory. **Propranolol** (a non-selective β-ADR antagonist) can also inhibit penile reflexes in animals and in humans. This mechanism is unclear, since, besides its dual antagonistic activity on adrenergic receptors, it has some 5-HT$_{1A}$ blocking effects (which induce the release of serotonin from serotonergic nerve terminals into the synaptic cleft with a consequent increased inhibition of major neuronal activities).

7.3 Ejaculation

Supposed mechanism and various agents that can affect retrograde ejaculation

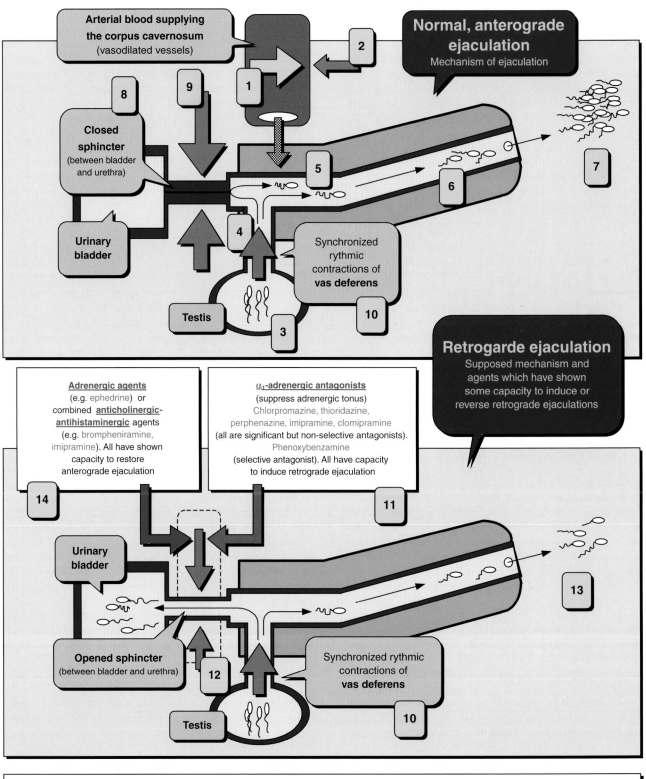

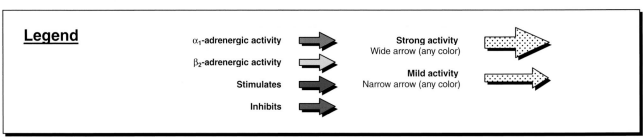

Notes about the numbered items in the scheme

1-5. Ejaculation, as erection, is also regulated by both central and peripheral mechanisms. This section discusses mainly the peripheral mechanism of ejaculation. For ejaculation to take place, the penis has to be, at least partially, erect. For proper erection to take place the arterial blood vessels supplying the corpus cavernosum must be dilated, allowing blood to enter and fill the corpus cavernosum. For such vasodilatation the β_2-adrenergic tonus (**1**) must predominate over the α_1-ADR activity (**2**). For further details concerning the mechanism of erection see former pages. A normal ejaculatory process is based on transporting the semen from the testis (**3**), through the vas deferens (**4**), into the proximal (**5**) and then to the distal urethra (**6**), to be finally ejaculated extraurethally (**7**).

8. During ejaculation the sphincter between the urinary bladder and the urethra is fully constricted. This inhibits the passage of urine from the bladder to the urethra, and at the same time, prevents the contents of the ejaculate to retrogradally enter the bladder (when this happens it is termed retrograde ejaculation).

9. The sphincter between the urinary bladder and the urethra is innervated predominantly by adrenergic fibers and both clinical and animal studies suggests that it is mostly regulated by α_1-adrenergic (ADR) activity. The sphincter is under the tonic stimulation of α_1-ADR activity, which in non-erect and not during ejaculatory process, is dilated enough to enable urine to pass distally into the urethra. Further stimulation of α_1-ADR receptors located on adrenergic nerve fibers innervating the sphincter (during erection, ejaculation or due to effect of various agents) leads to full sphincter constriction, with a consequent inability of the ejaculate to pass retogradally into the urethra.

10. Another process necessary for a proper ejaculation is the transition of sperms located in the testis (**3**) into the urethra (**5,6**). This process is initiated and maintained by synchronized rythmic contractions of the vas deferens (**10**). Most data suggests that the vas deferens is innervated predominantly by sympathetic nerves which are under the primary control of α_1-ADR activity.

11-13. Retrograde ejaculation is almost always the consequent of surgical procedures or following the use various drugs (**11**) acting on and altering the sympathetic tonus of the sphincter between the bladder and the urethra (**12**). The common effect of such agents, which most of them are non-selective drugs, is their α_1-ADR antagonistic properties (e.g. **thioridazine, chlorpromazine, perphenazine, imipramine** in relative high doses, **clomipramine**). However, a selective α_1-ADR antagonist such as **phenoxybenzamine** has also been reported to induce retrograde ejaculation. All these drugs reduce the sphincter's tonus, allowing semen to pass retrogradally during ejaculation and into the urinary bladder. Even so, some of the ejaculate's content may still pass anterogradally to be finally expeled outward of the urethra (**13**). Clinically, an individual with retrograde ejaculation experiences, usually, a normal sense of orgasm but the content of the ejaculate (as seen by the individual) is usually minimal or even completely dry. The ultimate diagnosis is based on finding sperms in the first urine sample collected following an ejaculatory process. The incidence of retrograde ejaculation is unknown but several reports suggest that it could affect about 20-50% of individuals treated with antipsychotic agents and especially with **thioridazine.**

14. Few agents have been reported to reverse retrograde ejaculation caused by drugs (mostly by **thioridazine**, see Section 7.4 for further details) or by surgical procedures which demaged the sympathetic fibers innervating the genitalia. Among these agents are **imipramine** (see Section 7.4) and sympathomimetics (e.g. **ephedrine**) which enhance the adrenergic transmission including the α_1-ADR activity. Other agents which have, beside their adrenergic properties, a significant anticholinergic and antihistaminergic capacities, were also shown to restore anterotrograde ejaculation in individuals with retrograde ejaculation.

7.4 Phenothiazine's – induced retrograde ejaculation

Suggested mechanism of phenothiazine's – induced retrograde ejaculation and treatment options

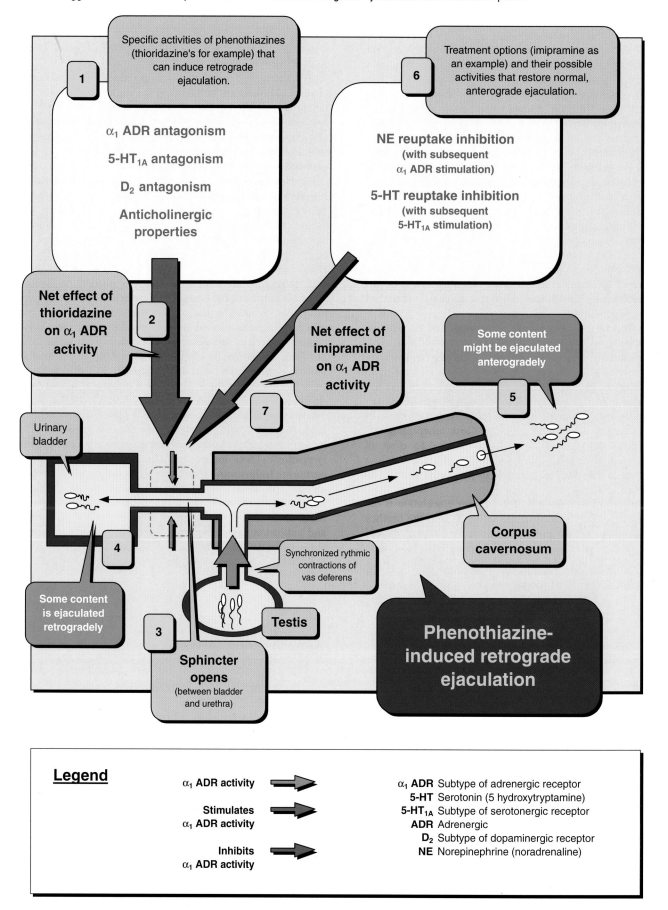

Chronic treatment with antipsychotic drugs is often associated with various symptoms of sexual dysfunction that might affect all domains of sexual activity. Among the antipsychotic drugs, **phenothiazines**, and especially **thioridazine**, are the most commonly associated with adverse sexual side effects. **Thioridazine** can cause various ejaculatory dysfunctions including retrograde, painful or delayed ejaculation in 20-50% of men treated with this agent. How **thioridazine** induces its adverse sexual side effects is unclear. There is no one specific interaction which could account for such impairments, and it presumably involves multireceptor interactions and probably via both central and peripheral mechanisms. **Thioridazine's** profile and the possible mechanism by which it induces retrograde ejaculation are brought in order to provides a schematic and logical approach to further understanding similar phenomena which might be evident with other psychotropic agents.

There are only few reports about drugs that can restore anterograde ejaculation following **phenothiazine**-induced retrograde ejaculation. **Ephedrine** and **imipramine** ($\geq$50 mg/day) have been shown to restore anterograde ejaculation in 14-43% of cases where retrograde ejaculation was caused by diabetes mellitus or following retroperitoneal lymph node dissection. Other preliminary data demonstrated the good efficacy of **imipramine** in restoring anterograde ejaculation following **thioridazine**- induced retrograde ejaculation. About 60% of patients receiving **imipramine** (25-50 mg/day) described full restoration of anterograde ejaculation within a few days of adding **imipramine** to **thioridazine**. Both **imipramine** and **ephedrine** seem to exert their effects via, mainly, enhancement of the adrenergic activity that regulates the tonus of the bladder-urethral sphincter. **Imipramine's** effect on retrograde ejaculation is explained in order to provide detailed information about a drug which is the most commonly associated with restoration of this phenomenon and to present a rational approach that can aid in seeking other pharmacological agents for the treatment of antipsychotics-induced retrograde ejaculation.

Notes about the numbered items in the scheme

1. Thioridazine binds with various affinities to several receptor complexes. It has the highest affinity for blocking various adrenergic (e.g. α_1 adrenergic), D_2 dopaminergic, acetylcholine muscarinic, various 5-HT serotonergic and histaminergic receptors (see sections 3.4-3.5 for further details).

2-5. Up to date, there is not enough data which can associate a specific receptor interaction of **thioridazine** with the induction of retrograde ejaculation. It is assumed that the ultimate effect of **thioridazine** that causes retrograde ejaculation is the decreased muscle tonus which constricts the sphincter between the urinary bladder and the urethra. Consequently, the sphincter dilates and it enables contents of the ejaculate to pass retrogradely into the bladder during sexual activity. The sphincter's tonus is regulated, mainly, by α_1-adrenergic activity, thus it is assumed that the net effect of **thioridazine** is associated with the suppression of such activity. **Thioridazine** can affect α_1-adrenergic activity both directly (as a central α_1-adrenergic antagonist) or indirectly via its other receptor interactions which might serve as central or peripheral modulators of α_1-adrenergic activity. The weight of each receptor interaction and its total contribution to the decreased α_1-adrenergic activity is, as of yet, a matter to speculations. We could only relate to the fact that **thioridazine's** antagonistic properties of the α_1-adrenergic, 5-HT$_{1A}$ serotonergic and various subtypes of dopaminergic receptors has been proposed (see further details in Section 7.1) to suppress various types of sexual behaviors and that it might likewise decrease the peripheral sympathetic tone of the sphincter between the bladder and the urethra (e.g. via reduced α_1-adrenergic activity), with a consequent evolvement of retraograde ejaculation. **Thioridazine** antagonizes, also, the 5-HT$_{2A}$ and 5-HT$_{2C}$ receptors. It is believed that this activity might have a net stimulatory effect on several sexual behaviors and it probably increases central and peripheral α_1-adrenergic activity. Hence, even though the latter effect might oppose the induction of retrograde ejaculation, it seems, empirically, that the other receptor interactions of **thioridazine** predominate, eventually, at the level of the bladder-urethral sphincter. It is not clear how **thioridazine's** anticholinergic properties affect the α_1-adrenergic activity. One possible explanation is that **thioridazine** blocks the peripheral postganglionic cholinergic receptors which are part of the sympathetic nerve fibers which innervate the bladder-urethral sphincter. These fibers, under normal control, are stimulated by acetylcholine to produce and release norepinephrine, which is then released to the synaptic cleft at the nerve terminal. When **thioridazine** interferes with such cholinergic stimulation it can cause a net decrease in norepinephrine release with a consequent suppression of the α_1-adrenergic activity at the level of the bladder-urethral sphincter. The net effect of **thioridazine's** multireceptor interaction is the inhibition of the α_1-adrenergic activity (**2**) which controls the tonus of the bladder-urethral sphincter. As a result, the tonus is reduced (**3**), allowing some (**4**) or all of the ejaculate to pass retrogradely into the bladder instead of anterogradely into the urethra. In case when only part of the ejaculate passes retrogradely, the rest might advance anterogradely (**5**) and the individual could experience a 'wet' ejaculation.

6,7. Imipramine has the highest affinity for blocking the α_1-adrenergic receptor and the norepinephrine (NE) and serotonin (5-HT) transporters (**6**) (Its other receptoral interactions are described in Sections 2.3, 2.10 and 2.11). Altogether, **imipramine** increases the availability of NE and 5-HT in the synaptic cleft with a consequent increased adrenergic and serotonergic activities. Consequently, central and peripheral α_1-adrenergic and 5-HT$_{1A}$ serotonergic receptors are stimulated and this can be associated with enhancement of certain sexual behaviors (see Section 7.1). Since the tonus of the bladder-urethral sphincter is regulated, mainly, by α_1-adrenergic activity, it is assumed that net effect of **imipramine** is associated with the enhancement of such activity (**7**) and the consequent constriction of the sphincter, preventing some or all of the ejaculate to pass retrogradely into the bladder. Instead, most of the ejaculate passes anterogradely into the urethra. **Imipramine** can affect α_1-adrenergic activity both directly (as a central adrenergic stimulator) or indirectly via its other receptor interactions which might serve as central or peripheral modulators of α_1-adrenergic activity. **Imipramine** also blocks, directly, the central and peripheral α_1-receptors, it has major anticholinergic properties (similar to **thioridazine's**) and it stimulates, indirectly, the 5-HT$_{2A}$ and 5-HT$_{2C}$ receptors. These activities might bring about an inhibitory effect on certain sexual behaviors, however, they are, presumably, less significant in the case of restoring anterograde ejaculation.

7.5 Female sexual behavior
Suggested modulators

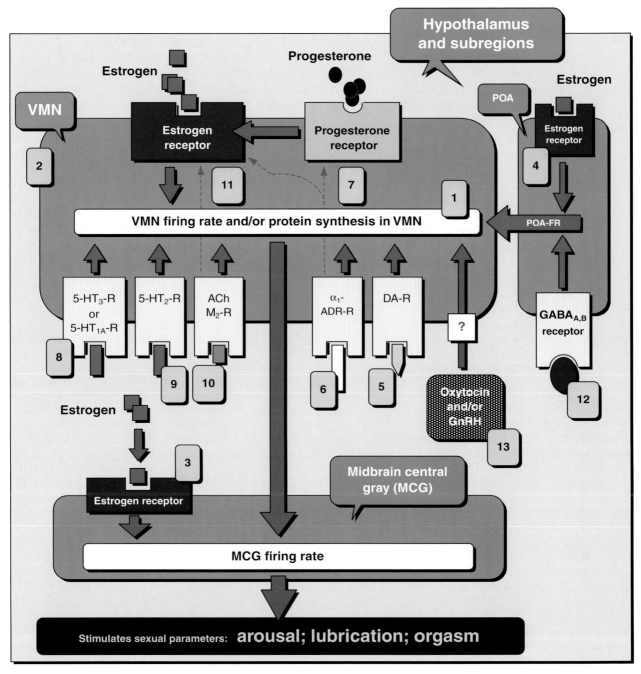

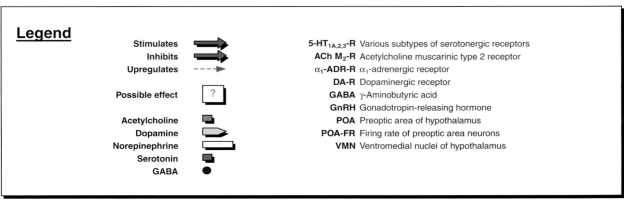

Notes about the numbered items in the scheme

1–4. In human females, baseline **estrogen** (mainly) and **progesterone** levels are essential to maintain adequate sexual behavior. Furthermore, no pharmacological agent has been shown to stimulate female sexual behavior in the absence of **estrogen**. The role of **progesterone** is somewhat more complex. There is some evidence that **progesterone** modulates the effects of **estrogen** while exerting dual effects, depending on the timing of secretion or administration. It might enhance **estrogen**-dependent sexual behavior in some instances while suppressing sexual behavior at other times. Nevertheless, it seems that **progesterone** has diminished effect on sexual behavior when given without the presence of **estrogen**. **Estrogen's** effects on sexual behavior have been demonstrated, mainly, in animal studies, where two major activities are evident: it stimulates protein synthesis at the genomic level [such as preproenkephalins, gonadotropin-releasing hormone (GnRH) and E170 proteins] and it alters membrane electrical activity of central nervous system (CNS) neurons (**1**). **Estrogen's** capacity to regulate sexual behavior is due to its affinity for multiple CNS sites, particularly hypothalamic regions such as the ventromedial nucleus (VMN) (**2**) and the midbrain central gray (MCG) (**3**). These areas are considered to be the major regions responsible for modulating sexual behavior. In these regions, **estrogen** enhances sexual behavior by increasing the firing rate of neurons projecting from the VMN to the MCG, or originating from the MCG itself. In other regions, such as the preoptic (POA) or septal areas, **estrogen** exerts inhibitory effects on sexual behavior (**4**). The E170 protein whose synthesis **estrogen** stimulates, has been shown to stimulate sexual behavior by enhancing axonal transport and the by stimulating the secretion of metenkephalin in VMN neurons projecting to the MCG (in rodents, metenkephalin stimulates lordosis). The exact mechanism of **estrogen**-induced stimulation of sexual behavior in humans is still unclear.

5. Dopamine has been shown to both increase and decrease sexual behavior in females, depending on its site of action and administered dose. It appears that it has stimulatory effects in the VMN (**5**), but opposite effects in areas such as the arcuate or median eminence. However, increased dopaminergic activity has consistently been shown to stimulate sexual arousal in human females.

6,7. Norepinephrine (NE) stimulates female sexual activity possibly via activating the α_1-adrenergic receptors in the VMN (**6**). It is possible that NE mediates the effects of **estrogen** and **progesterone** on sexual behavior, since it was found to increase **estrogen**- and **progesterone**-receptor densities in the hypothalamus of various animals (**7**). The role of α_1-adrenergic receptors is based mainly on animal studies, where **prazosin**, a relatively selective α_1-adrenergic antagonist, has been shown to inhibit lordosis. The role of the β-adrenergic receptors in sexual behavior is unclear since there are a few contradictory reports of both inhibitory and stimulatory effects when these receptors are activated.

8,9. Serotonin probably has inhibitory effects on female sexual behavior. The activation of 5-HT_{1A} receptors in the VMN (it is unclear whether these are predominantly presynaptic or postsynaptic) presumably inhibits sexual behavior (**8**), and activation of 5-HT_3 receptors might exert similar properties on sexual behavior, since 5-HT_3 antagonists (**ondansetron**, **MDL 7222**) have been shown to stimulate receptivity in animals, while **mirtazapine** exerts fewer sexual adverse effects than other antidepressant agents in humans. Even so, $5\text{-HT}_{2A,2C}$ activation might exert stimulatory effects when it affects the VMN or regions such as the median eminence (**9**).

10,11. Acetylcholine stimulates sexual behavior, probably via activating M_2 muscarinic receptors in the VMN, with a consequent increased firing rate of neuronal projections to the MCG (**10**). Acetylcholine may also increase the sensitivity of hypothalamic regions to **estrogen** since cholinergic agents (e.g. **bethanecol**) have been shown to upregulate **estrogen** receptors in the hypothalamus (**11**).

12. γ-Aminobutyric acid (GABA) inhibits female sexual behavior via, presumably, both $GABA_A$ and $GABA_B$ receptors located mainly in the POA. Most studies have shown that the POA has inhibitory effects on female sexual behavior. GABAergic activity, as well as increased **estrogen** binding to **estrogen** receptors in the POA, have been shown to attenuate the normal inhibitory effects of the POA on the VMN.

13. The role of oxytocin and gonadotropin-releasing hormone (GnRH) is not well established. However, they have all been shown to increase sexual behavior (especially by stimulating lordosis in rodents). Their mode of action is assumed to be via an increased neuronal firing rate in the VMN.

7.6 Sexual dysfunctions (I)
Antidepressants-induced sexual dysfunctions

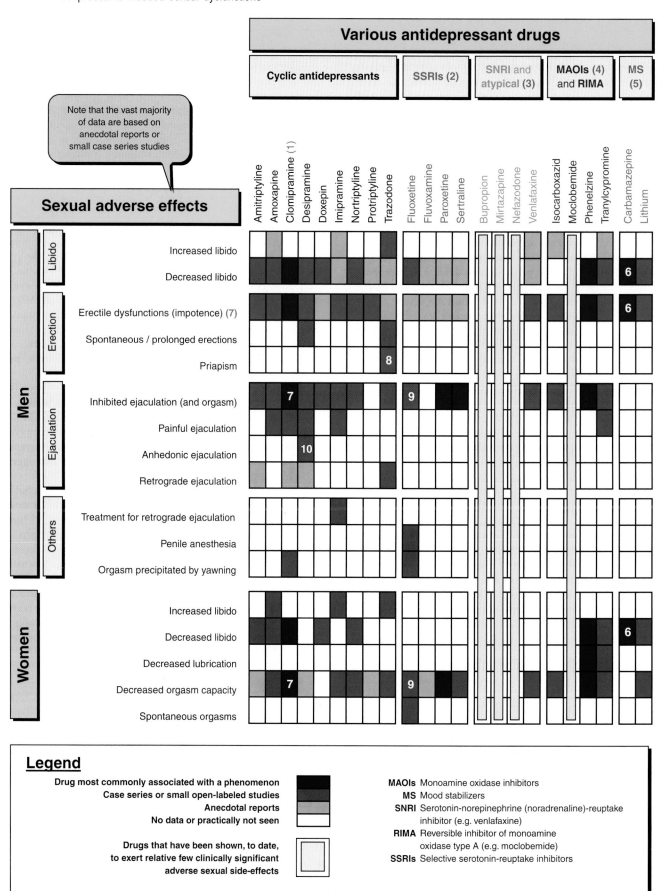

Data about antidepressant-induced sexual adverse effects are limited, and consist mainly of case reports and small open-labeled studies. Practically all cyclic antidepressants (tricyclic and tetracyclic) have been shown to cause sexual adverse side-effects, as well as the selective serotonin reuptake inhibitors (**SSRIs**) and the monoamine oxidase inhibitors (**MAOIs**). The most commonly reported side-effects are as follows:

1. Decreased libido.
2. Impotence.
3. Inhibited ejaculation in men.
4. Anorgasmia or decreased orgasmic capacity in women.

Notes about the numbered items in the scheme

1. Clomipramine is the tricyclic antidepressant (**TCA**) most commonly asssociated with the induction of sexual adverse effects. Between 33% and 95% of patients treated with **clomipramine** complained of some sexual adverse effects.

2. The incidence of sexual adverse effects with the **SSRIs** is unclear, as is their relative incidence compared with the cyclic antidepressants. As a group, all the **SSRIs** can cause sexual adverse effects, especially anorgasmia in women and delayed ejaculation in men. Among the **SSRIs**, **paroxetine** seems to be the most commonly associated with these adverse effects.

3. Preliminary data with **mirtazapine** and relatively well-established data with **bupropion** indicate that they are comparable to placebo in inducing sexual adverse effects. Up to 95% of people who suffered sexual adverse effects due to various antidepressant drug treatments (**tricyclics**, **SSRIs** or **MAOIs**) reported complete or near complete resolution of their dysfunction following the substitution of their drug with **bupropion**. Several reports suggest that **nefazodone** is also comparable to placebo in causing sexual adverse effects. Other data imply that it might cause minimal sexual adverse effects, though much less than **TCAs** or **SSRIs**.

4. MAOIs cause sexual adverse effects in about 5-30% of treated patients. As a group, **MAOIs** cause more sexual adverse effects than the cyclic antidepressants or the **SSRIs**. **Phenelzine** causes more sexual adverse effects than the other **MAOIs**. Its main effects are decreased libido, impotence and anorgasmia in both men and women. The estimated incidence of sexual adverse effects is about 20–30% with **phenelzine**, 5–10% with **isocarboxazid** and 2–3% with **tranyl-cypromine**. It seems that the reversible inhibitor of monoamine oxidase type A (**RIMA**) **moclobemide** is less associated with sexual dysfunctions.

5. Lithium is considered to be a relatively benign agent concerning its sexual adverse effects. Even so, a few reports of **lithium** induced decreased libido and reversible orgasmic dysfunction in women have been published.

6. Carbamazepine can cause decreased libido and impotence in about 10–15% of patients treated for seizure disorders. This might be due to **carbamazepine's** capacity to decrease free serum testosterone levels.

7. Many suggestions concerning the mechanisms involved in antidepressant-induced sexual dysfunctions have been proposed in the literature, and some contradict the others. The following mechanisms are mostly accepted:

a. Erectile dysfunction. Several neurotransmitter interactions are believed to induce erectile dysfunctions in men. The most frequently encountered and presumably one of the major causes of erectile dysfunction induced by antidepressants is their capacity to stimulate central and peripheral α_1-adrenergic receptors (indirect stimulation via enhancement of adrenergic transmission). Stimulated α_1-adrenergic receptors impair the antagonizing ratio between α_1-adrenergic versus β_2-adrenergic and cholinergic antagonism of the peripheral vasculature supplying the penis. This followed by peripheral vasoconstriction and the consequent erectile dysfunctions (see Sections 7.1 and 7.2 for further details).

b. Anorgasmia. There are several possible etiological mechanisms that might impair orgasm in women:

1. α_1-**adrenergic antagonism.** Since all **TCAs** share the capacity to antagonize (to some extent) the α_1-adrenergic receptors, and all **TCAs** have been reported to cause orgasmic dysfunctions, this leads to the assumption that α_1-adrenergic blockade might play a role in impairing orgasm capacity.

2. **Anticholinergic properties. Clomipramine**, which has one of the most potent anticholinergic capacities of all antidepressants, is the agent most frequently associated with anorgasmia.

3. **Enhanced serotonergic (5-HT) and/or reduced norepinephrine activities**. An agent that causes relatively less orgasmic dysfunction is **desipramine**, especially when compared with antidepressants that are less potent agonists of 5-HT or less potent reuptake inhibitors of norepinephrine. This suggests that enhanced 5-HT activity and/or reduced norepinephrine activity might cause orgasmic dysfunction. Note that **cyproheptadine**, a potent 5-HT and histaminergic antagonist, has been shown in a few cases to reverse anorgasmia related to the use of several antidepressive agents.

c. Priapism. The mechanism that induces priapism is unclear. It is speculated to be via very similar factors that cause erectile dysfunctions, mainly a high ratio of α_1-adrenergic versus cholinergic antagonism. Such an antagonizing profile is characteristic and a relative unique property of **trazodone**, which might explain why this agent is mostly associated with priapism (compared with the other antidepressants).

8. The incidence is between 1:1000 and 1:10 000 and usually within the first month of treatment. It is almost always associated with the use of doses above 150 mg/day.

9. Causes anorgasmia in about 8–16% of patients. **Cyproheptadine** and **mianserin** (both of which are non-selective 5-HT$_{2A,2C}$ blockers) have shown beneficial effects in treating and reversing anorgasmia in some of these patients.

10. Isolated cases of 'anhedonic ejaculation' (ejaculation that is not accompanied by the unique feeling of orgasm) have been reported with **desipramine**.

7.7 Sexual dysfunctions (II)
Antipsychotics-induced sexual dysfunctions

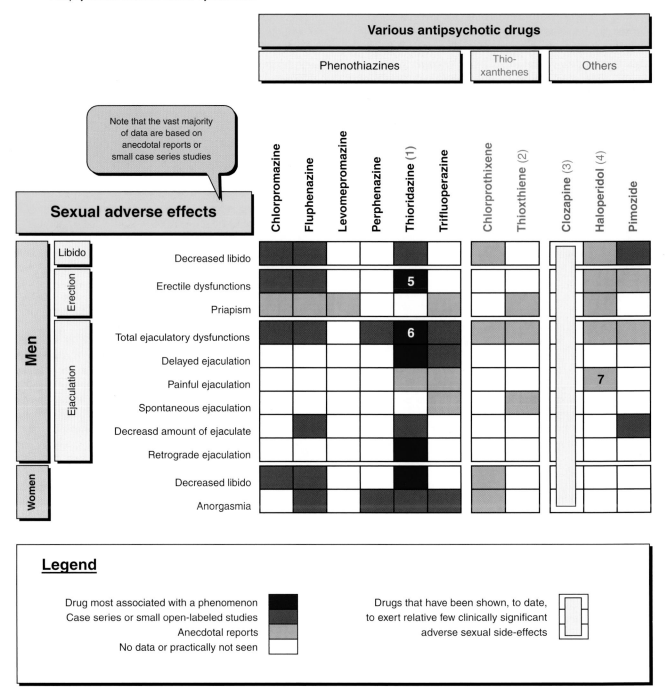

As in the case of most psychotropic agents, data about the role of antipsychotic drugs (**APDs**) in inducing sexual dysfunctions are limited and based mainly on case reports or small open-labeled studies. There are many methodological difficulties associated with most of the relevant studies and it is difficult to distinguish in many cases between the role of the antipsychotic medication and that of other parameters such as the the primary psychiatric disorder, concurrent drug treatment, baseline sexual functioning and non-specific stress (unrelated to a psychiatric disorder) in inducing the dysfunction.

The incidence of sexual dysfunctions induced by **APDs** is unclear. Most data suggest that between 30% and 60%

of people treated with **APDs** exhibit some sexual impairment related directly to the drug they receive. The incidence of some specific adverse effects (partial or complete impotence, decreased amount of ejaculate or retrograde ejaculation and priapism) varies according to the **APD** in use and the study performed. However, these adverse effects are quite abundant, and are estimated to occur in 20–65% of **APD**-treated patients. Other adverse effects (painful ejaculation, spontaneous ejaculation and anorgasmia) are considered less frequent, and are evident in less than 20% of **APD**-treated patients. Altogether, it seems that the **phenothiazines** (especially the aliphatics) have the biggest capacity to cause sexual adverse effects, followed by the thioxanthenes and butirophenones (haloperidol). The atypical APDs might prove to be the most benign in terms of inducing sexual adverse effects although current data are only partially established and mainly concern clozapine.

Antipsychotic drugs (APDs) can modulate sexual parameters via several mechanisms:

A. All APDs act as dopamine type 2 antagonists, and since increased dopaminergic activity in central nervous system regions (especially in the hypothalamus) is a major contributor to intact sexual behavior, it is likely that antagonizing such effects could cause sexual dysfunctions. Clozapine, a relatively weak dopamine type 2 antagonist, has fewer sexual adverse effects than the other APDs, presumably due to this unique receptor-antagonizing profile.

B. All APDs, except clozapine and possibly the other atypical agents, induce chronic hyperprolactinemia secondary to their dopamine receptor blockade in the tubero-infundibular pathway. Chronic hyperprolactinemia suppresses all aspects of human sexual behavior, especially libido and erection (see Section 7.1). Nevertheless, hyperprolactinemia itself is not usually sufficient to induce sexual dysfunctions (mainly decreased libido) and there has to be another coexisting abnormality in order to induce full impairment.

C. APDs that have a substantial α_1-adrenergic blocking capacity (trifluoperazine) cause erectile impairments, including spontaneous erections and/or priapism. Cholinergic activity has some role in modulating and enhancing the α_1-adrenergic activity. This means that agents that exert a dual action of both suppressing the α_1-adrenergic activity and decreasing the cholinergic transmission (agents with anticholinergic properties) might also induce spontaneous erections and/or priapism. The validity of this hypothesis was further strengthened when agents with combined anti-α_1-adrenergic and anticholinergic effects were found to induce spontaneous erections (e.g. chlorpromazine, thioridazine). There are no reports, to date, of agents with predominant anticholinergic properties without a concomitant anti α_1-adrenergic activity that cause spontaneous erection.

D. Some APDs have a known capacity to either decrease serum testosterone levels (thioridazine) or to increase it (haloperidol). The incidence of this effect is not known, although it is estimated to be about 15% of APD-treated patients. It is not clear if these alterations in testosterone levels are centrally or peripherally mediated, although there is some evidence to support the view that the dominant mechanism is peripheral. Testosterone is probably the most important hormone modulating male sexual behavior, and it is assumed to exert its effects on the central nervous system following aromatization to estradiol (see Section 7.1 for details). Thus, the fact that thioridazine is the drug mostly associated with sexual dysfunctions might be attributed to its unique capacity to decrease serum testosterone levels (along with its other effects such as dopaminergic and α_1-adrenergic blockade, anticholinergic effects and the chronic hyperprolactinemia it causes).

Notes about the numbered items in the scheme

1. Thioridazine is the neuroleptic most commonly associated with sexual adverse effects. These effects are believed to be present in about 60 - 85% of treated patients. Only about 25% of patients on other antipsychotic agents are reported to have sexual adverse side effects.

2. Thioxthienes usually cause fewer sexual adverse effects than phenothiazines.

3. Clozapine usually cause fewer sexual adverse effects than other antipsychotic drugs. It is assumed to be the result of its relative low antagonism capacity of the D_2 dopaminergic receptors and/or to its diminished capacity to increase serum prolactin levels.

4. Haloperidol usually cause fewer sexual adverse effects than phenothiazines.

5. In about 35% of patients.

6. Up to 50% have ejaculatory difficulties or changes in orgasm qualities.

7. In very rare cases.

8.1 Electroconvulsive therapy (ECT)

Supposed mechanism of action

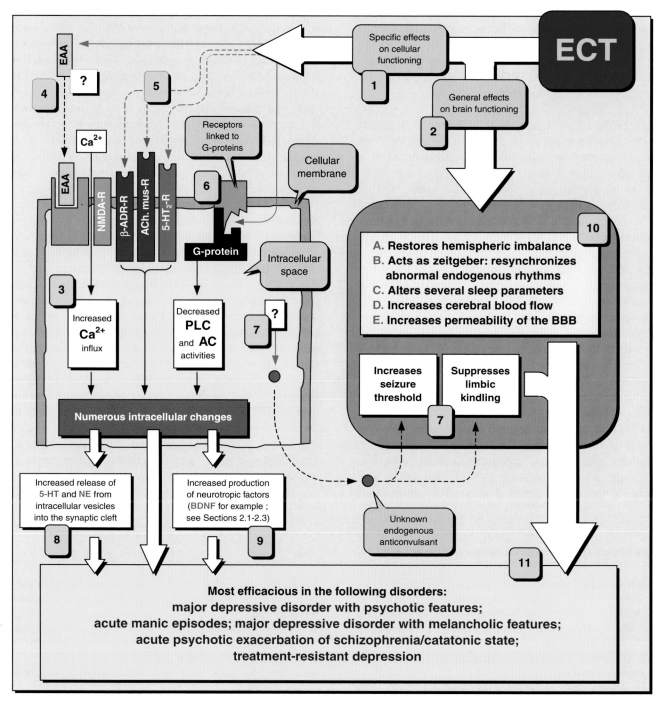

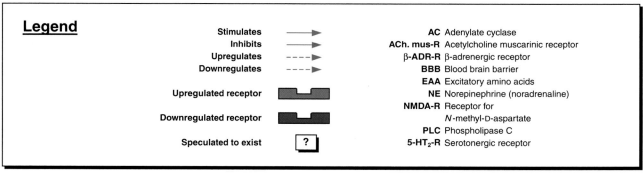

Most efficacious in the following disorders:
major depressive disorder with psychotic features;
acute manic episodes; major depressive disorder with melancholic features;
acute psychotic exacerbation of schizophrenia/catatonic state;
treatment-resistant depression

Legend

Stimulates	→	
Inhibits	→	
Upregulates	--→	
Downregulates	--→	
Upregulated receptor	▬	
Downregulated receptor	▬	
Speculated to exist	?	

AC	Adenylate cyclase
ACh. mus-R	Acetylcholine muscarinic receptor
β-ADR-R	β-adrenergic receptor
BBB	Blood brain barrier
EAA	Excitatory amino acids
NE	Norepinephrine (noradrenaline)
NMDA-R	Receptor for N-methyl-D-aspartate
PLC	Phospholipase C
5-HT$_2$-R	Serotonergic receptor

Electroconvulsive therapy (**ECT**) is one of the most effective treatments in psychiatry. It is assumed that 80–90% of depressed patients respond to it (compared with 60–80% response rates with tricyclic antidepressants or selective serotonin-reuptake inhibitors). The mortality rate for **ECT** is estimated to be about 1:10 000 of treated patients, and is almost always associated with preexisting cardiac disorder. Both anterograde and retrograde amnesias might occur following **ECT**, but are usually transient, and cognitive capacity is fully restored within a few months at the most (6–9 months). Seizure induction is the most relevant and necessary event that has to take place in order to achieve the therapeutic effects of **ECT** (studied with depressive episodes, but presumed to be so with other clinical entities as well). The exact mechanism of action of **ECT** is unclear, although much data are available regarding its secondary intra- and intercellular effects.

Notes about the numbered items in the scheme

1,2. **ECT** affects both intracellular (**1**) and intercellular (**2**) functioning, and changes are induced either directly or indirectly following **ECT**.

3–9. The most consistent alterations in intracellular functions following **ECT** are certain modulations of receptor functioning. **ECT** has been shown to increase calcium influx (**3**). This is due to stimulation of the N-methyl-D-aspartate (NMDA) receptor for glutamate. It is unclear how **ECT** stimulates the NMDA activity, although it presumed to be via the increased production of an endogenous excitatory amino acid that binds with high affinity to the NMDA receptor (**4**). At the same time, **ECT** downregulates postsynaptic β-adrenergic and acetylcholine muscarinic receptors (**5**) and upregulates the postsynaptic 5-HT$_{2A,2C}$ (serotonergic) receptors (**5**). **ECT** inhibits the coupling of various neurotransmitters to their corresponding G-proteins, with a consequent decrease in phospholipase C and adenylate cyclase activities (**6**). **ECT** might also induce the production of an endogenous anticonvulsant (**7**) that, when released into the synaptic cleft, might increase the seizure threshold and/or suppress limbic kindling (see Sections 2.7 and 2.9).

Animal studies support the observation that **ECT** stimulates the release of various cathecholamines (especially norepinephrine and serotonin) into the synaptic cleft, with a consequent increase in their availability for neuronal transmission (**8**). Chronic **ECT** treatment, as with most other of the various antidepressive modalities [**tricyclic antidepressants (TCAs)**, **selective serotonin reuptake inhibitors**, **monoamine oxidase inhibitors**] is associated with the increased and continuous expression of certain factors, such as brain-derived neurotropic factor (**BDNF**) (**9**). The role of these factors in depression is discussed in detail elsewhere.

10. Alterations in global brain functioning or with interneural transmission are also evident following **ECT** (**2**). Some data, based mainly on neuropsychological testing, suggest that major depressive disorder might be associated with right-hemispheric dysfunction. **ECT** has been shown to enhance right-hemispheric functions and it could be relevant to its antidepressive effects (**10A**). Mood disorders are usually associated with desynchronization of certain circadian rhythms (such as the '24-hour biological clock'). **ECT** has been shown to normalize such dysregularities, thus serving as an exogenous zeitgeber (**10B**). Several abnormal sleep parameters are normalized following **ECT**, especially the short rapid-eye-movement sleep latency, the reduced slow-wave sleep and the high nocturnal temperature associated with depressive disorders (**10C**). Other and less consistent evidence suggests that **ECT** is associated with increased cerebral blood flow (**10D**) and increased permeability of the blood brain barrier (**10E**).

11. **ECT** has been shown to possess superior efficacy over **TCAs** or other regularly indicated drugs in several psychiatric disorders. The most beneficial effects of **ECT** (compared with other agents) are in major depressive disorder with psychotic features (efficacious in 80–90% of cases, versus only about 30% efficacy of the **TCAs**). In acute manic episodes, **ECT** is efficacious in about 80% of cases versus only about 60% efficacy of **lithium**. Other disorders respond relatively well to **ECT**, although well-established data concerning the response rates are lacking (major depressive disorder with melancholic features, acute psychotic exacerbation of schizophrenia/catatonic state and treatment-resistant depression).

8.2 Light therapy

Supposed mechanism of action in major depressive disorder with seasonal pattern

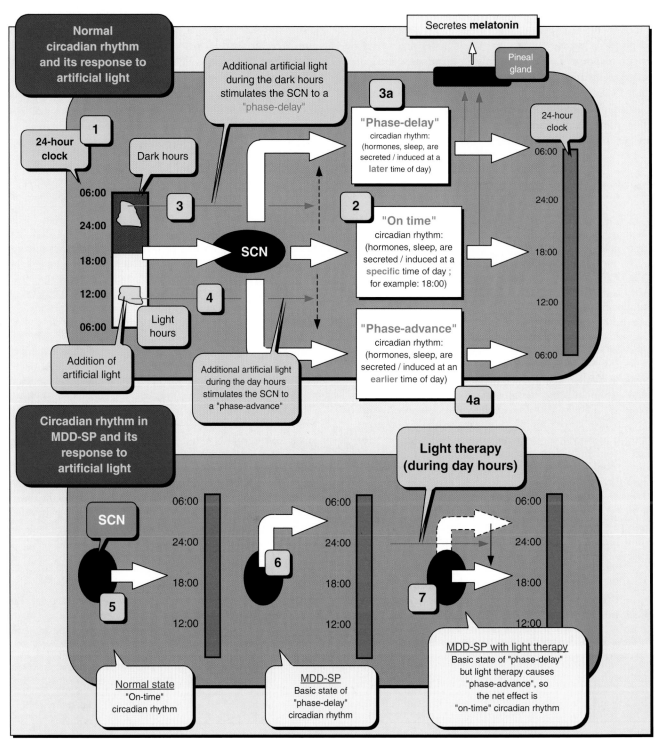

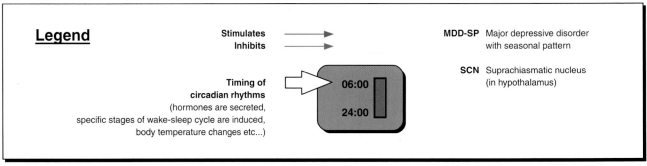

Major depressive disorder with seasonal pattern (MDD-SP) is characterized, clinically, by a depressed mood which occurs at the same time each year, virtually every year since the disorder was first experienced. These depressive states are often termed "winter depressions" since it worsens as the duration of light hours is reduced during the year (which extremes in the winter, usually during January and February). The mood change is usually modest and is characterized by depressed mood, low self esteem, hypersomnia (patients wake later than usual, hence the circadian rhythm is in a "phase-delay" status), fatigue, increased appetite and weight gain, negativism and an impaired social, occupational and other daily functioning. The prevalence of MDD-SP is estimated to be around 5% in the US and women are affected 5 times more than men. As the population is located further from the equator, more people are affected by the disorder. This has to do, probably, with shortening of the light hours in the 24 hours day cycle. The role of melatonin in MDD-SP is under intensive research. Present data suggests that it does not have a direct part in inducing the disorder and it may only serve as a marker associated with changes related to MDD-SP.

Major aspects of light therapy in MDD-SP

1. MDD-SP patient should be exposed 2 hours to light (2500 lux) immediately upon awakening.
2. Significant response should be observed in about 5 days and a full response in 1-2 weeks.
3. Maintenance treatment should be given all winter, 30 minutes of 2500 lux per day or every 2 days.
4. Patients should avoid exposure to strong light during the night hours.

Notes about the numbered items in the scheme

1. Basic circadian rhythms are regulated by several pacemakers which can be either endogenous or exogenous. The major endogenous pacemaker is located, probably, in the suprachiasmatic nucleus (SCN) of the hypothalamus. One of the major exogenous pacemakers is the light-dark cycle, in which different durations of light or dark hours affect the timing of sleep induction, hormone secretion and many more biological rhythms. Normal status, in a person without MDD-SP, is associated with a specific duration of light hours and dark hours during a 24 hour cycle. This ratio of light to dark hours triggers the SCN to induce certain activities, including sleep, hormone secretion and the secretion of melatonin via stimulating the pineal gland.

2. The normal state, described above, triggers the SCN to induce certain activities at a specific time of the 24 hour day cycle. For methodological reasons, the specific time is termed: 'on-time'.

3. Empirical data suggests that when a person is exposed to bright light during the dark hours, the SCN is stimulated to induce its activities at a later time in the 24 hour cycle. This is termed 'phase-delay' circadian rhythm (**3a**). This exposure to light was found to suppress the secretion of melatonin by inhibiting, probably, the necessary stimulus of the pineal gland.

4. Empirical data suggests that when a person is exposed to bright light during the light hours, the SCN is stimulated to induce its activities at an earlier time in the 24 hour cycle. This is termed 'phase-advance' circadian rhythm (**4a**). This exposure to light does not affect the secretion of melatonin by the pineal gland.

5. As mentioned above, a normal status is characterized by certain activities triggered by the SCN in a specific time in the 24 hour clock cycle ('on-time' circadian rhythm').

6. MDD-SP is characterized, among others, by a basic state of 'phase-delay' circadian rhythm. This means that the same triggered activities (by the SCN) are induced at a later time in day (24 hour clock) than in non-MDD-SP patients.

7. When light therapy is administered (during the light hours of day) a 'phase-advance' is triggered. If it is administered to a MDD-SP patient, the 'phase-advance' is superimposed on a 'phase-delay' status, which, in many cases, brings the system (the SCN) to an equilibrium, causing a net effect of 'on-time' circadian rhythm. This could have a role in ameliorating the depressive symptoms of MDD-SP.

SECTION B

ABUSED SUBSTANCES

9.1 Abused substances

Direct effects as first messengers

Abused substances

Direct effect as first messenger
(on membrane receprors / ion channels / transporters)

Neurotransmitters involved

Legend: ■ = Presumed main effect · ▨ = Presumed secondary effect · ? = Possible mechanism

Direct effect as first messenger	Opioids	Amphetamines	Cocaine	PCP	Alcohol	Cannabis	LSD	BDZs	Nicotine
DA — Stimulate the 'reward system' (1)	■	■	■	■		▨	▨		■
DA-reuptake inhibition		▨	■						
Direct postsynaptic DA agonism			?						
Inhibit DA autoreceptor (presynaptic)									
Inhibit MAO$_B$		▨							
Inhibit the release of DA into the synaptic cleft									
Stimulate the release of DA into the synaptic cleft	▨	■							
NE — Decrease NE firing rate	▨								2
NE-reuptake inhibition		▨	▨						
Inhibit the release of NE into the synaptic cleft	▨								
Stimulate the release of NE into the synaptic cleft		▨	▨	?					
5-HT — 5-HT-reuptake inhibition		▨	▨	▨					
Inhibit the release of 5-HT into the synaptic cleft	▨								
Postsynaptic 5-HT$_2$ agonism							■		
Glut. — Inhibit the release of glutamate into the synaptic cleft						▨			
Postsynaptic NMDA antagonism				■	▨				
ACh — Inhibit the release of ACh into the synaptic cleft	▨								
Postsynaptic nicotinic ACh agonism									■
Misc. — Postsynaptic GABA$_A$ agonism					▨			3	
Inhibit calcium influx						▨			
Inhibit MAO$_A$		▨							
Inhibit tyrosine hydroxylase						▨			
Postsynaptic opiate (μ, δ) agonism	■								?
Stimulate calcium influx						?			
Stimulate canabinoid receptors (CB$_1$)						■			

Legend

■ Presumed main effect

▨ Presumed secondary effect

? Possible mechanism

5-HT Serotonin (5-hydroxytryptamine)
ACh Acetylcholine
BDZs Benzodiazepines
DA Dopamine
GABA$_A$ γ-Aminobutyric acid receptor type A
Glut. Glutamate
LSD Lysergic acid diethylamide
MAO$_{A/B}$ Monoamine oxidases type A or B
Misc. Miscellaneous
NE Norepinephrine (noradrenaline)
NMDA N-Methyl-D-Aspartate
PCP Phencyclidine
VTA Ventral tegmental area. Gives rise to the mesolimbic/cortical pathways (arises from the substantia-nigra, terminates in the ventral striatum, amygdaloid body, frontal lobe, and some other basal forbrain areas)

Notes about the numbered items in the scheme

1. The dopaminergic projections from the ventral tegmental area to major cortical and limbic structures.

2. Possibly via stimulating the opiate receptors.

3. Via stimulating the benzodiazepine receptor.

9.2 Abused substances – acute effects

Frequently encountered non-psychiatric symptoms

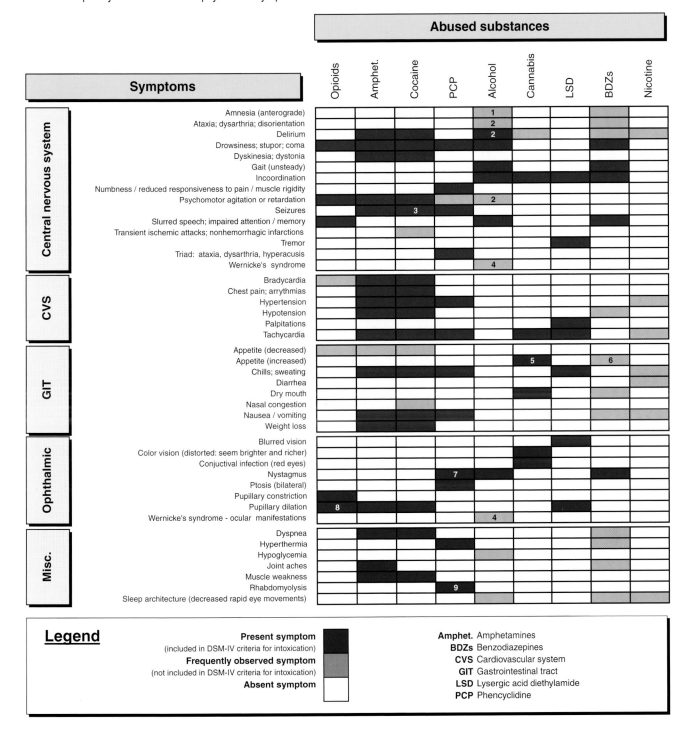

Legend

Present symptom (included in DSM-IV criteria for intoxication)	■ (dark)
Frequently observed symptom (not included in DSM-IV criteria for intoxication)	■ (gray)
Absent symptom	□ (white)

Amphet. Amphetamines
BDZs Benzodiazepines
CVS Cardiovascular system
GIT Gastrointestinal tract
LSD Lysergic acid diethylamide
PCP Phencyclidine

Notes about the numbered items in the scheme

1. Referred to as 'blackouts'.

2. Could be also part of 'idiosyncratic **alcohol** intoxication'. It is characterized by severe behavioral and psychotic symptoms following ingestion of very small amounts of **alcohol**.

3. **Cocaine** is the number one seizure inducer among the described substances, followed by **amphetamines**.

4. Wernicke's syndrome – cluster of acute neurologic symptoms, such as gait ataxia, confusion, horizontal nystagmus, lateral rectal palsy, gaze palsy, anisocoria and impaired reaction to light. It is, in part, due to thiamine defficieny (secondary to malabsorbtion or poor nutrition) which serves as a co-factor for major enzymatic reactions. The cardinal feature is the evident impairment in short-term memory.

5. Also termed 'munchies'.

6. Accompanied by weight gain.

7. Vertical or horizontal.

8. Pupillary dilation can be secondary to severe anoxia.

9. In up to 2%.

9.3 Abused substances – acute effects

Frequently encountered psychiatric symptoms

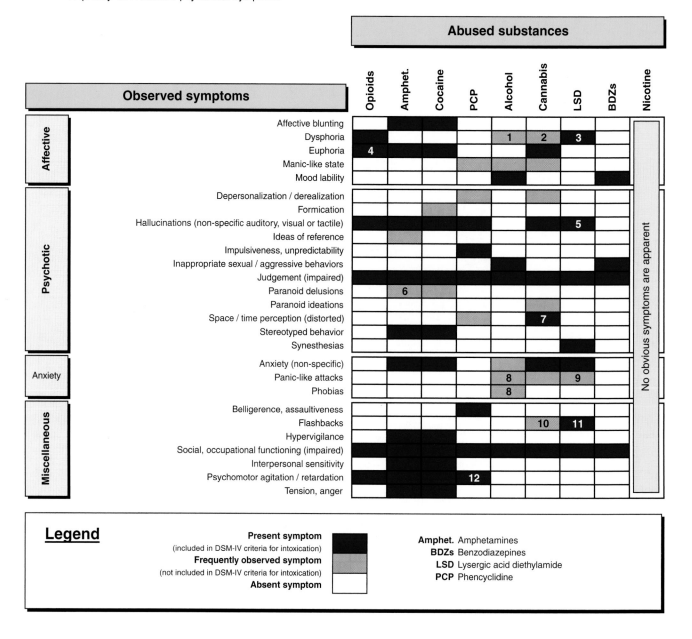

Abused substances — Observed symptoms chart comparing Opioids, Amphet., Cocaine, PCP, Alcohol, Cannabis, LSD, BDZs, Nicotine across Affective, Psychotic, Anxiety, and Miscellaneous symptom categories.

Numbered cells: Dysphoria — Alcohol (1), Cannabis (2), BDZs (3); Euphoria — Opioids (4); Hallucinations (non-specific auditory, visual or tactile) — LSD (5); Paranoid delusions — Amphet. (6); Space / time perception (distorted) — Cannabis (7); Panic-like attacks — Alcohol (8), LSD (9); Phobias — Alcohol (8); Flashbacks — LSD (10), BDZs (11); Psychomotor agitation / retardation — PCP (12).

Nicotine column: No obvious symptoms are apparent.

Legend

- Present symptom (included in DSM-IV criteria for intoxication) — black
- Frequently observed symptom (not included in DSM-IV criteria for intoxication) — grey
- Absent symptom — white

Amphet. Amphetamines
BDZs Benzodiazepines
LSD Lysergic acid diethylamide
PCP Phencyclidine

Notes about the numbered items in the scheme

1. About 35% suffer (sometimes during the disorder) from mood disorders, mostly bipolar I. Women are more prone to experience unipolar depressions.

2. Termed 'amotivational syndrome'.

3. Often marked.

4. Often followed by apathy.

5. Especially a sensation of slowed time.

6. Resembles schizophrenic delusions. The differential diagnosis is based on the absence of other schizophrenia-like signs (disorganized thought, inappropriate affect auditory hallucinations).

7. Usually transient (resolves within a week).

8. About 25–50% of alcohol abusers suffer (sometimes during the disorder) from anxiety disorders, mostly phobias and panic attacks.

9. Termed 'bad trip'. Resembles the panic attacks experienced with cannabis abuse.

10. Controversial. Was found to exert these effects when co-administered with phenyclidine.

11. Flashbacks are usually evident following abstinence from hallucinogen abuse. They are the re-experiencing of perceptual symptoms that were experienced during intoxication: geometric hallucinations, flashes of colors, moving objects are seen with trails behind them, colors might seem intense, objects are surrounded by halos, macroscopia, microscopia.

12. Only psychomotor agitation is part of DSM-IV criteria.

9.4 Abused substances

Frequently encountered withdrawal symptoms

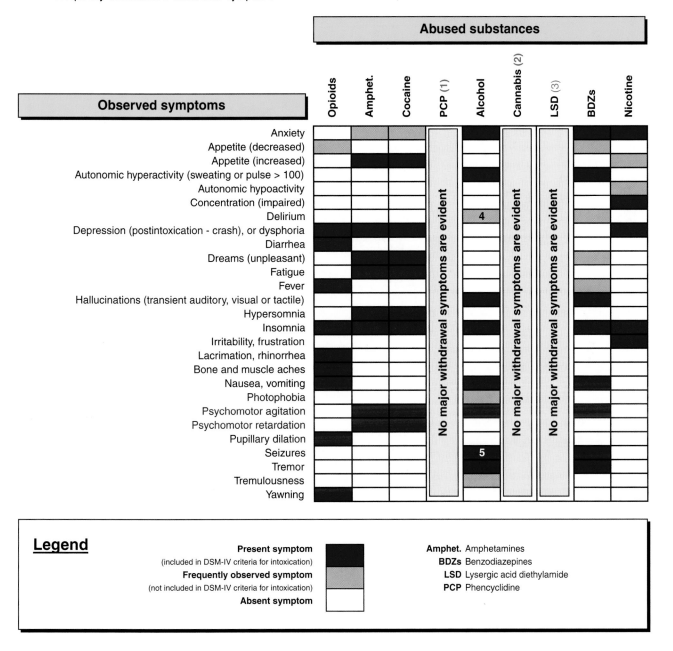

Legend

Present symptom
(included in DSM-IV criteria for intoxication)

Frequently observed symptom
(not included in DSM-IV criteria for intoxication)

Absent symptom

Amphet. Amphetamines
BDZs Benzodiazepines
LSD Lysergic acid diethylamide
PCP Phencyclidine

Notes about the numbered items in the scheme

1. Withdrawal symptoms are evident only in animals.

2. Withdrawal symptoms are rare and usually very mild. The syndrome might include decreased appetite, gastrointestinal discomfort, nausea, vomiting, diarrhea, hyperthermia, sweating, and insomnia.

3. Anxiety or depressive episodes are sometimes reported following hallucinogen (or LSD) withdrawal, but hallucinogen abstinence has not been shown to be the direct cause of these episodes.

4. Delirium tremens (DT) is the most severe form, and it is a medical emergency due to its high rate of mortality (up to 20%). Death usually results from concurrent medical illness (pulmonary, renal or hepatic). DT is almost always preceded by withdrawal seizures. It occurs within the first week of alcohol abstinence, and its main features are autonomic hyperactivity, and visual, auditory or tactile hallucinations (transient, lasting less than a week). DT follows, almost always, at least 10 years of chronic alcohol consumption.

5. Usually precedes the delirium.

10.1 Abused substances – opioids

Supposed mechanism of dependence, withdrawal symptoms and treatment options

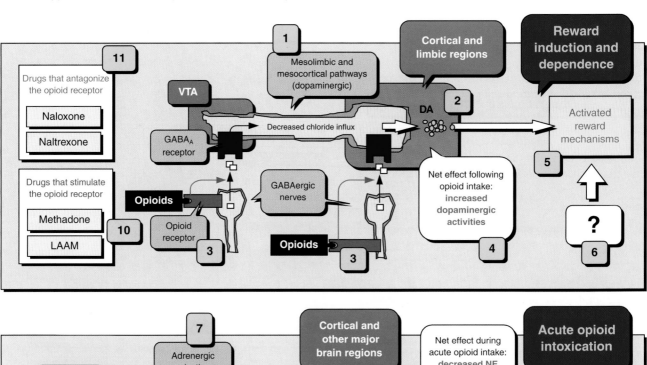

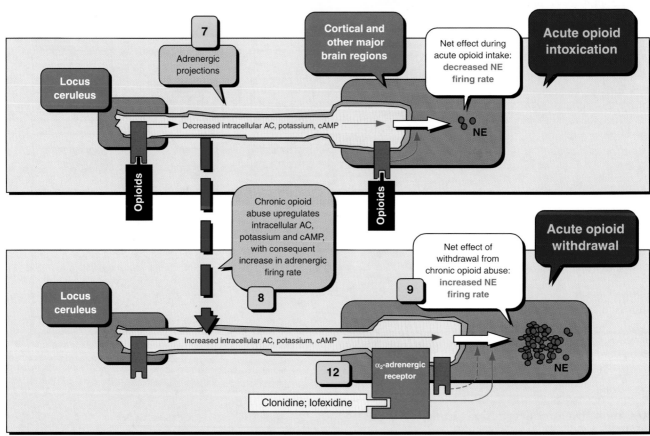

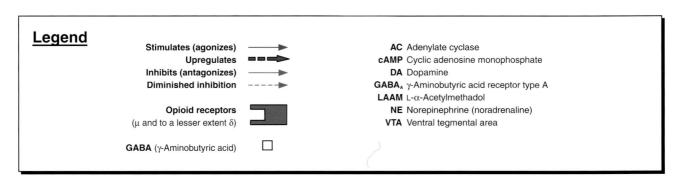

Legend

Stimulates (agonizes)	⟶	AC	Adenylate cyclase
Upregulates	⤏	cAMP	Cyclic adenosine monophosphate
Inhibits (antagonizes)	⟶	DA	Dopamine
Diminished inhibition	⤍	GABA$_A$	γ-Aminobutyric acid receptor type A
		LAAM	L-α-Acetylmethadol
Opioid receptors		NE	Norepinephrine (noradrenaline)
(μ and to a lesser extent δ)		VTA	Ventral tegmental area
GABA (γ-Aminobutyric acid)	□		

Opiates [**heroin** (diacetylmorphine), **morphine**, **codeine**, **hydromorphone**] are derivatives of the naturally occuring compound opium. They have high affinity for receptors that are most abundant in limbic and cortical regions and termed μ, δ and κ. **Opioids (meperidine, methadone, pentazocine, propoxyphene)** are synthetic narcotics with opiate-like properties. A number of endogenous ligands (**endorphins, enkephalins**) have also high affinity to the opiate receptors but their exact physiological role is as yet unclear. Substance dependence refers to a compulsive drug-seeking behavior that is characterized by a withdrawal syndrome when the abused substance is abruptly discontinued. The charac-

teristic symptoms lead to a significant impairment in daily, occupational, recreational and social functioning. It is assumed that no single element or brain region is responsible for the production of the typical substance-dependence syndrome, although enhanced reward mechanisms, triggered by **opioids** and most other abused substances, are key factors. Tolerance is a state in which an increasing amount of a substance is required to achieve the same effect. Tolerance can result, mainly, from reduced absorption, increased metabolism, downregulation of receptors with high affinity to the specific substance, and/or impaired distribution of the specific substance.

Notes about the numbered items in the scheme

1,2. Dopamine (DA) is viewed as the most important neurotransmitter mediating substance dependence and it is believed to exert its effects mainly via stimulating a reward mechanism. The mesolimbic and mesocortical (MLMC) dopaminergic pathways are relatively well-established elements involved in reward induction (**1**). These pathways constitute dopaminergic projections from the ventral tegmental area (VTA) to certain cortical and limbic regions. The main limbic regions involved in reward induction are the nucleus accumbens, olfactory bulb, striatum and the amygdala, while the frontal cortex is the main cortical region involved (**2**).

3. Opiates bind predominantly to the μ, δ and κ receptors. The μ and, to a lesser extent the δ receptors mediate the reward-inducing and reinforcing properties of **opioids**. These receptors are abundant in both limbic and cortical regions, a similar distribution to the dopaminergic projections from the VTA. Stimulation of the κ receptors does not generate reinforcing properties and the distribution of these receptors is quite different from that of the μ and the δ receptors. Stimulation of μ and δ opiate receptors decreases (via G-protein) adenylate cyclase's (AC) activity, with a consequent decrease in intracellular cyclic adenosine monophosphate (cAMP) concentrations and GABA release from GABAergic interneurons. This latter effect results in diminished stimulation of GABA receptors located on dopaminergic neurons, increased excitability of these neurons, and consequent increased release of DA.

4–6. The exact mechanism of reinforcement or reward induction is unknown, but, practically all substances with a significant dependence potential were found in animal studies and in human clinical trials to stimulate the MLMC dopaminergic pathways (**4**). This leads to substance dependence, manifested mainly by rewarding properties, compulsive self-administration and withdrawal symptoms (**5**). Even so, it is quite clear that dependence induction is a complex phenomena, and other intra- and interneural interactions, as well as behavioral, psychological and different modulating variables such as genetics, social and environmental factors, are probably vital and contribute to the typical substance-dependence symptoms (**6**).

7,8. During acute opiate intoxication, opiate receptors located on noradrenergic projections from the locus ceruleus (LC) to almost all brain regions are stimulated, with consequent secondary intracellular changes, mainly decreased adenylate

cyclase (AC) and cyclic adenosine monophosphate (cAMP) activities and potassium concentrations (**7**). These changes induce a decrease in LC firing rate. The chronic abuse of opiates upregulates certain intra-cellular components, especially the AC, along with a significant reduction in potassium conductance (**8**).

9. The upregulated compounds increase the NE firing rate to normal while opiates are consumed. When opiates are withdrawn and the opiate receptors are not stimulated, the upregulated components are still active and they exert a net increase in neuronal NE firing rate, leading to a hyper-excitability state with a concomitant withdrawal syndrome.

10. Methadone is a relatively long acting orally administered synthetic **opioid** ($t_{1/2}$ about 24 hours), with less dependence potential than **heroin**, which can be used once per day. **L-α-acetylmethadol (LAAM)** is a derivative of **methadone**, with a longer duration of action (up to 3 days). It is less abused, and less sedative than **methadone**. **LAAM** is particularly appealing for individuals who can not attend a clinic on a daily basis.

11. Naloxone is a short-acting μ receptor antagonist ($t_{1/2}$ 2–4 hours). It is mostly used intravenously to reverse the effects of opiate agonists. In opioid-dependent subjects, small doses (0.4 mg) of **naloxone** can precipitate a withdrawal syndrome so aiding in diagnosis of physical dependence. Fatal adverse effects following **naloxone** administration have been reported in opioid-dependent people, presumably due to the acute release of NE into synaptic clefts and its greater availability for neuronal transmission. **Naltrexone** is a long acting, orally administered μ receptor antagonist (half-life up to 24–72 hours). It is used to maintain abstinence in already detoxified persons, 7-10 days following a documented abstinence, or alternatively following a negative **naloxone** challenge test. If **naltrexone** is administered before abstinence is completed, profound aversive reactions can appear, which is very difficult to reverse due to **naltrexone's** high affinity for the μ receptors, along with its long duration of action.

12. Clonidine and **lofexidine** are α₂-adrenergic agonists that decrease NE release into the synaptic cleft. They have been used with some success in reducing the characteristic hyper-adrenergic withdrawal symptoms.

10.2   Abused substances – amphetamines

Supposed mechanism of dependence, adverse effects and treatment options

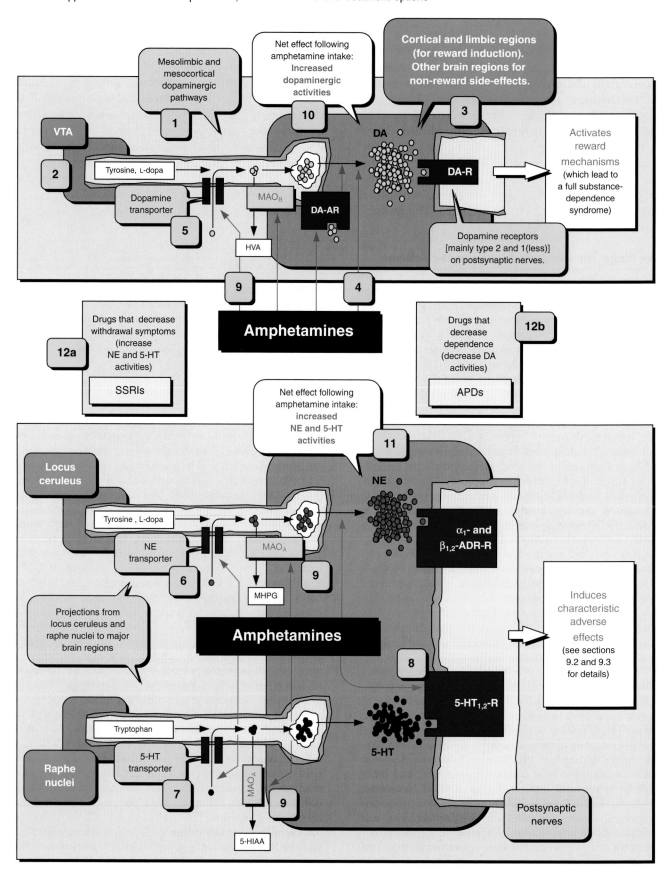

Legend

Stimulates →		DA-AR	Dopaminergic autoreceptor
Inhibits →		DA-R	Dopaminergic receptor
		DA	Dopamine
5-HT	Serotonin (5-hydroxytryptamine)	$MAO_{A,B}$	Monoamine oxidases type A or B
$5-HT_{1,2}$	Serotonergic receptors type 1A,1D,2A,2C	MHPG	3-Methoxy-4-hydroxyphenylglycol
5-HIAA	5-hydroxyindole acetic acid	NE	Norepinephrine (noradrenaline)
ADR-R	Adrenergic receptor	SSRIs	Selective serotonin reuptake inhibitors
APDs	Antipsychotic drugs	VTA	Ventral tegmental area

Amphetamines are synthetic psychostimulants, which are subdivided into 'classic amphetamines' (**dextroamphetamine**, **methamphetamine**, and **methylphenidate**) and 'designer amphetamines' (**Adam**, **MDEA**, **MDMA**, **MMDA**, **DOM**, **XTC**), which have, besides their euphoric effects, some hallucinogenic properties. **Amphetamines**, like **cocaine**, are though to exert rewarding effects via stimulating the mesolimbic and mesocortical dopaminergic pathways (see Section 10.1 for details). They are less addictive than **cocaine**. **Amphetamines** also block the reuptake of norepinephrine (NE) and, at high doses, serotonin (5-HT) (**designer amphetamines**' have more effects on 5HT). All **amphetamines** increase the availability of catecholamines for synaptic transmission. Typical **amphetamines** are often termed by street names such as crystal, ice and speed.

Notes about the numbered items in the scheme

1–3. Amphetamines induce their rewarding and reinforcing effects via stimulating the mesolimbic and mesocortical dopaminergic pathways (**1**). These are dopaminergic projections originating from the ventral tegmental area (**2**) to different limbic (nucleus accumbens, amygdala, olfactory tubercle) and cortical regions, especially the frontal cortex (**3**). **Amphetamine's** adverse effects (other than its stimulatory/rewarding effects) are induced by its similar cathecholamine-enhancing properties in other major brain regions.

4–11. The main stimulatory effects of most **amphetamines** are achieved by stimulation of dopamine release from presynaptic vesicles into the synaptic cleft (**4**) and by inhibiting dopamine reuptake by its transporter at the presynaptic nerve endings (**5**). They also block the reuptake of NE into presynaptic vesicles (**6**) and some, mostly '**designer amphetamines**', also block the reuptake of serotonin at its transporter site (**7**). **Amphetamines** may also exert direct agonistic activities at postsynaptic serotonergic receptors (**8**). Most **amphetamines** have a relatively minor capacity to block monoamine oxidases type A and B (**9**) and thus further increase the concentrations of catecholamines in the synaptic cleft. The net effect of **amphetamines** abuse is the increased concentrations of dopamine (**10**), norepinephrine and serotonin (**11**) in the synaptic cleft, with their subsequent increased availability for neuronal transmission.

Treatment options

Amphetamine intoxication and withdrawal share many similarities with symptoms of **cocaine** intoxication and withdrawal. Intoxicated persons should be under careful cardiovascular and respiratory monitoring. Antipsychotic drugs (**APDs**) should also be administered very carefully especially in cases with hyperthermia (due to the increased risk of developing neuroleptic malignant syndrome) and seizure disorder (**APDs** lower seizure threshold). When **APDs** are administered, low doses should be used due to their possible adverse side-effect profile (mainly extrapyramidal) and the addict's usual unwillingness to experience such adverse effects in order to suppress their craving for **amphetamines**. The treatment of **amphetamine** abuse is much less studied than that of **cocaine**. Because the many similarities, both in pharmacological effects and in the overall clinical syndrome, most treatment regimens for **amphetamine** abuse are based on established treatment strategies for **cocaine** abuse (see Section 10.3). These treatments are aimed at either decreasing the acute withdrawal symptoms (by increasing dopaminergic and other biogenic amines activities) or blocking the effects of the psychostimulant at the receptor site, and thus reducing the rewarding or reinforcing properties of the **amphetamines**.

Drugs that decrease reward and reinforcing properties of amphetamines

12a. Selective serotonin reuptake inhibitors (SSRIs). **Fluoxetine** was found to decrease self-administration of **amphetamines** in animal studies and is often taken by users to prolong the 'high' and decrease the 'crash' from Ecstacy.

12b. Pimozide has shown inconsistent antagonistic effects on euphoria and drug-seeking induced by **amphetamines**. **Flupenthixol** has been shown to reduce some of the rewarding and reinforcing properties of **cocaine**.

10.3 Abused substances – cocaine

Supposed mechanism of dependence, adverse effects and treatment options

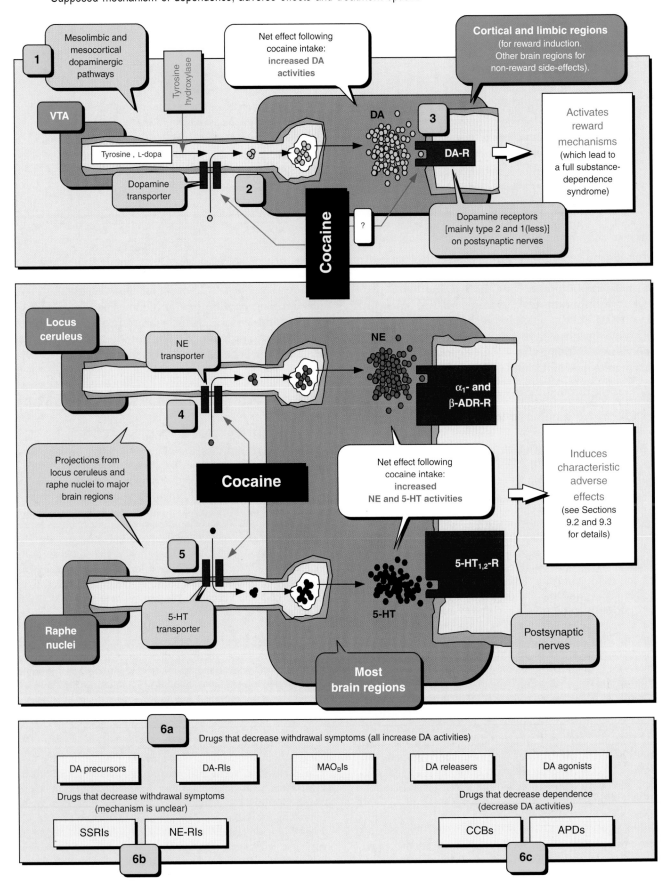

Legend

Stimulates ⟶		**DA**	Dopamine
Inhibits ⟶		**DA-R**	Dopaminergic receptor
		DA-RIs	Dopamine-reuptake inhibitors
5-HT	Serotonin (5-hydroxytryptamine)	**MAO$_B$Is**	Monoamine oxidase inhibitors type B
5-HT$_{1,2}$	Serotonergic receptors type 1A,1D,2A,2C	**NE**	Norepinephrine
APDs	Antipsychotic drugs	**SSRIs**	Selective serotonin-reuptake inhibitors
CCBs	Calcium channel blockers	**VTA**	Ventral tegmental area

Cocaine is an alkaloid derived from the shrub *Erythroxylon coca*. It exerts its rewarding effects via stimulating the mesolimbic and mesocortical dopaminergic pathways (see Section 10.1 for details). **Cocaine** also blocks the reuptake of norepinephrine (NE), and serotonin (5-HT), leading to increased availability of these substances for synaptic transmission. **Cocaine** is referred to by several street names such as coke, crack, girl, lady and snow.

Notes about the numbered items in the scheme

1. Cocaine induces its rewarding and reinforcing effects via stimulating the mesolimbic and mesocortical dopaminergic pathways. These are dopaminergic projections originating from the ventral tegmental area (VTA) to different limbic and cortical regions, especially to the nucleus accumbens, amygdala, olfactory tubercle and the frontal cortex. **Cocaine's** adverse effects (other than its stimulatory/rewarding effects) are induced by its similar catecholamine-enhancing properties on other major brain regions.

2–5. The main stimulatory effects of **cocaine** result from inhibiting dopamine reuptake (**2**). It may also act as a direct agonist at the postsynaptic dopaminergic receptors, where **cocaine** preferentially stimulates the postsynaptic DA$_1$ and DA$_2$ dopaminergic receptors (**3**). **Cocaine** also blocks the reuptake of both norepinephrine (**4**) and serotonin (**5**) into presynaptic nerves. Some data suggests that it might also inhibit the uptake of acetylcholine into the presynaptic nerves.

Treatment strategies – intoxication
Acute **cocaine** intoxication commonly resolves quickly due to the drug's short duration of action. Thus intoxicated individuals can be usually handled by careful monitoring (especially cardiovascular), supportive and symptomatic treatments. **β-adrenergic antagonists** should be avoided in cases where acute myocardial infarction or angina are suspected to be the result of **cocaine** intoxication, as they might further intensify **cocaine**-induced ischemia by allowing greater unopposed α-adrenergic stimulation. Antipsychotic drugs (**APDs**) should also be administered very carefully, especially in cases of **cocaine**-induced hyperthermia (due to the increased risk of developing neuroleptic malignant syndrome) and seizure disorder (**APDs** lower seizure threshold). If **APDs** are to be given, they should be administered in low doses due to their possible adverse side-effect profile (mainly extrapyramidal side-effects) and the addict's usual unwillingness to experience such adverse effects in order to suppress their craving for **cocaine**.

6a–6c. Withdrawal. Most treatment regimens are aimed at either decreasing the acute withdrawal symptoms (by increasing dopaminergic activities) or blocking the effects of **cocaine** at the receptor site, and thus reducing its rewarding or reinforcing properties at the mesolimbic and mesocortical pathways.
Drugs that decrease withdrawal symptoms. Agents that increase DA activity have shown some capacity to decrease **cocaine**-withdrawal symptoms (**6a**). The effect is presumably mediated by their ability to compensate for the lost **cocaine**-induced dopaminergic stimulation. Among the agents that have been reported to exert some beneficial effects are the DA reuptake inhibitors (**bupropion**), DA precursors (**ʟ-tyrosine** and **ʟ-dopa**), DA agonists (**bromocriptine**), monoamine oxidase inhibitors type B (MAO$_B$Is ; **selegiline** and to a lesser extent **phenelzine**), DA releasers [**amantadine** (also a dopamine reuptake inhibitor)] and stimulants (**methamphetamine**, **methylphenidate**, **pemoline** ; mainly due to their dopamine reuptake inhibition properties and some dopamine releasing capacities).
Norepinephrine-reuptake inhibitors (NE-RIs; **desipramine**, **imipramine**, **maprotiline**) and selective serotonin reuptake inhibitors (**SSRIs; fluoxetine**) have also shown some beneficial effects in reducing **cocaine**-induced withdrawal symptoms. The effect is presumed to be associated with their capacity to enhance adrenergic and serotonergic transmission, but the exact mechanism of action is unclear (**6b**).
Drugs that decrease reward and reinforcing properties (**6c**). These agents suppress dopaminergic transmission, thus opposing the enhanced dopaminergic transmission associated with the reward-inducing properties of **cocaine**. Among these are antipsychotic drugs (**flupenthixol**) that are direct DA antagonists and calcium-channel blockers (CCBs ; **nifedipine**, **nimodipine**). Increased intracellular calcium concentrations following numerous stimuli enhance the activities of tyrosine hydroxylase, with a consequent increased in dopamine synthesis and transmission. **CCBs** inhibit such effects and suppress dopaminergic transmission.

10.4 Abused substances – phencyclidine (PCP)

Supposed mechanism of dependence, adverse effects and treatment options

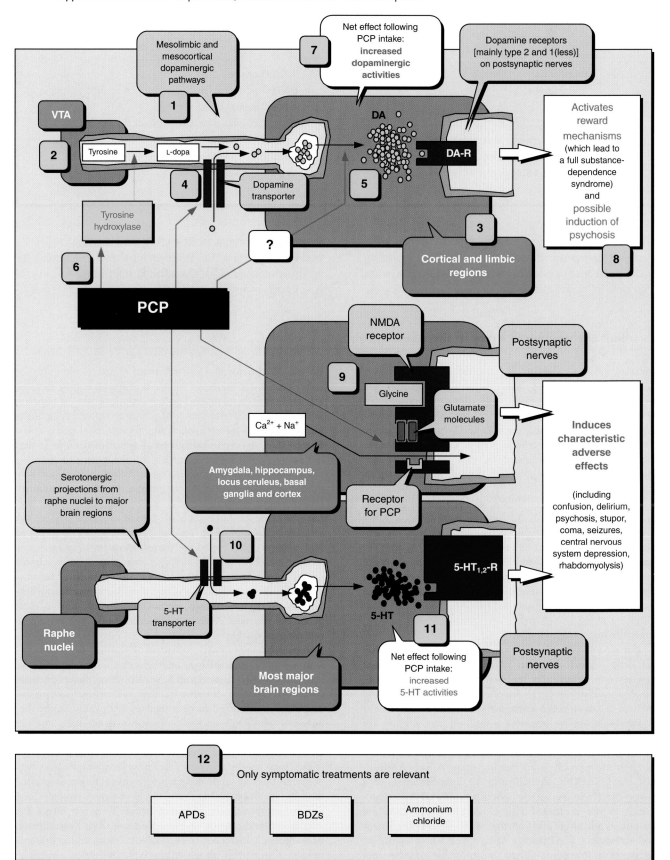

Legend

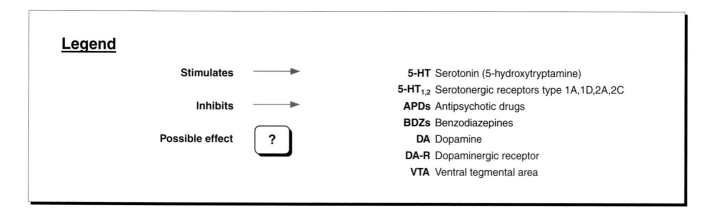

Stimulates →

Inhibits →

Possible effect ?

5-HT Serotonin (5-hydroxytryptamine)
5-HT$_{1,2}$ Serotonergic receptors type 1A,1D,2A,2C
APDs Antipsychotic drugs
BDZs Benzodiazepines
DA Dopamine
DA-R Dopaminergic receptor
VTA Ventral tegmental area

Phencyclidine (**PCP**) is a synthetic psychoactive substance that was originally developed as a general anesthetic. The medical use of PCP is presently contraindicated due to its severe adverse side-effect profile – mainly delirium (in about 33%), agitation, hallucinations and rhabdomyolysis (in about 2%). **PCP** exerts its effects via several neurotransmitter systems, especially the glutamatergic, dopaminergic and serotonergic. **PCP** can induce a clinical syndrome quite similar to schizophreniform psychosis and, at the same time, it greatly increases the risk of schizophrenic patients to develop prolonged psychotic episodes. Even so, It often causes nystagmus and cardiovascular or renal complications that are distinct and are not usually present in other psychiatric disorders. Physical dependence with **PCP** is less common than with other abused substances (**opioids**, **amphetamines**, **cocaine**, **alcohol**), but it can occur. Withdrawal symptoms are rare, possibly due to the lack of a direct effect of **PCP** on the adrenergic system.

Notes about the numbered items in the scheme

1–8. PCP has an enhancing effect on the dopaminergic system including on the mesolimbic-mesocortical pathways (**1**) thus playing a major role in activating the brain reward mechanisms. **PCP** increases the dopaminergic transmission in neuronal projections from the ventral tegmental area (VTA ; **2**) to major cortical and limbic regions (**3**). **PCP** exerts its effects via several main mechanisms:

a. It inhibits the reuptake of dopamine into the presynaptic neurons (**4**), leading to an increase in dopamine availability for neuronal transmission.

b. It probably stimulates the release of dopamine from presynaptic vesicles into the synaptic cleft (**5**).

c. It inhibits tyrosine hydroxylase (**6**), the rate-limiting enzyme in the synthesis of dopamine. This effect opposes the enhancing effects described previously. However, the net effect of **PCP** on the dopaminergic system is stimulatory by increasing dopamine concentrations in the synaptic cleft (**7**). The dopaminergic stimulation induces the typical rewarding properties of **PCP**, and is possibly associated with the emergence of characteristic schizophreniform psychotic symptoms (**8**).

9. PCP antagonizes the N-methyl-D-aspartate (NMDA) subtype of glutamatergic receptors by binding with high affinity to a site within the coupled cationic channel. **PCP's** binding to the ion channel reduces sodium and calcium influx and decreases the intracellular concentration of these compounds. The glutamatergic neurons are mostly excitatory; thus **PCP's** antagonistic properties induce inhibitory effects, which are spread to major brain regions, causing central nervous system depression.

10,11. PCP has been found to exert complex effects on the serotonergic system. It blocks the uptake of serotonin into the presynaptic nerves (**10**) with a consequent increase in its synaptic concentrations (**11**) and its availability for further neuronal transmission. On the other hand, several studies have demonstrated the capacity of **PCP** to reduce the firing rate of serotonergic nerves, with a consequent suppression of the serotonergic transmission. **PCP's** effects on the serotonergic system might explain the similarities in clinical symptoms often found between **PCP** and lysergic acid diethylamide (**LSD**).

12. No antidote has been found beneficial, to date, for **PCP** intoxication. Treatment is symptomatic, and includes careful monitoring of the patient's level of consciousness, cardiovascular and respiratory functioning. Activated charcoal is indicated if the patient reaches the hospital soon enough. The use of antipsychotic drugs (**APDs**) in cases of psychotic episodes or severe agitation should be limited as much as possible due to their capacity to lower the seizure threshold and induce convulsions. If the patient is severely psychotic or aggressive, use high-potency **APDs**, which have a reduced potential to induce seizures compared to the low-potency agents. **Benzodiazepines** are used to treat autonomic instability, muscle spasms and seizures induced by **PCP**, and may also aid in controlling aggressive behavior or agitation.

10.5 Abused substances – alcohol

Abnormal findings in acute intoxication and withdrawal. Treatment options

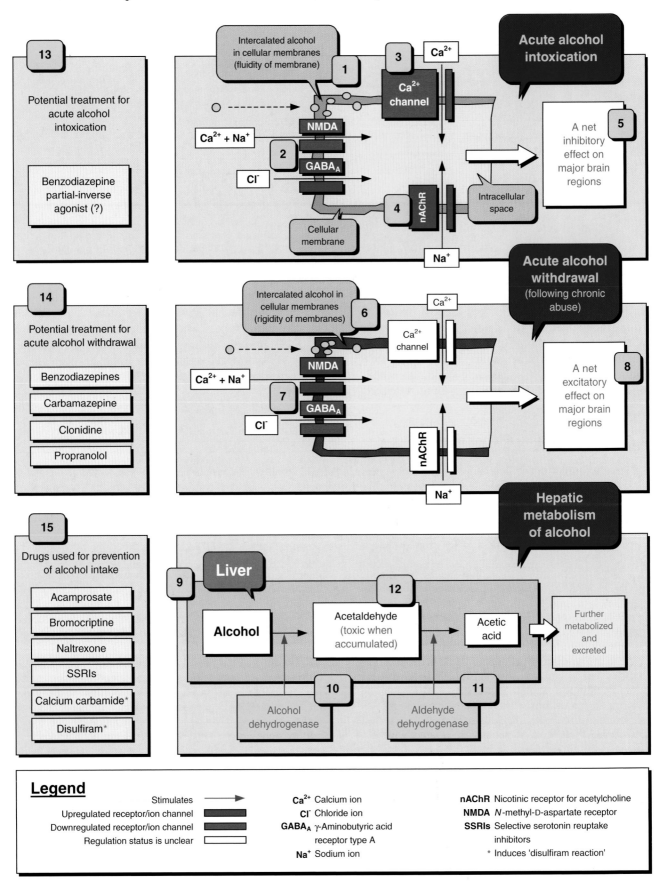

The psychiatric and neurological symptoms associated with ingestion of **ethanol** (the most common form of **alcohol**) are related both to the last-consumed drink and to the total amount of **alcohol** consumed over a lifespan. Characteristic symptoms are often observed at blood alcohol levels (BAL) of 0.01–0.1%, although parameters such as the chronicity of alcohol consumption, concomitant drug intake, hepatic insufficiency, genetic predisposition and rate of absorption (an empty stomach enhances absorption) might greatly affect the clinical presentation. For a non-tolerant person, BAL of 0.01–0.1% often cause a mild decline in coordination, decreased anxiety, disinhibited behavior, euphoric mood and anterograde amnesia. Moderate intoxication (poor coordination, ataxia, dysarthria, impaired judgment and clumsy motor functioning) is apparent at levels between 0.1% and 0.2%, and severe toxicity is observed at 0.2% BAL (diplopia, incoherence, confusion and markedly impaired coordination). At BAL of 0.3–0.4% conscious alternates between stupor to coma. At BAL higher than 0.5%, fatal coma, cardiac and respiratory collapse could predominate. **Alcohol** exerts its effects via numerous neuronal mechanisms, and the apparent clinical picture is usually the consequence of many interactions.

Notes about the numbered items in the scheme

1–5. Alcohol's effects on neuronal functioning are quite different during an acute intoxication from when superimposed on chronic abuse. **Alcohol** intercalates itself into the cellular membrane (**1**), and acute intoxication brings about membrane modifications (fluidity), including an impairment in ion-channel or receptor functioning. The exact intra- or extracellular effects of **alcohol** are unclear, although some receptor modifications are evident, especially decreased sensitivity of N-methyl-D-aspartate (NMDA) receptors and increased sensitivity of the γ-aminobutyric acid (GABA) receptors (**2**). Downregulation of calcium-channel activities (**3**) and upregulation of sodium-ion channels activated by nicotinic acetylcholine receptors (**4**) are also evident. All these changes exert a net significant inhibitory effect on most major brain regions (**5**).

6–8. Alcohol withdrawal syndrome can be seen, even in people only recently abusing **alcohol**, but is usually more pronounced if the abuse is chronic. Chronic **alcohol** abuse causes the cell membrane to be more rigid (**6**), it upregulates NMDA receptors and downregulates GABAergic receptors (**7**). These receptor changes exert an excitatory effect, but as long as **alcohol** is consumed its inhibitory effects counteract the excitatory tendencies. When **alcohol** is withdrawn, the excitatory effects predominate (**8**) and a characteristic 'hangover' is seen, manifested by tremulousness (6–8 hours following cessation), mild autonomic hyperactivity, irritability, photophobia, headaches and gastrointestinal discomfort. Perceptual disturbances, including psychosis, are classically evident within 8–12 hours. Seizures can complicate the clinical picture within the first 24 hours and delirium tremens can be evident during the first 3–7 days following acute abstinence from **alcohol**.

9–12. Alcohol metabolism is primarily hepatic (**9**). Alcohol dehydrogenase (**10**) converts **alcohol** into acetaldehyde and aldehyde dehydrogenase (**11**) metabolizes acetaldehyde into acetic acid. Acetic acid is further metabolized, to be finally excreted. Acetaldehyde (**12**) is toxic when accumulated and if **alcohol** is ingested along with an aldehyde-dehydrogenase inhibitor, the characteristic 'disulfiram reaction' appears.

13. No specific agent has shown significant beneficial effect in suppressing symptoms of acute **alcohol** intoxication. Partial-inverse agonists of the benzodiazepine receptor have shown beneficial effect in animal studies. Their application for **alcohol** intoxication in humans is currently unclear.

14. Benzodiazepines (**BDZs**) suppress autonomic hyperactivity and reduce seizure potential. Long-acting **BDZs** with active metabolites are preferred (**chlordiazepoxide, diazepam**). They allow less-frequent dosing and induce less drug-seeking behavior. **Lorazepam**, which has an intermediate half-life and no active metabolites, is often advantageous because it is less sedative and it can be given parenterally (better dose monitoring). **Clonidine**, an α_2-adrenergic agonist that decreases norepinephrine transmission has also shown some beneficial effects. **Propranolol**, a β-adrenergic antagonist, improves the anxiety, tachycardia and tremor associated with withdrawal. **Carbamazepine** has a similar efficacy to **BDZs** in improving withdrawal symptoms when given in doses of 800 mg/day. It has much less abuse potential than **BDZs**.

15. Several drugs have some limited capacity to prevent **alcohol** intake. **Disulfiram** inhibits aldehyde dehydrogenase, leading to a 5–10 times higher rate of acetaldehyde accumulation when **alcohol** is simultaneously consumed. Consequently, a 'disulfiram reaction' appears, characterized by flushing, chest pain, palpitations, headaches, nausea, vomiting, weakness, agitation, sweating and confusion. This reaction is aversive so putting people off drinking. The problem with **disulfiram** is compliance and it only works if taken regularly, but preferably under supervision. **Calcium carbamide** is a more selective and rapidly acting aldehyde dehydrogenase inhibitor than **disulfiram**. It has a shorter half-life than **disulfiram,** and probably exerts fewer adverse effects. **Acamprosate** is a synthetic indirect GABA agonist that has been shown to reduce **alcohol** intake and is licenced in a number of countries. **Naltrexone** is a μ opiate receptor antagonist that has been shown to reduce **alcohol** consumption in humans when used in a multi modal regimen. **Bromocriptine** and selective serotonin reuptake inhibitors (**SSRIs**) have been reported anecdotally to reduce **alcohol** intake.

10.6 Abused substances – cannabis

Supposed mechanism of dependence and adverse effects

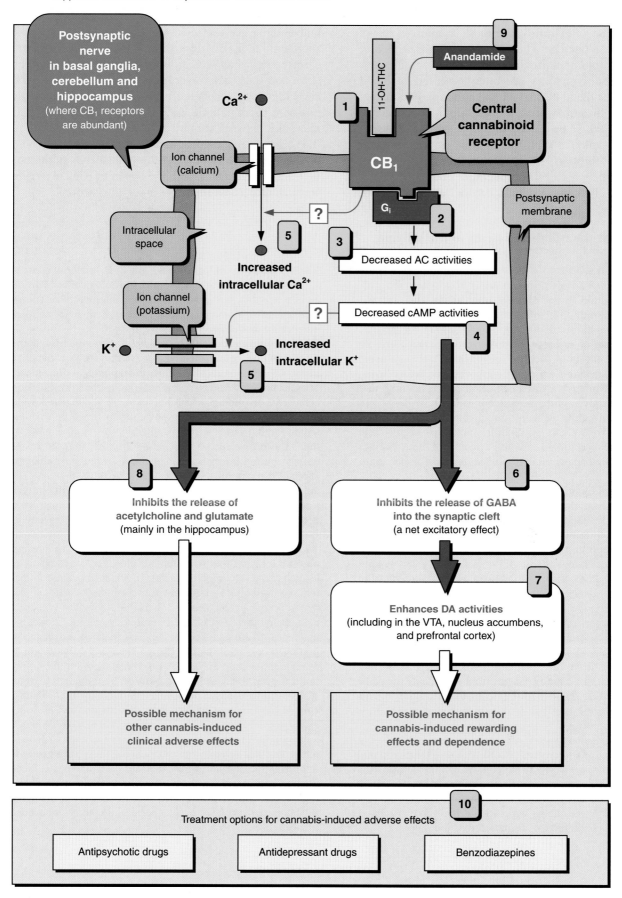

Legend

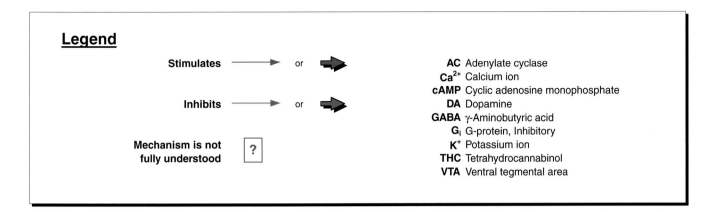

Stimulates ——→ or ⮕	**AC** Adenylate cyclase
	Ca²⁺ Calcium ion
	cAMP Cyclic adenosine monophosphate
Inhibits ——→ or ⮕	**DA** Dopamine
	GABA γ-Aminobutyric acid
	Gᵢ G-protein, Inhibitory
Mechanism is not [?]	**K⁺** Potassium ion
fully understood	**THC** Tetrahydrocannabinol
	VTA Ventral tegmental area

Cannabis, commonly termed bhang, grass, hash, hashish, marijuana and pot, represents various psychoactive substances that are produced from the hemp plant *Cannabis sativa*. The most abundant of them is Δ^9-tetrahydrocannabinol (**THC**), which is converted in the human body to a more psychoactive substance **11-OH-THC**. A number of synthetic cannabinoids also exist and some have medicinal indications. **Cannabis** abuse is associated with many short- and long-term adverse effects. The symptoms of acute intoxication are usually moderate and it is not fatal in cases of acute intoxication. Long-term effects, though highly controversial may include permanent brain damage (atrophy, lowered seizure threshold), impaired testosterone regulation and chromosomal damage. **THC** and other cannabinoids have some analgesic, antiemetic and anticonvulsant properties, and are currently marketed for the treatment of nausea and vomiting secondary to cancer chemotherapy.

Notes about the numbered items in the scheme

1. Two cannabinoid receptors have been found to exist, the CB₁ and CB₂ receptors. The CB₁ is the central cannabinoid receptor that binds **11-OH-THC** and consequently leads to numerous intra- and intercellular reactions that exert the characteristic clinical and adverse effects of **cannabis** and related compounds. CB₂ is the human peripheral cannabinoid receptor found especially in spleen and thymus.

2–5. Stimulation of CB₁ leads to secondary intracellular reactions mediated by inhibitory G-proteins (**2**). The CB₁-G protein interaction suppresses the activities of adenylate cyclase (**3**), with a consequent decrease in intracellular cyclic adenosine monophosphate (cAMP) concentrations (**4**). This has an immediate effect on both calcium and potassium channels, and increased intracellular concentrations of both components are evident (**5**).

Neurotransmitter Interactions
6,7. Alterations in a few neurotransmitter systems are evident as a consequence of **cannabinoid** abuse. **11-OH-THC** inhibits the release of γ-aminobutyric acid (GABA) into the synaptic cleft (**6**), especially, but not exclusively, in the substantia nigra. GABAergic neurons act as inhibitory neurons in the central nervous system, so the suppressed GABAergic transmission leads to a net excitatory effect on certain brain regions, e.g. the dopaminergic projections from the ventral tegmental area (VTA) to limbic structures (primarily to the nucleus accumbens) and to the prefrontal cortex (**7**). This dopaminergic overactivity in the so called 'reward system' can explain some of the rewarding effects of cannabis abuse, and the physical dependence it can cause. Nevertheless, the dependence potential of **cannabis** is much less than that of most other abused substances, and it seems that **cannabis**-induced enhancement of the reward system is not as prominent as its other central nervous system interactions.

8. There is relatively good evidence that **11-OH-THC** can inhibit the presynaptic release of acetylcholine and of glutamate into the synaptic cleft. These effects are evident mostly in the hippocampus. Their clinical significance is uncertain.

Endogenous Cannabinoids
9. Recently, a novel derivative of arachidonic acid, **anandamide** (arachidonylethanolamide) was identified as the endogenous ligand for the cannabinoid receptors, and it was shown to produce similar effects as **11-OH-THC** following stimulation of the cannabinoid receptor. The physiological role of **anandamide** in regular cell functioning is unknown.

Treatments
10. The major treatment strategies are abstinence and supportive therapy. Drugs are used only for symptomatic relief of the mild anxiety that might be experienced during withdrawal (**benzodiazepines**), or for the treatment of depressive episodes (**antidepressants**) or the characteristic paranoid ideations (**antipsychotics**). To date, no specific regimen has been shown to be beneficial in reducing the rewarding properties of **cannabis** abuse, although CB₁ receptor antagonists now exist and might have such a role.

10.7 Abused substances - hallucinogens (lysergic acid diethylamide – LSD)

Proposed mechanism of action and treatment options

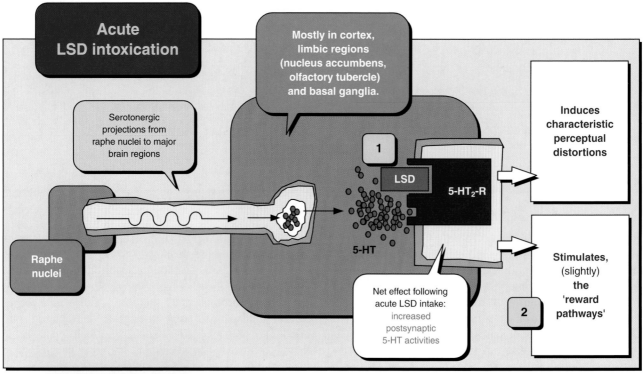

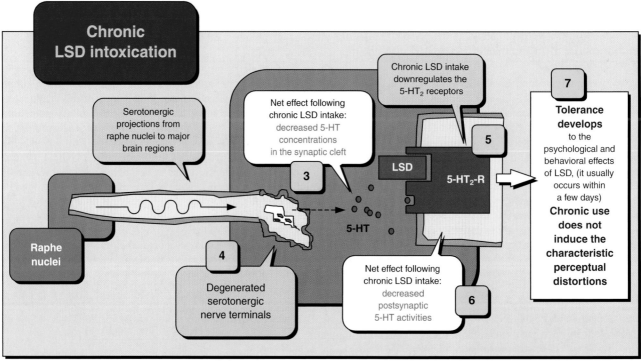

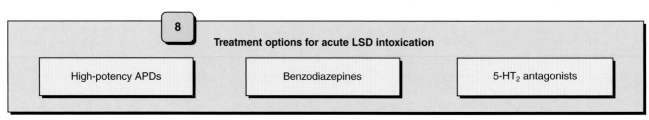

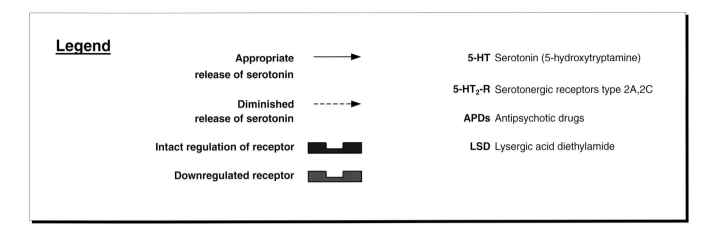

Hallucinogens are chemically diverse compounds that induce, as their primary effect, perceptual distortions (depersonalization, derealization, synesthesias), hallucinations (usually visual) and heightening of consciousness. Many natural and synthetic hallucinogens are abused by humans. The natural substances most commonly abused are N,N-dimethyltryptamine (**DMT**), **mescaline** and **psilocybin**. The most studied and the first abused (prototypic) synthetic hallucinogen is lysergic acid diethylamide (**LSD**). Hallucinogens' mechanism of action is unclear, but it involves, presumably, an enhancement of the serotonergic system (as the primary effect) and a relative minor effect of stimulating the dopaminergic and possibly other cathecholaminergic systems. Hallucinogens are taken orally, although some such as **DMT**, are usually smoked. **LSD's** mental effects occur within an hour after ingestion and last for about 12 hours (peak effect in 2–4 hours). Hallucinogen abuse can lead to fatal outcome and death have been reported, usually from cardiovascular complications (hypertension) or hyperthermia. Tolerance to the psychological and behavioral effects of **LSD** develops quite rapidly (2–4 days of repeated use), and it reverses in about a week following complete abstinence. Hallucinogens or **LSD** do not induce physical dependence and no clinically significant withdrawal syndrome is apparent.

Notes about the numbered items in the scheme

Mode of action

1,2. It is relatively well established that **LSD** enhances the activities of postsynaptic 5-HT$_2$ serotonergic receptors as its primary effect (**1**). **LSD** either binds with high affinity to the serotonin binding site itself or to an adjunct site on the serotonergic receptor. Serotonergic antagonists prevent animals from identifying **LSD** in drug discrimination tests. **LSD**, and probably some of the other hallucinogens can also stimulate (probably indirectly) dopaminergic transmission, including the mesolimbic and mesocortical pathways, which have been termed the 'reward system' (**2**). These are dopaminergic neurons, originating from the VTA (ventral tegmental area) and projecting to major limbic structures (nucleus accumbens, olfactory tubercle), and to the frontal cortex (see Sections 10.1–10.4). In contrast to other abused drugs (**heroin, cocaine**) the stimulation of these reward mechanisms is relatively slight, and it does not produce the classic reinforcing effects, or dependence, as other substances do. **3–7.** Little data are available about the inter- or intraneuronal changes following chronic abuse of hallucinogens. There are some animal data, implying that chronic **LSD** abuse causes depletion of serotonin from presynaptic nerve terminals (**3**), due possibly to degenerative processes at these neuron endings (**4**). Repeated administrations of **LSD** in rats was also found to downregulate the 5-HT$_2$ receptors (**5**). The net effect of these changes is tolerance to the drug effects and decreased serotonergic transmission in the affected regions (**6,7**). The effects of chronic **LSD** abuse on the dopaminergic system is unclear. Tolerance develops rapidly to the behavioral and psychological effects of hallucinogens, and reverses almost as rapidly following abstinence (**7**), probably due to the decreased serotonergic transmission mentioned earlier.

Treatment of Intoxification

8. Reassurance, reduction of sensory input, and supportive care are the hallmarks in the treatment of hallucinogen intoxication. To date, no antidote has been found beneficial in reducing or eliminating hallucinogen-induced clinical symptoms. The use of **antipsychotics** is usually not indicated, but if the patient is severely agitated, psychotic or possibly aggressive, low doses of **high-potency antipsychotic** drugs might be administered. Low-potency agents such as **chlorpromazine** have been shown to induce seizures and to cause cardiovascular collapse when co-administered with hallucinogens. Anxiety states might be treated with **benzodiazepines**. Controlled studies of the use of **5-HT$_2$ antagonists** as possible antidotes for hallucinogens have not been done though animal studies have demonstrated that such compounds can antagonize some of the effects of **LSD**.

10.8 Abused substances – benzodiazepines

Supposed mechanism of dependence, withdrawal symptoms and treatment options

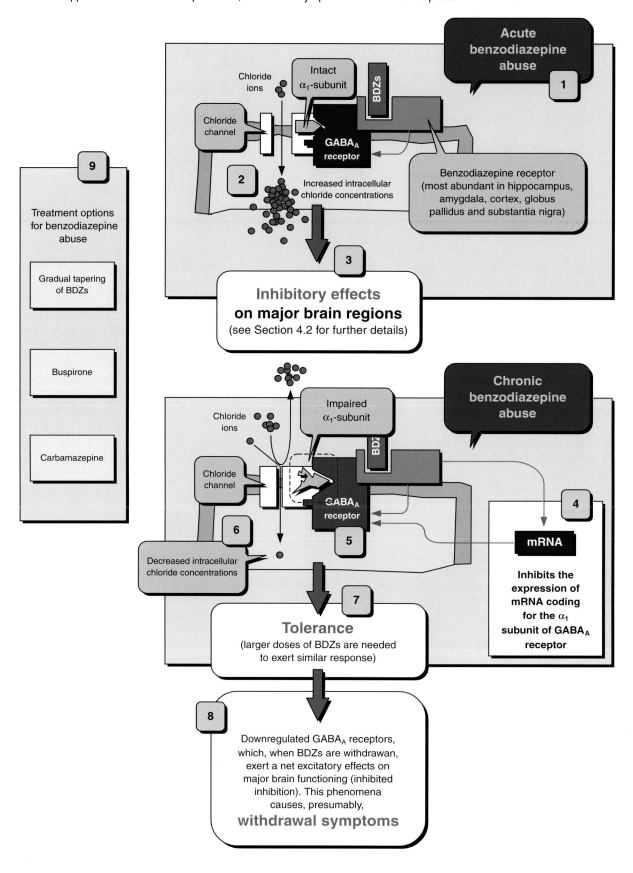

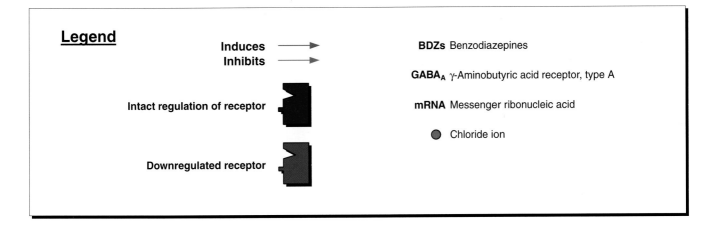

Legend

Induces ⟶

Inhibits ⟶

Intact regulation of receptor

Downregulated receptor

BDZs Benzodiazepines

GABA$_A$ γ-Aminobutyric acid receptor, type A

mRNA Messenger ribonucleic acid

● Chloride ion

Benzodiazepines exert their therapeutic effects by increasing the affinity of γ-aminobutyric acid (GABA) to the GABA$_A$ receptor, and thus increasing chloride influx into the intracellular space (see Section 4.2). The increased influx hyperpolarizes the neuron and further enhances the inhibitory effects of the GABAergic neuron. Therefore **benzodiazepines** act as neuromodulators that enhance the inhibitory effects of GABA.

Notes about the numbered items in the scheme

Benzodiazepine abuse

1. Benzodiazepine abuse is different from other substance-abuse disorders (**opioids, amphetamines, nicotine**) because **benzodiazepines** exert much less euphoria and do not activate the 'classic' reward systems that are activated with the other substances (mainly the mesolimbic and mesocortical dopaminergic projections) (see Sections 10.1–10.4). In fact, most people do not find the subjective effects of **benzodiazepines** pleasant beyond their therapeutic anxiolytic or sleep-inducing effects. Therefore, the abuse of **benzodiazepines** is usually secondary to other substance-abuse disorder when the **benzodiazepine** is taken for relief from symptoms induced by the use of another drug.

Mode of action

2–6. Benzodiazepines enhance the activities of GABA at its receptor site, increase chloride influx (**2**) and further generate inhibitory effects on major brain regions (**3**). At the same time and when **benzodiazepines** are chronically abused, they suppress the expression of the specific messenger ribonucleic acid (mRNA) coding for the production of the α$_1$ subunit of the GABA$_A$ receptor (**4**). This subunit is one of the major components responsible for the sufficient coupling between the GABA$_A$ receptor and the adjunct chloride channel. Thus chronic **benzodiazepine** abuse impairs the effective coupling leading to downregulation of the GABAergic receptors (**5**) and a decrease in chloride influx (**6**).

7. Because of the decreased chloride influx into the intracellular GABAergic nerves that follows chronic **benzodiazepine** abuse, larger doses of **benzodiazepine** are needed to exert the same clinical effects. This is the physiological basis for the development of tolerance.

Withdrawal

8. When **benzodiazepines** are withdrawn, the GABA$_A$ receptors are still downregulated and their activities are relatively suppressed compared with their baseline status. Since GABAergic nerves exert inhibitory effects on major brain regions, when they are suppressed the affected brain regions are in a relatively hyperexcitable state. This excitability might play a major role in the induction of the characteristic withdrawal symptoms.

Treatment

9. Several treatment options are relevant in the case of **benzodiazepine** abuse. Gradual tapering of **benzodiazepines** is probably the hallmark and the most effective modality for **benzodiazepine** abuse. The tapering schedule should include a reduction of about 20–25% of the consumed dosage per week. Detoxification can be accomplished within 7–21 days. For short-acting **benzodiazepines**, (e.g. **alprazolam**), a more-conservative detoxification plan should be taken, e.g. **alprazolam** should be tapered at a maximum of 0.5 mg every 3 days. Alternatively, replace with a long acting **benzodiazepine** and then withdraw it. The gradual tapering enables the downregulated GABA$_A$ receptors to recover parallel with the decrease in **benzodiazepine** dose. **Buspirone** or antidepressants [(especially selective serotonin reuptake inhibitors (**SSRIs**)] should be considered if tapering is not fully successful and there is still a need for an anxiolytic agent. Both are used primarily as anxiolytic agents, and their main advantages are diminished abused potential, the absence of withdrawal syndromes during acute abstinence, non-impaired psychomotor performance and no anterograde amnesia. **Buspirone** was found beneficial in reducing the craving for **benzodiazepines**, probably due to its anxiolytic effects. The main drawback in using **buspirone** or **SSRIs** is the relative long time needed before the anxiolytic effects are achieved (at least 1–2 weeks). **Carbamazepine** is only effective for withdrawal-induced convulsions.

10.9 Abused substances - nicotine

Supposed mechanism of dependence, withdrawal symptoms and treatment options.

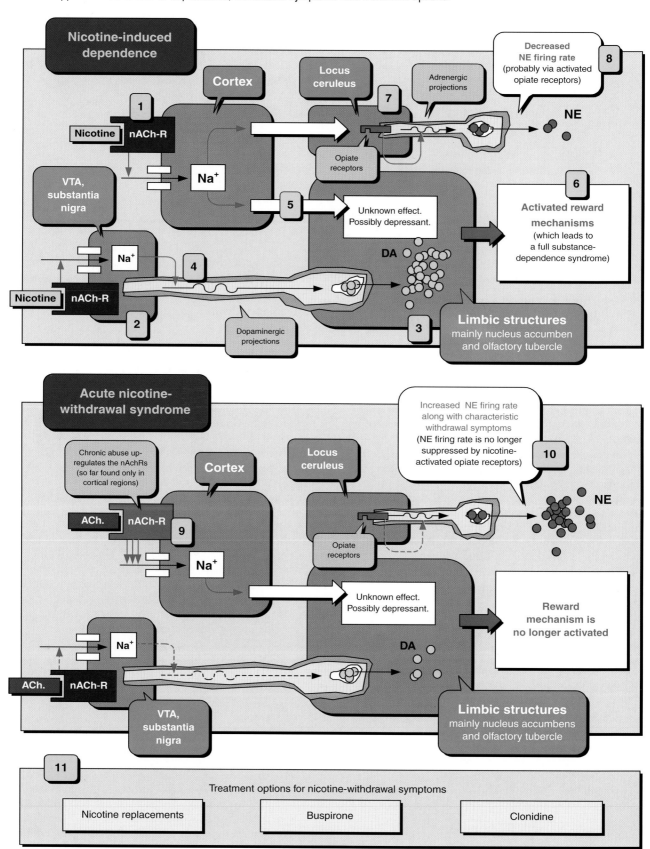

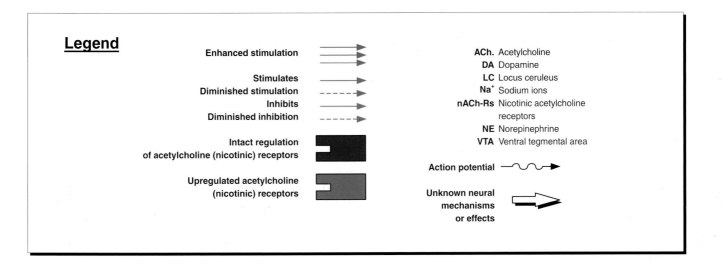

Addiction to **nicotine** appears mainly in the form of cigarette smoking. **Nicotine** rapidly enters the bloodstream via the pulmonary vascular system and reaches the brain faster than it would if it were administered intravenously. The major adverse effect of **nicotine** abuse (in the form of tobacco smoking) is death from lung cancer, emphysema and ischaemic cerebrovascular or cardiovascular diseases. **Nicotine** abuse causes both depressant and stimulatory effects, but tolerance develops to the depressant effects while the stimulatory effects are unaffected. The mechanism for this dual effect is unclear, and probably involves several different receptor interactions (as well as other modalities).

Notes about the numbered items in the scheme:

Mode of action

1-6. Nicotine binds to nicotinic acetylcholine receptors (nAChRs) which are highly concentrated in the interpenduncular nucleus, medial habenula, thalamus and cerebral cortex (**1**). Nicotinic receptors are also present in midbrain regions such as the ventral tegmental area (VTA) and the substantia nigra (**2**) and in limbic structures (**3**). **Nicotine** stimulates the nAChRs that are attached to a rapidly responding ligand-gated sodium channel, and it consequently increases intracellular sodium concentrations and depolarizes the neuronal membrane (**4**). As a result of this **nicotine**-induced depolarization, the mesolimbic dopaminergic pathway and cortical projections to the same limbic structures are activated. The effect of the latter is unclear, although it is assumed to be depressant (**5**). The net effect of these activities is to induce the characteristic **nicotine**-dependence syndrome (**6**).

7,8. The interaction of **nicotine** with nAChRs is believed to be the major element in inducing dependence, but chronic changes in other neurotransmitter systems, especially opiate receptors, are thought to contribute to the characteristic behavioral and psychological changes that are evident when **nicotine** is withdrawn. It is possible that nicotine indirectly stimulates the opiate receptors located in the lucus ceruleus (LC) (**7**), which leads to a decrease in the norepinephrine (NE) firing rate from the LC to major brain regions (**8**).

Withdrawal

9,10. Chronic **nicotine** abuse upregulates the nAChRs located in cortical regions (**9**). When **nicotine** is withdrawn, the nAChRs are stimulated by the endogenous acetylcholine. At the same time, the absence of **nicotine** does not generate the typical **nicotine**-induced stimulatory effects on the opiate receptors and so the LC firing rate is no longer suppressed. The net effect is an increase in NE release from the LC (**10**). This increase in LC firing rate might play a role in the induction of the characteristic withdrawal symptoms of impaired concentration and sleep, anxiety, irritability, and craving for **nicotine**.

Treatment

11. Nicotine replacement by **nicotine** chewing gum or by transdermal patches is the most effective treatment for **nicotine** dependence in the form of cigarette smoking. These modalities are estimated to induce a 1-year abstinence rate of 20–50% (a 10–20% drug–placebo difference). **Clonidine** is an α_2-adrenergic agonist that reduces the release of NE into the synaptic cleft. **Clonidine** was found to double the short-term abstinence rates from smoking as compared with placebo, and it is effective in minimizing the craving for cigarettes and some other withdrawal symptoms. The long-term effects of **clonidine** are yet to be ascertained. The main disadvantage of **clonidine** is its sedative effects, which often worsen the impairments in concentration associated with **nicotine** abuse. **Buproprion** is an antidepressant (see Section 2.4) that increases dopamine levels in the synaptic cleft. It has recently been licenced in the USA for the treatment of smoking cessation and can double the 1-year abstinence rates. This is presumably because a deficiency of dopamine in the mesolimbic/mesocortical pathway contributes to the low mood, loss of pleasure and drive found during **nicotine** withdrawal and **buproprion** helps reverse this.

SECTION C

DRUG INTERACTIONS

11.1 Tricyclic and tetracyclic antidepressants
Drug interactions

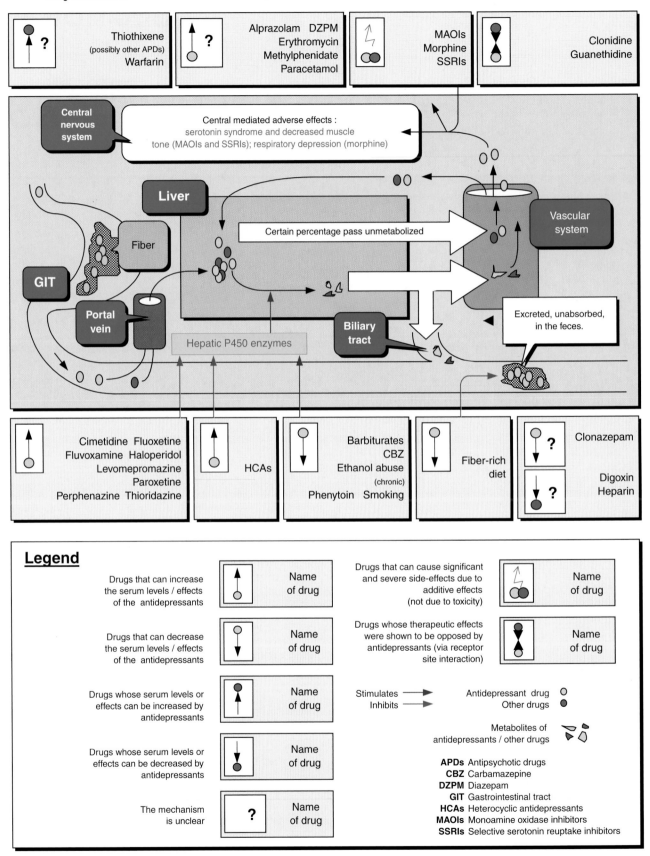

Significant Drug Interactions

Anticoagulants. There are anecdotal reports of *trazadone* decreasing **heparin** serum levels (20%). *Clomipramine, nortriptyline,* and *trazodone* can raise **warfarin's** serum levels, leading to the need for a 30% dose.

Anticonvulsants. **Phenytoin**, a liver enzyme inducer, decreases serum levels of tricyclic antidepressants (*TCAs*) (especially *desipramine* and *clomipramine*). An increase in serum levels of *nortriptyline* and *trazodone* has also been reported. In these cases, presumably the net effect of enzyme induction (by **phenytoin**) and enzyme inhibition (by *TCAs*) was 'in favor' of the inhibitory effects. **Carbamazepine** also induces liver enzymes, with a consequent reduction in serum levels of *TCAs* (*amitriptyline, desipramine, doxepin* or *nortriptyline*). These effects of **carbamazepine** were not observed with *clomipramine*, but have been reported with selective serotonin reuptake inhibitors (*SSRIs*).

Antihypertensive agents. **Clonidine's** antihypertensive effects were reduced by about 50% when co-administered with *clomipramine* or *desipramine*. The antihypertensive effects of **guanethidine** can be reduced by *doxepin, amitriptyline* or *desipramine*, but not by *maprotiline*.

Antipsychotic drugs (APDs). Most **APDs**, as well as *TCAs*, are inhibitors of the P450 enzymes, thus potentially increasing each other's serum levels. For **haloperidol**, an increase in serum levels of *TCAs* (by about twice) is found in up to 10% of patients treated with *clomipramine* and *nortriptyline* (not with *desipramine*). **Levomepromazine** can significantly increase *clomipramine's* serum levels. **Perphenazine** was found to increase serum levels of *amitriptyline, desipramine* and *nortriptyline*, while **thioridazine** was reported to increase *desipramine's* serum levels. **Thiothixene** levels are usually increased by *TCAs* such as *doxepin, nortriptyline* and *clomipramine* (the latter combination increases the risk for tardive dyskinesia).

Barbiturates. These induce liver catabolic enzymes with a consequent reduction in serum levels of *TCAs* (evident with *amitriptyline, clomipramine, desipramine,* and *nortriptyline*).

Benzodiazepines. Most studies revealed no significant interactions with a combined **benzodiazepine–TCA** regimen. Anecdotal reports suggest that **alprazolam** might increase the serum levels of *imipramine* by up to 30% and that **clonazepam** can decrease serum levels of *desipramine*. **Diazepam** was reported to increase *amitriptyline's* serum levels in few cases.

Cimetidine. This inhibits liver catabolic enzymes, with a consequent increase of up to 35% in serum levels of *TCAs* (reported with *amitriptyline, clomipramine, desipramine, doxepin* and *nortriptyline*) and up to 50% increase in patients considered to be 'rapid hydroxylators'.

Digoxin. A few cases were reported of decreased serum **digoxin** levels by up to 3-fold (mainly with *trazodone*).

Ethanol. Chronic abuse of **alcohol** can lead to enhanced activity of the P450 enzymes and a consequent decrease in *TCA* serum levels. Central receptor interactions between **ethanol** and *TCAs* can cause impaired motor abilities (evident with *amitriptyline, clomipramine, doxepin* and *nortriptyline*).

Fiber-rich diet. This lowers serum levels of *TCAs* (*desipramine, doxepin*). It is probably due to a decreased gastro-intestinal absorption of the *TCAs*.

Monoamine oxidase inhibitors (MAOIs). Co-administration is usually safe and effective, although rare cases of serotonin syndrome are documented patients. *Amitriptyline* and *nortriptyline* are safer as compared with *clomipramine, desipramine,* or *imipramine*. *Clomipramine* should be avoided. Additive toxicity is rare, and could be evident by hyperpyrexia, convulsions, cardiac collapse, disseminated intravascular coagulation, and death. No significant interactions were found with *amitriptyline* or *desipramine* and **moclobemide.**

Methylphenidate. This can increase *TCA* serum levels (*clomipramine, nortriptyline*). *Desipramine's* levels were not found to be impaired, although an additive adverse effect profile is evident (nausea, tremor, tachycardia).

Morphine. *Amitriptyline, clomipramine, desipramine,* and *doxepin* can enhance **morphine's** analgesic and respiratory effects possibly mediated by serotonergic stimulation.

Selective serotonin reuptake inhibitors (SSRIs). **Fluoxetine** inhibits the P450 liver catabolic enzymes leading to increased *TCA* serum levels by 2–4 fold (can be toxic). This is evident with *amitriptyline, clomipramine, desipramine* and *nortriptyline*. Such changes were not found, even though tested, with a combined *doxepin–***fluoxetine** regimen. More modest increases are found when *trazodone* is administered with **fluoxetine** compared with the *TCA–***fluoxetine** regimens. **Fluvoxamine** also inhibits the P450 liver catabolic enzymes leading to increased *TCA* serum levels by 1–2 fold. This is evident with *amitriptyline, clomipramine, desipramine* and *nortriptyline*. **Paroxetine** – *TCA* levels could increase by up to 5-fold via inhibition of the P450II catabolic enzyme. **Paroxetine** levels might also be increased (mainly with *amitriptyline, desipramine* and *nortriptyline*).

Smoking. Many components of cigarettes/tobbaco are hepatic enzyme inducers, leading to a decrease in *TCA* serum levels (up to 50% reduction in serum levels of *amitriptyline, clomipramine* or *desipramine*) though not evident with *nortriptyline*.

> Note: Lack of stated interaction mean studies not reported, not that such combinations are safe.

11.2 Selective serotonin reuptake inhibitors (SSRIs) – fluoxetine
Drug interactions

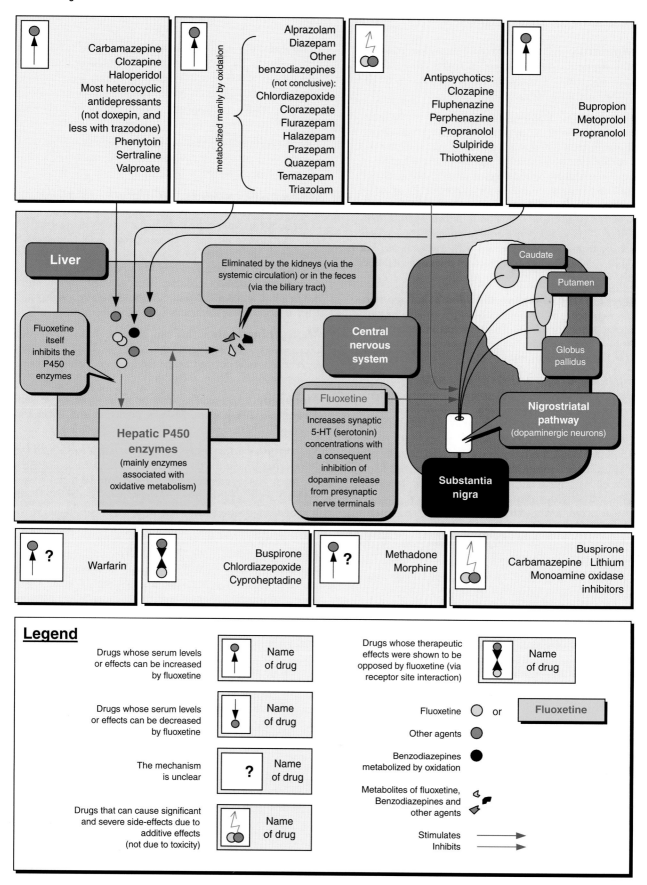

Significant Drug Interactions

Antidiabetic drugs. There are anecdotal data of enhanced hypoglycemic capacity when *fluoxetine* is added to hypoglycemic agent or given to insulin-dependent patients.

Anticonvulsants. *Fluoxetine* inhibits the metabolism of **carbamazepine** (up to 30% increase in its serum levels) and of **valproate** (up to 50% increase in serum levels). Some significant adverse effects were reported with **carbamazepine** (parkinsonism, serotonin syndrome) which are presumably related to the enhanced serotonergic transmission. Anecdotal reports are available of **phenytoin** intoxication following the addition of *fluoxetine* to the regimen.

Antidepressants. *Fluoxetine* inhibits the P450 liver catabolic enzymes, leading to increased tricyclic antidepressant (**TCA**) serum levels by 2–4 fold. This is mostly evident with **amitriptyline, clomipramine, desipramine, imipramine** and **nortriptyline** (increased serum levels of up to about 10 times were reported with the latter, with possible severe adverse effects such as prolonged PR, QRS and QT intervals, seizure induction, and anticholinergic delirum). Such changes were not found, even though tested, with a combined **doxepin**–*fluoxetine* regimen. Much more modest increases are found when **trazodone** is administered with *fluoxetine* compared with the **TCA**–*fluoxetine* regimens. *Fluoxetine* might also inhibit the metabolism of other selective serotonin reuptake inhibitors (**SSRIs**), with a subsequent increase in their serum levels (**sertraline**).

Antipsychotic drugs. In a few cases, marked extrapyramidal side-effects (akathisia, dystonia, parkinsonism) have been reported with **fluphenazine, perphenazine, sulpiride** or **thiothixene** when *fluoxetine* was added to the regimen. The mechanism is speculated to be the result of *fluoxetine's* further suppression of dopaminergic activity in the nigrostriatal pathways (serotonergic stimulation leads to decreased dopamine release). *Fluoxetine* was shown to increase **haloperidol** serum levels by about 20%, presumably via inhibition of the P450 enzymes. *Fluoxetine* can increase the risk of seizure induction when added to **clozapine** due to an increase in **clozapine** serum levels, or by additive effects.

Benzodiazepines. *Fluoxetine* inhibits the hepatic microsomal enzymes associated with oxidative metabolism, thus potentially increasing the serum levels of **alprazolam, chlordiazepoxide, clorazepate, diazepam, flurazepam, halazepam, prazepam, quazepam, temazepam** and **triazolam. Benzodiazepines** metabolized mainly by glucuronidation (**clonazepam, lorazepam** and **oxazepam**) should not be affected. In practice, *fluoxetine* has been shown to raise the serum levels of **alprazolam** and **diazepam**, without any apparent effect on the pharmacokinetics of **clonazepam** or **triazolam**. *Fluoxetine's* oxidative metabolite norfluoxetine inhibits the metabolism of **alprazolam** to a greater extent than *fluoxetine* itself; thus **alprazolam's** serum levels can remain high for a prolonged time following the decline in *fluoxetine* serum levels (norfluoxetine's half-life is longer).

β-adrenergic antagonists. *Fluoxetine* has some capacity to inhibit the oxidative metabolism of **β-adrenegic antagonists** (especially the lipophilic ones: **metoprolol, pindolol, propranolol**), thus raising their serum levels. There are rare reports of severly enhanced antiadrenergic activity (could lead to consequent sinus arrest) with a combined *fluoxetine*–**propranolol** regimen, possibly related to increased serum levels of **propranolol**.

Bupropion. A few cases were reported suggesting that **bupropion** metabolism might be inhibited by *fluoxetine*, which could eventually lead to abrupt emergence of psychosis and seizure disorder.

Buspirone. *Fluoxetine* can antagonize the anxiolytic effects of **buspirone**. The emergence of serotonin syndrome and seizure disorder have also been reported with this combination.

Cyproheptadine. This can antagonize the antidepressant effects of *fluoxetine*, probably via **cyproheptadine's** antiserotonergic properties, which might oppose the enhanced serotonergic transmission induced by *fluoxetine*.

Ethanol. The pharmacokinetics of **alcohol** are not significantly affected by *fluoxetine* (or fluvoxamine).

Lithium. Evidence is not conclusive. The combined **lithium**–*fluoxetine* regimen was found to be safe in many studies and is generally considered as safe. Even so, a few isolated reports describe the emergence of **lithium** toxicity, seizure induction, delirous state and serotonin syndrome with the combined **lithium**–*fluoxetine* regimen.

Methadone. *Fluoxetine* may increase the serum levels of **methadone**.

Monoamine oxidase inhibitors (MAOIs). The concurrent use of *fluoxetine* and **MAOIs** (**phenelzine, tranylcypromine**) has been found to induce a high incidence (up to 50% according to some reports) of toxic reactions including fatal serotonin syndrome. No such severe interactions were found, to date, with the combined use of *fluoxetine* and **moclobemide**.

Morphine. *Fluoxetine* may increase the serum levels of **morphine**.

Warfarin. Most data suggest that there are no significant interactions between these two agents. A few cases have been reported in which an apparent increase in **warfarin** serum levels or activities led to decreased prothrombin time and spontaneous bleeding when *fluoxetine* was added to the regimen.

Note: Lack of stated interaction mean studies not reported, not that such combinations are safe.

11.3 Selective serotonin reuptake inhibitors (SSRIs) – fluvoxamine and paroxetine
Drug interactions

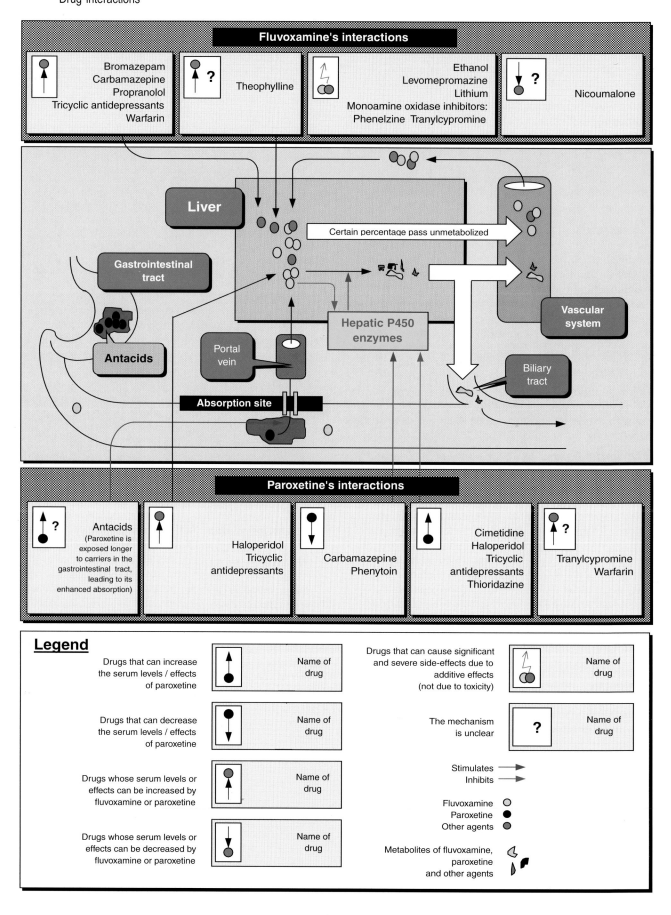

Fluvoxamine's interactions

↑ Bromazepam
Carbamazepine
Propranolol
Tricyclic antidepressants
Warfarin

↑ ? Theophylline

⚡ Ethanol
Levomepromazine
Lithium
Monoamine oxidase inhibitors:
Phenelzine Tranylcypromine

↓ ? Nicoumalone

Liver

Certain percentage pass unmetabolized

Gastrointestinal tract

Antacids

Portal vein

Hepatic P450 enzymes

Absorption site

Vascular system

Biliary tract

Paroxetine's interactions

↑ ? Antacids
(Paroxetine is exposed longer to carriers in the gastrointestinal tract, leading to its enhanced absorption)

↑ Haloperidol
Tricyclic antidepressants

↓ Carbamazepine
Phenytoin

↑ Cimetidine
Haloperidol
Tricyclic antidepressants
Thioridazine

↑ ? Tranylcypromine
Warfarin

Legend

Drugs that can increase the serum levels / effects of paroxetine — ↑● Name of drug

Drugs that can decrease the serum levels / effects of paroxetine — ●↓ Name of drug

Drugs whose serum levels or effects can be increased by fluvoxamine or paroxetine — ↑ Name of drug

Drugs whose serum levels or effects can be decreased by fluvoxamine or paroxetine — ↓ Name of drug

Drugs that can cause significant and severe side-effects due to additive effects (not due to toxicity) — ⚡ Name of drug

The mechanism is unclear — ? Name of drug

Stimulates →
Inhibits →

Fluvoxamine ○
Paroxetine ●
Other agents ●

Metabolites of fluvoxamine, paroxetine and other agents

Significant Drug Interactions

Fluvoxamine's interactions

Anticoagulants. There are anecdotal reports of bleeding disorder with a concomitant use of **nicoumalone** (a coumarin derivative), *fluvoxamine* and ibuprofen (which can also interact with the anticoagulant). *Fluvoxamine* inhibits **warfarin** metabolism which could result in about a 65% increase in serum levels and a concomitant prolongation of the prothrombin time.

Anticonvulsants. Co-administration with *fluvoxamine* may result in increased **carbamazepine** serum levels by up to 60%.

Antidepressants. *Fluvoxamine* inhibits the P450 liver catabolic enzymes (predominantly inhibition of N-demethylation), leading to an increase in tricyclic antidepressant (**TCA**) serum levels by 1–2-fold. This is evident, mostly, with **amitriptyline, clomipramine, desipramine, imipramine, maprotiline** and **nortriptyline**.

Antipsychotic drugs. *Fluvoxamine* can increase the risk of seizure induction when added to **levomepromazine**.

Benzodiazepines. There is little evidence, to date, of clinically significant interactions with **benzodiazepines.**

β-adrenergic blockers. *Fluvoxamine* was reported to increase **propranolol** serum levels by up to 5-fold, without major impairments in blood pressure or cardiac transmission. The mechanism involves the inhibition of cytochrome P450 activities generated by *fluvoxamine*.

Ethanol. The pharmacokinetics of **alcohol** are not significantly affected by fluoxetine or *fluvoxamine*.

Lithium. Established data are lacking. **Lithium** may enhance the serotonergic effects of *fluvoxamine*, and a few cases of hyperpyrexia and/or induction of seizure disorder were reported with a combined **lithium**–*fluvoxamine* regimen.

Monoamine oxidase inhibitors (MAOIs). Few data are available about *fluvoxamine's* interactions with **MAOIs,** even though they might be similar to those of fluoxetine. Clinically significant or severe interactions were not found to date (in several well-controlled trials) with the combined use of *fluvoxamine* and **moclobemide**.

Theophylline. *Fluvoxamine* can raise **theophylline** serum levels with consequent intoxication.

Paroxetine's interactions

Anticonvulsants. Serum levels of *paroxetine* can decrease when co-administered with **anticonvulsants** (some are enzyme inducers). The data are limited but it seems that **phenytoin** may cause the greatest decrease followed by **carbamazepine**. **Valproate's** serum levels are unchanged by *paroxetine* co-administration.

Antidepressants. *Paroxetine* levels might be increased (**TCAs** inhibit its metabolism); this is evident mainly with **amitriptyline, desipramine** and **nortriptyline**. Note that **TCA** levels could also increase since *paroxetine* concomitantly inhibits their metabolism. Studies so far have confirmed this with **imipramine** and **desipramine** (whose half-life can increase by 5-fold).

Antipsychotic drugs. A mutual increase in serum levels of both **thioridazine** and *paroxetine* is evident when these agents are combined. *Paroxetine* inhibits P450IID6, which metabolizes **thioridazine** and other antipsychotics. *Paroxetine* was also shown to increase **haloperidol** serum levels, presumably via inhibition of these hepatic enzymes.

Benzodiazepines. *Paroxetine* was not found to alter the pharmacokinetics of **diazepam** or **oxazepam**.

Cimetidine. This can increase *paroxetine* serum levels by up to 50% (due to its inhibitory effects on hepatic microsomal enzymes), though the clinical significance is questionable.

Ethanol. A minor (probably insignificant) decrease in attentiveness can be induced when **alcohol** is added to *paroxetine*.

Lithium. No significant pharmacokinetic interactions have been found to date with *paroxetine*.

MAOIs. Few data are available about *paroxetine's* interactions with **MAOIs**, even though they might be similar to those of other selective serotonin reuptake inhibitors (SSRIs). Clinically significant or severe interactions have not been found to date, although anecdotal data might indicate that *paroxetine* can potentially increase **tranylcypromine's** serum levels by about 10-15%.

Propranolol. Isolated reports suggest no interactions.

Warfarin. No significant pharmacokinetic interactions between *paroxetine* and **warfarin** were found, although some individuals may experience prolonged prothrombin time or mild hematuria.

Note: Lack of stated interaction mean studies not reported, not that such combinations are safe.

11.4 Selective serotonin reuptake inhibitors (SSRIs) – sertraline and citalopram
Drug interactions

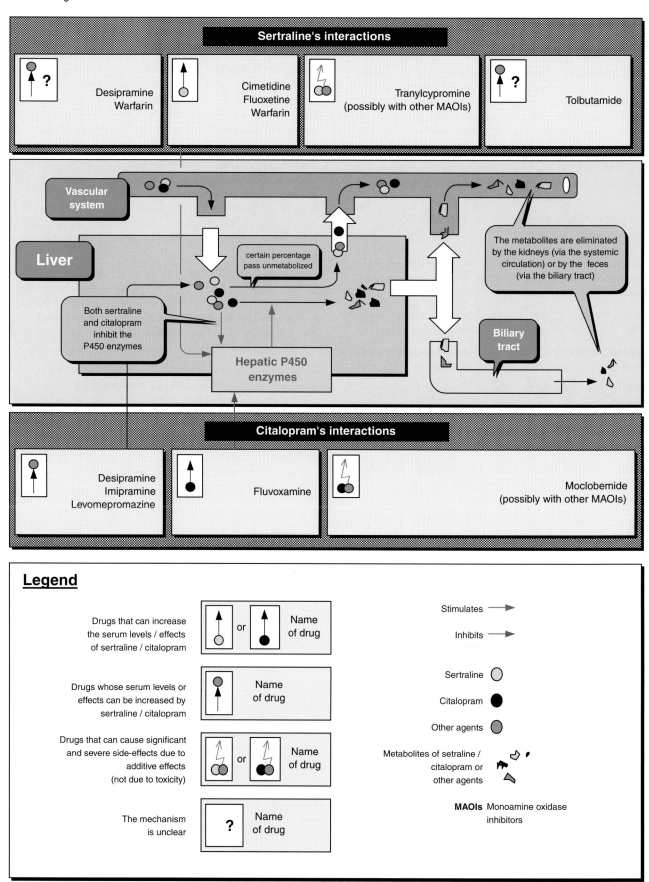

Significant Drug Interactions

Sertraline's interactions

Antidepressants. To date, *Sertraline* has not been found to increase tricyclic antidepressant (**TCA**) serum levels as much as the other selective serotonin reuptake inhibitors (SSRIs) (fluoxetine, fluvoxamine or paroxetine).

Benzodiazepines. *Sertraline* did not alter, in healthy volunteers, the pharmacokinetics of ***diazepam***. Anecdotal data suggest no clinically significant interactions with ***clonazepam***.

β-adrenergic antagonists. *Sertraline* has no significant interaction with ***atenolol***. Data concerning other ***β-antagonists*** are lacking.

Cimetidine. This can increase *sertraline* serum levels by about 25% (due to its inhibitory effects on hepatic microsomal enzymes). The data are limited, and the clinical significance of such an effect is questionable.

Hypoglycemic drugs. In most studies, no clinically significant interactions were described with the combined use of ***tolbutamide*** and *sertraline*. Anecdotal data suggests increased serum levels of ***tolbutamide*** when co-administered with *sertraline*. The mechanism is unknown. A similar study did not find any pharmacokinetic interactions between ***gliben-clamide*** and *sertraline*, so it seems that co-administration of *sertraline* with ***hypoglycemic agents*** is safe.

Ethanol. Preliminary data suggests no interactions.

Lithium. Most studies found that *sertraline* does not or only negligibly decreases ***lithium*** serum levels, so the co-administration is considered safe. The most serious reported effect with the combined regimen was the enhancement of ***lithium***-induced tremor.

Monoamine oxidase inhibitors (MAOIs). Few data are available about *sertraline's* interactions with ***MAOIs*** even though they are expected to be similar to those of other SSRIs i.e. the risk of serotonin syndrome reported with ***tranyl-cypromine*** (and clonazepam). This combination should be avoided.

Warfarin. There are probably no clinically significant pharmacokinetic interactions between *sertraline* and ***warfarin***.

Citalopram's interactions

Antidepressants. Several reports indicate that *citalopram* does not alter serum levels of tricyclic antidepressants (***amitriptyline, clomipramine, maprotiline*** or ***nortripty-line***). There are isolated data that suggest that *citalopram* (presumably via inhibiting the P450 enzymes) might increase the AUC of ***desipramine***, the primary metabolite of ***imipramine***, with a possible increase in therapeutic effects, adverse effects or the induction of toxicity. The co-administration of *citalopram* and other ***SSRIs*** has not been sufficiently studied. Preliminary data describe the ability of ***fluvoxamine*** to increase the serum levels of *citalopram* when co-administered.

Antipsychotic drugs. Well-controlled studies revealed no clinically significant alterations in serum levels of various commonly used ***antipsychotic drugs*** when co-administered with *citalopram*. In these cases the serum levels of *citalopram* itself seem not to be altered by the concomitant use of the antipsychotics. Anecdotal reports describe the ability of *citalopram* to increase the serum levels of ***levomepromazine*** by about 10–20%.

Ethanol. No significant interactions reported.

Lithium. No pharmacokinetic interactions were observed in a small study.

MAOIs. A few cases of fatal and rapidly developing serotonin syndrome were reported with the combined use of *citalopram* and ***moclobemide***. Other ***MAOIs*** should be avoided as with other SSRIs. Recent data suggest the main metabolite of *citalopram* may be toxic (prolonged QT_c interval) in high doses (e.g. after overdose). Some fatalities reported.

> Note: Lack of stated interaction mean studies not reported, not that such combinations are safe.

11.5 Mood stabilizers – lithium

Drug interactions

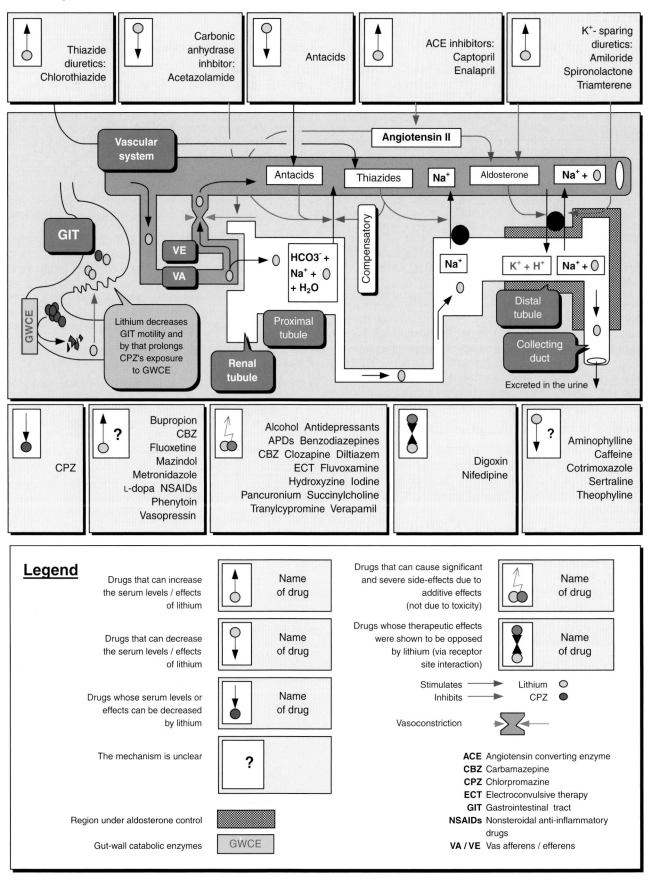

Significant Drug Interactions

Angiotensin converting enzyme (ACE) inhibitors. *Lithium* toxicity may occur with **captopril** or **enalapril** (both inhibit angiotensin II production with consequent enhanced aldosterone activity and intensified sodium and *lithium* reabsorbtion in the distal tubule).

Antacids. May contain sodium bicarbonate, which enhances the renal excretion of *lithium*.

Anticonvulsants. **Carbamazepine** and *lithium* can elevate each other's serum levels (mechanism unknown). *Lithium's* diuretic effects outweighs **carbamazepine's** antidiuretic effect, so **Carbamazepine** does not protect from *lithium*-induced diabetes insipidus. *Lithium* can enhance **carbamazepine**-induced hyponatremia.

Antidepressants. The combined use is regarded as safe. Even so, **bupropion** was shown, in isolated cases, to increase *lithium* serum levels and to induce seizure activity when given as a combined regimen. **Fluoxetine** was reported, in some cases to increase *lithium* serum levels by 25–50%. **Sertraline** was shown to have the opposite effect. The mechanisms are unknown and their clinical significance is questionable.

Antipsychotic Drugs (APDs). A sudden emergence of extrapyramidal symptoms was reported to occur when *lithium* was co-administered with **flupenthixol, fluphenazine, loxapine, sulpiride, thioridazine** or **thiothixene**. Some data suggest that the concurrent use of *lithium* and certain antipsychotics (**chlorpromazine, perphenazine, thioridazine, thiothixene**) increases the prevalence of sleepwalking episodes (up to 10%). *Lithium* can lower the serum levels of **chlorpromazine** by up to 40% presumably via delaying its gastric emptying with a consequent longer exposure of **chlorpromazine** to gut wall catabolic enzymes. There are some isolated reports of irreversible brain damage following co-administration of *lithium* and **fluphenazine**. The use of *lithium* and **haloperidol** is considered safe and effective but isolated reports of severe neurotoxicity (fever, extrapyramidal symptoms, delirium, tremmulousness, hyperglycemia) were noted. Anecdotal cases of neuroleptic malignant syndrome, delirium, seizures and agranulocytosis were reported with the use of **clozapine** and *lithium*. The blood count analysis might be misleading and ineffective in monitoring patients on *lithium* and **clozapine**.

Benzodiazepines. Co-administration does not usually impair *lithium* serum levels.

Caffeine. **Caffeine** intake can enhance *lithium's* renal excretion to subtherapeutic levels.

Calcium-channel blockers. **Diltiazem** might cause acute extrapyramidal symptoms and delirium when co-administered with *lithium*. Both agents decrease calcium influx into neurons and *lithium* may also compete with intracellular calcium ions on target organelles (due to similar ionic properties). **Verapamil**, when given with *lithium*, can cause neurotoxicity (nausea, vomiting, ataxia, dysarthria, dyskinesia) and cardiotoxicity (*lithium* levels could remain within normal ranges). Cases of decreased *lithium* serum levels and other cases of uneventful concurrent use of *lithium* and **verapamil** were also reported.

Cotrimoxazole. 'Paradoxical intoxication' (*lithium* intoxication while its serum levels decrease) may occur.

Digoxin. This may antagonize the acute antimanic effects of *lithium*. Severe bradycardia has also been reported.

Diuretics. **Thiazides** (**chlorothiazide, hydrochlorothiazide**) can increase *lithium* serum levels by depleting sodium in the distal tubule. This leads to increased sodium uptake from the proximal tubules (and *lithium* uptake as well because it is concomitantly absorbed with that sodium) leading to increased serum levels of *lithium* by up to 2-fold. When **thiazides** and *lithium* are co-administered, a 50% reduction in *lithium* dosage is therefore recommended. **Potassium-sparing diuretics** (**amiloride, spironolactone**) either unchange or slightly increase the serum levels of *lithium*. **Loop diuretics** (**ethacrinic acid, furosemide**) do not usually alter *lithium* serum levels. **Carbonic anhydrase inhibitors** (**acetazolamide**) decrease bicarbonate reabsorption from the proximal tubule, leading to increased excretion of bicarbonate, sodium, water and *lithium* and a consequent decrease in *lithium* serum levels.

Electroconvulsive therapy (ECT). Co-administration of *lithium* with **ECT** (given a week before or after the **ECT**) increases the risk of developing organic brain syndrome (prolonged delirium, seizure activity and non-convulsive status epilepticus).

Ethanol. The combined **ethanol**–*lithium* regimen exerts synergistic depressant effects.

Monoamine oxidase inhibitors (MAOIs). There are isolated cases of tardive dyskinesia induced by the combined **tranylcypromine**–*lithium* regimen. No apparent interactions were observed with **phenelzine** or **moclobemide**.

Metronidazole. There are isolated reports of *lithium* intoxication, with up to a 2-fold increase in its serum levels.

Neuromuscular blocking agents. There are several reports of prolonged neuromuscular blockade with a potential for developing a delirious state following the combined use of *lithium*, **succinylcholine** or **pancuronium** and ECT. Other data suggest the concurrent use is usually safe but caution is advised.

Non-steroidal anti-inflammatory drugs (NSAIDs). **Ibuprofen, diclofenac** and **naproxen** are reported to increase *lithium* serum levels by about 40%, while **indomethacin** has, a greater effect on *lithium* serum levels (up to 65% increase). Other **NSAIDs** (**ketoprofen, mefenamic acid, phenylbutazone**) are also associated, occasionally, with a rise in *lithium* serum levels. **Aspirin** was found not to exert any significant changes on *lithium* serum levels. The mechanism of such changes is not fully understood.

Theophylline. Serum levels of *lithium* can decrease by 20–30% when combined with *lithium*.

> Note: Lack of stated interaction mean studies not reported, not that such combinations are safe.

11.6 Mood stabilizers – carbamazepine and valproate

Drug interactions

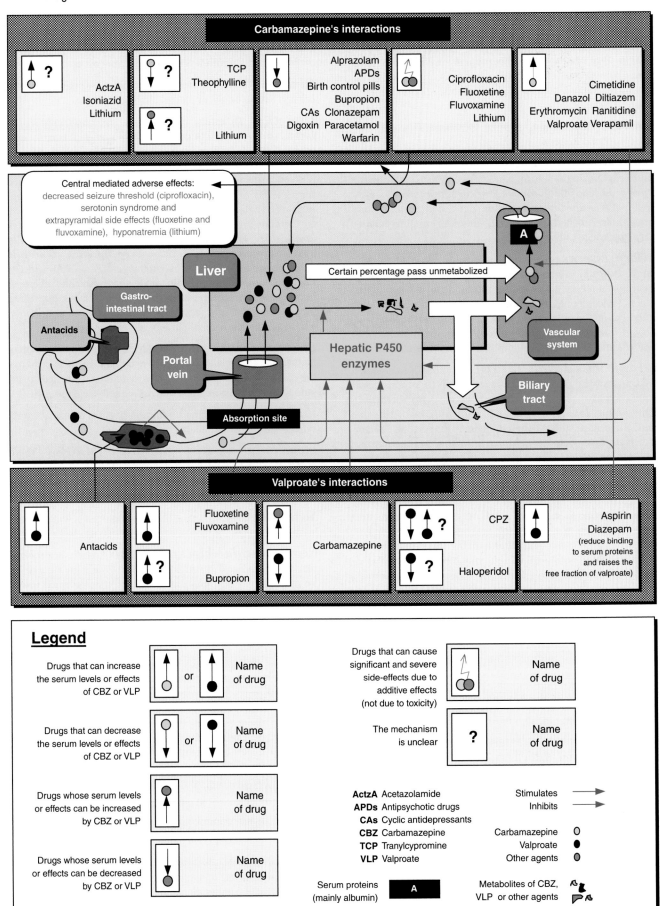

Significant Drug Interactions

Acetazolamide. Can increase the serum levels of *carbamazepine* (CBZ) by up to 50%, with the possible development of toxicity (mechanism unclear).

Antacids. **Aluminum/magnesium hydroxide** can slightly enhance the absorption of *valproate*, with a parallel increase in its serum levels or effects. The clinical significance is limited.

Antibiotics. **Ciprofloxacin** can greatly increase the risk of seizure induction in patients taking anticonvulsants. **Erythromycin** markedly inhibits the hepatic metabolism of CBZ (data are well established), but it has a diminished interaction with *valproate*.

Anticoagulants. **Warfarin** serum levels and anticoagulant effects may be decreased due to CBZs hepatic metabolism of **warfarin**.

Anticonvulsants. Valproate has inhibitory effects on hepatic metabolism, and when co-administered with CBZ it can increase its serum levels and effects. CBZ can reduce *valproate* serum levels by about 60%.

Antidepressants. CBZ induces hepatic liver catabolic enzymes, with a consequent reduction in serum levels of antidepressants (up to a 40% reduction with **amitriptyline, desipramine, doxepin, imipramine** and **mianserin**, and up to a 67% reduction with **nortriptyline**). A decrease in **bupropion** serum levels was also reported with CBZ. These effects were not observed with **clomipramine**. **Fluoxetine** and **fluvoxamine** inhibit the metabolism of CBZ and *valproate* (up to 30% and 50% increases in serum levels respectively). No significant interaction has yet been found between **paroxetine** and CBZ or *valproate*. **Bupropion** is reported to increase the serum levels of *valproate*.

Antipsychotic drugs (APDs). CBZ was found to decrease the plasma levels of **phenothiazines** by as much as 50% (**chlorpromazine, perphenazine, fluphenazine**). CBZ has also been reported to decrease the serum levels of non-phenothiazines by about 50% (**haloperidol**) and 60–85% (**clozapine**) due to their hepatic P450-inducing properties. **Haloperidol** itself can decrease the serum levels of *valproate*. **Chlorprothixene** was found to increase the serum levels of CBZ, due, probably, to its inhibition of hepatic mono-oxygenase activities. **Haloperidol** pharmacokinetics are not affected by *valproate*.

Benzodiazepines (BDZs). **BDZs** have complex interactions with anticonvulsants – the consequence of both inhibitory and stimulatory effects of **BDZs** on the hepatic metabolism of anticonvulsants. The co-administration of CBZ can (infrequently) cause significant (up to 50%) decreases in serum levels of **clonazepam** or **alprazolam**. Valproate displaces **diazepam** from

plasma protein binding, and possibly inhibits its metabolism, leading to increased serum levels by up to 50%.

Birth control pills. CBZ has shown to increase the hepatic metabolism and to decrease the effects and safety of **birth control pills**. Higher doses of estrogen are vital to secure safety (about 50–100 μg) (or use other methods).

Calcium channel blockers (CCBs). **Diltiazem** and **verapamil** have inhibitory effects on hepatic microsomal enzymes, and so can increase anticonvulsant serum levels. **Diltiazem** and **verapamil** can increase the serum levels of CBZ. **Nifedipine** has not been studied as well as the other **CCBs**, but probably does not interact significantly with CBZ.

Danazol. This inhibits the hepatic microsomal enzymes. CBZ serum levels can increase by up to 2-fold.

Digoxin. CBZ increases the risk of cardiac conduction disturbances. **Digoxin** serum levels can decrease.

H_2 *blockers*. Transient elevation of CBZ plasma levels is evident with **cimetidine** (due to the latter's P450 inhibition capacity). **Ranitidine** has little or no interaction with CBZ.

Isoniazid. This increases CBZ serum levels, and leads to the possible emergence of toxicity (disorientation, aggression).

Lithium. CBZ and **lithium** can elevate each other's serum levels (the mechanism is unknown). Toxicity is possible while blood levels are within normal range, and is partially associated with pre-existing brain abnormalities. The diuretic effect of **lithium** outweighs CBZ's antidiuretic effect. CBZ does not protect from **lithium**-induced diabetes insipidus. **Lithium** can enhance CBZ-induced hyponatremia.

Monoamine oxidase inhibitors. **Phenelzine, tranylcypromine** or **moclobemide** have no clinically significant interactions with CBZ.

Non-steroidal anti-inflammatory drugs (NSAIDs). The co-administration of **paracetamol** and CBZ might increase the risk of hepatotoxicity (the mechanism is unclear). **Aspirin** can displace *valproate* from protein-binding sites leading to increased serum levels and possible toxicity. **Aspirin** may also inhibit *valproate* hepatic metabolism.

Theophylline. Isolated data suggest that **theophylline** might decrease CBZ serum levels.

Note: Lack of stated interaction mean studies not reported, not that such combinations are safe.

11.7 Monoamine oxidase inhibitors (MAOIs)

Drug interactions

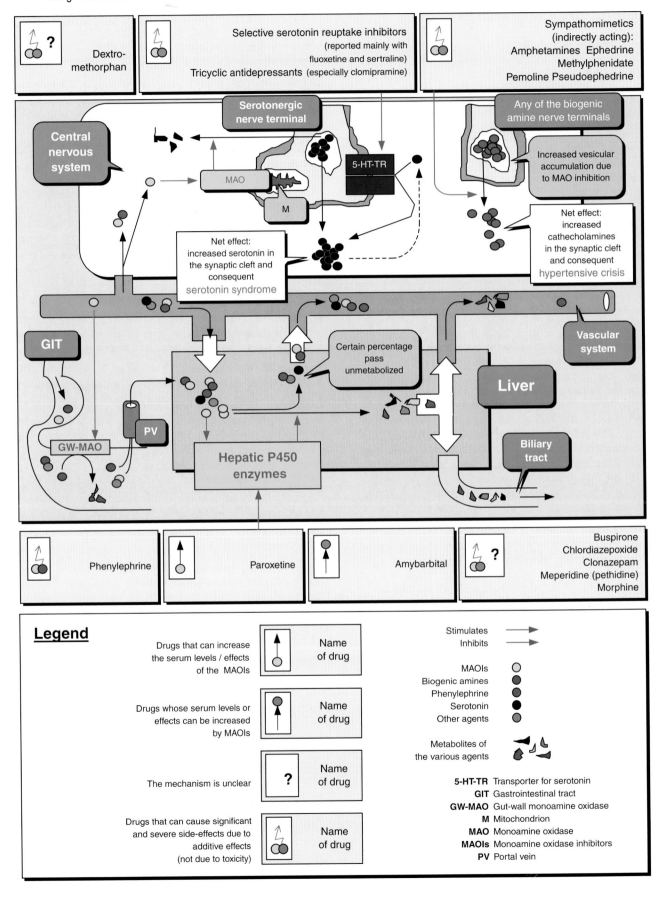

Significant Drug Interactions

Antidepressants. As a rule, antidepressant drugs should be avoided as adjuvants to monoamine oxidase inhibitors (*MAOIs*), due to the potential induction of the serotonin syndrome. Combined therapy should be restricted to refractory patients. Co-administration of *MAOIs* with tricyclic antidepressants (**TCAs**) is usually safe and effective but the relatively rare cases of adverse interactions can often become fatal. **Amitriptyline** and **nortriptyline** are safer than **clomipramine**, **desipramine** or **imipramine**. Additive toxicity is rare, and could be evidenced by hyperpyrexia, convulsions, cardiac collapse, disseminated intravascular coagulation and death. Little data are available about newly introduced drugs and *MAOIs* [due, most likely, to the relative avoidence in clinical practice of regimens consisting a combined **serotonin reuptake inhibitor** (**SRI**) with a *MAOI* in view of the potentially high incidence of serotonin syndrome]. **Sertraline** was shown to induce serotonin syndrome (combined with *tranylcypromine* and clonazepam). **Paroxetine** can increase the serum levels of *tranylcypromine* by about 15%. The concurrent use of **fluoxetine** and *MAOIs* (*phenelzine, tranylcypromine*) has been found to induce a high percentage (up to 50% according to some reports) of toxic reactions including fatal serotonin syndrome. Few data are available about **fluvoxamine's** interactions with *MAOIs*, although they might be similar to those of **fluoxetine**.

Antipsychotic drugs. Many reports, including well-controlled studies, found no adverse interaction with **phenothiazines**, except rare reports of fatal adverse effects when a *MAOI* (*pargyline, tranylcypromine*) was given with **methotrimeprazine**.

Barbiturates. *MAOIs* (mainly *tranylcypromine*) have been shown, in isolated reports, to enhance the activities of **barbiturates** (mainly **amybarbital**), probably by inhibition of microsomal enzymes.

Benzodiazepines. There are isolated reports of severe adverse side-effects when *MAOIs* (*isocarboxazid, phenelzine*) were co-administered with **chlordiazepoxide** (severe edema, dyskinesias, dysarthria) or **clonazepam** (headaches).

β-adrenergic antagonists. Several cases of significantly slowed heart rate following the administration of *phenelzine* to **nadolol** or **metoprolol** were reported.

Buspirone. Isolated cases of non-fatal hypertensive reactions (with *phenelzine* or *tranylcypromine*) were reported. The mechanism is unclear but may be related to a metabolite of **buspirone**, I-pp, which is an α_2-adrenoreceptor antagonist that can increase noradrenaline release. Clinicians should closely monitor the patient when using this combination.

Dextromethorphan. A few fatal cases and a couple of severe adverse effects were reported with the combination of *phenelzine* and **dextromethorphan**. Hyperpyrexia, cardiovascular collapse/arrhythmias, nausea, tremor, muscle spasm, and impaired consciousness/coma developed within minutes to a few hours of ingesting agents containing **dextromethorphan**, eventually leading to death (in some of them). Similar, but less

severe and non-fatal effects were evidenced with *isocarboxazid*. The mechanism is presumably via serotonin syndrome.

Mazindol. There is an isolated report of a hypertensive episode when added to *phenelzine*. The mechanism is unclear, but may be related to increased dopaminergic activity.

Meperidine (pethidine). Many cases of serious (some fatal) adverse effects were reported when **pethidine** was added to a *MAOI* (*iproniazid, phenelzine, tranylcypromine*). The most-often encountered adverse and serious symptoms are hyperpyrexia, respiratory failure, impaired consciousness (including coma and death) and numerous neurological signs. Even so, there are many published cases and studies that did not reveal any interaction between *MAOIs* and **pethidine**. The combined therapy is relatively contraindicated. The mechanism of the potentially fatal reactions is unknown.

Morphine. Anecdotal data described marked hypotension and impaired consciousness when **morphine** was added to *tranylcypromine*. Many studies have shown no clinically significant interactions with *isocarboxazid, phenelzine, tranylcypromine* and **morphine**, including in patients with known adverse reactions to pethidine.

Phenylephrine. A marked and life-threatening hypertensive crisis can result when **phenylephrine** is given to a person using a *MAOI* (*phenelzine, tranylcypromine*). The catastrophic reaction is a consequence of the inhibited gut monoamine oxidases, which do not detoxify the ingested **phenylephrine** (the gut enzymes detoxify the vast majority of the **phenylephrine** when they are not inhibited).

Sympathomimetics (directly acting). *MAOIs* do not or only minimally enhance the pressor effects of directly acting amines such as **epinephrine** or **norepinephrine** (since *MAOIs* cause **norepinephrine** to accumulate in presynaptic vesicles and thus it does not directly stimulate the postsynaptic receptors).

Sympathomimetics (indirectly acting). Combining *MAOIs* with agents such as **amphetamines, ephedrine, pseudoephedrine, methylphenidate, pemoline, cocaine, phenylpropanolamine** and others (many cold and allergy medications) can cause a potentially fatal hypertensive crisis, since these sympathomimetic amines stimulate the presynaptic nerves to release the accumulated cathecholamines into the synaptic cleft, and some of them are direct agonists of the postsynaptic receptors for catecholamines.

Tranylcypromine. There are anecdotal reports of cerebral hemorrhages when patients were switched from *phenelzine* to **tranylcypromine**. The cause might involve the amphetamine-like properties of **tranylcypromine**.

> Note: Lack of stated interaction mean studies not reported, not that such combinations are safe.

11.8 Reversible inhibitors of monoamine oxidase type A (RIMAs) – moclobemide

Drug interactions

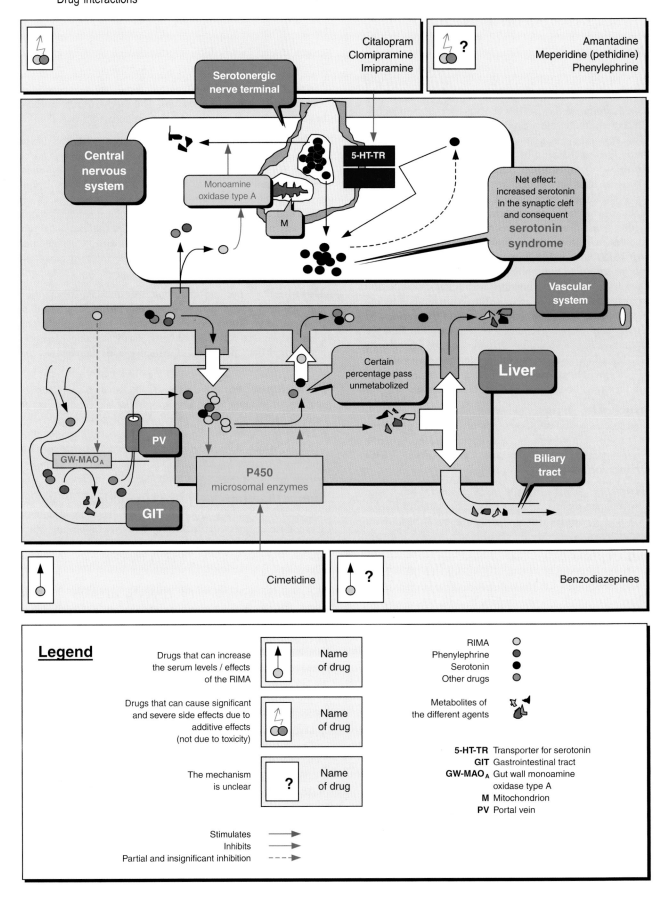

Significant Drug Interactions

Amantadine. Isolated report of hypertensive reaction when *amantadine* was combined with *moclobemide* and other agents. This effect was not confirmed in other studies. The mechanism is unknown and the clinical significance is questionable.

Anticonvulsants. Only few published cases concerning the combined use of **carbamazepine** and *moclobemide* were reported, up to date, and no clinically significant interactions were observed.

Antidepressants. Few cases of fatal and rapidly developing serotonin syndrome were reported with the combined use of **citalopram** and *moclobemide*. Clinically significant or severe interactions were not found up to date (in several well controlled trials) with the combined use of **fluvoxamine, fluoxetine** and *moclobemide* and not with **amitriptyline** or **desipramine** when given with *moclobemide*. One case was reported of a serotonin syndrome with the combined use of *moclobemide* and **imipramine** and another suspected serotonin syndrome when given with **clomipramine**.

Antipsychotic drugs. Many reports found no adverse pharmacokinetic interactions with most of the **phenothiazines, butyrophenones, clozapine** and others (**sulpiride, clopenthixol**).

β-adrenergic blockers. *Moclobemide* can further enhance the hypotensive properties of **metoprolol**, but the effect is usually mild and clinically insignificant.

Benzodiazepines (BDZs). Data about the co-administration of **BDZs** with *moclobemide* has revealed contradictory results - some reports suggest that there are no clinically significant interactions with the combined use, but other studies suggest a greater risk (incidence increases by up to 100%) of developing adverse effects usually related to *moclobemide* (mainly sedation).

Birth control pills (BCPs). Co-administration of *moclobemide* to several types of **BCPs** did not show any significant interaction and the efficacy of both agents did not seem to be altered.

Breast milk. *Moclobemide* is widely distributed in body fluids and tissues (lipophilic) and it is excreted in the **breast milk**, although in minimal amounts (less than 1% of maternal dose).

Calcium channel blockers (CCBs). Up to date, no clinically significant interactions were reported concerning the combined use of *moclobemide* and **CCBs** (mostly examined with **nifedipine**).

Cimetidine. Can increase *moclobemide's* serum levels by between 40-100%, due to its inhibitory effects on hepatic microsomal enzymes.

Dextromethorphan. Unlike the combined monoamine oxidase inhibitor (MAOI) and **dextromethorphan** regimen (were fatal interactions are well documented) there is only limited evidence from animal studies which supports the potentially dangerous interactions with **dextromethorphan** and *moclobemide*.

Digoxin. Preliminary data suggests that there are no significant pharmacokinetic interactions between *moclobemide* and **digoxin**.

Diuretics. Only few published cases concerning the combined use of **diuretics** and *moclobemide* were reported, up to date. The thiazide diuretics and especially **hydrochlorothiazide**, were shown to have no significant interactions with *moclobemide* and there are no significant changes in the efficacy of both regimens.

Ethanol. Up to date, no clinically significant interactions were reported concerning the combined use of *moclobemide* and **alcohol**.

Hypoglycemic agents. Numerous hypoglycemic agents (**chlorpropramide, glibenclamide, metformin**) were co-administered with *moclobemide* and no clinical significant interactions were noticed.

Ibuprofen. Has no clinically significant interactions with *moclobemide*, even though some inconsistent interactions were evident in animal studies.

L-dopa. *Moclobemide* has a negligible capacity to increase the dopaminergic transmission, but studies made so far revealed no significant interactions or major adverse side effects when *moclobemide* was co-administered with **L-dopa**.

Lithium. Preliminary data suggests that there are no significant pharmacokinetic interactions between *moclobemide* and **lithium**.

Meperidine (pethidine). Many cases of serious (some of them fatal) adverse effects were reported when **pethidine** was added to a MAOI (see drug interactions of MAOIs). Such serious effects were not reported, yet, with *moclobemide* but data from animals studies suggest that it can enhance the effects of **pethidine**. There are many published cases and studies which did not reveal any interaction between MAOIs and **pethidine**. The combined therapy is relatively contraindicated. The mechanism for the potentially fatal reactions is unknown.

Phenylephrine. A marked and life-threatening hypertensive crisis can result when **phenylephrine** is given to an individual using a MAOI. The catastrophic reaction is a consequence of the inhibited gut MAOs which do not detoxify the ingested **phenylephrine** (the gut enzymes detoxify the vast majority of the **phenylephrine** when not inhibited). Smaller, and probably insignificant elevation of blood pressure are evidenced with *moclobemide*.

Note: Lack of stated interaction mean studies not reported, not that such combinations are safe.

12.1   Typical antipsychotics – phenothiazines
Drug interactions

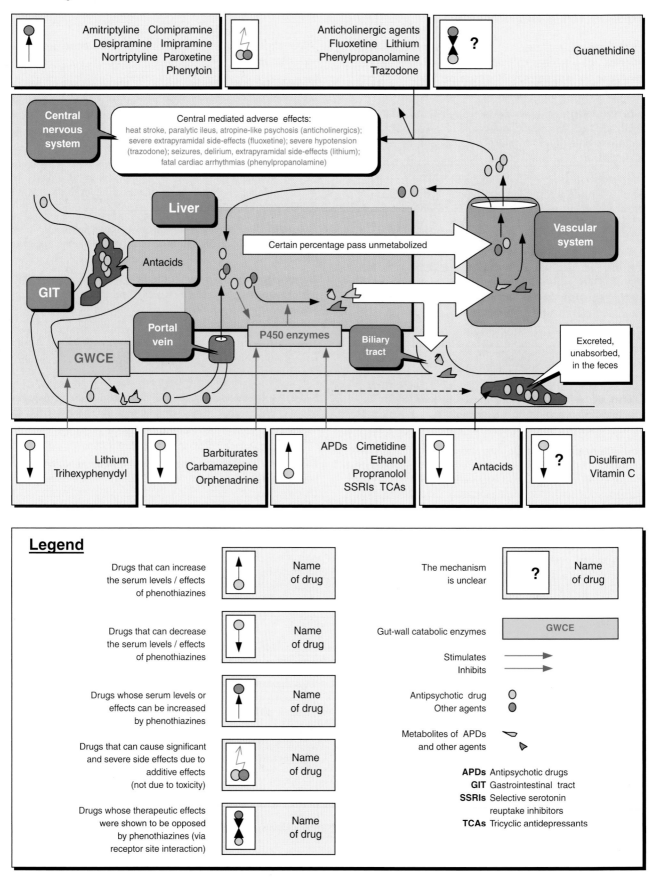

Significant Drug Interactions

Antacids. *Chlorpromazine* serum levels can be rapidly decreased by about 50% (due to its adsorption onto gel antacids) when co-administered with **antacids** such as **aluminum hydroxide** or **magnesium tricilicate**.

Anticholinergic drugs. The combined use of *phenothiazines* (reported mainly with *chlorpromazine*) that have marked anticholinergic properties with other **anticholinergic drugs** can induce heat stroke, especially in hot and humid conditions. The rise in body temperature might be the result of suppressed sweat gland activity regulated by parasympathetic cholinergic innervation. Other serious adverse and additive effects of such combined regimens are the induction of paralytic ileus and atropine-like psychosis. Some data suggest that **trihexyphenidyl** can lower serum levels of *chlorpromazine*, probably due to their additive anticholinergic impairment of gastric motility and absorption.

Anticonvulsants. **Carbamazepine** induces hepatic microsomal enzymes that can decrease the steady-state plasma levels of *phenothiazines* (reported mainly with *chlorpromazine, perphenazine* and *fluphenazine*). *Chlorpromazine* and *thioridazine* may increase the serum levels of **phenytoin** due to its inhibition of hepatic mono-oxygenase activities. Some reports claim that *chlorpromazine* may decrease the serum levels of *valproate*, while other reports suggest the opposite.

Antidepressants. Most *antipsychotic drugs* (*APDs*) as well as tricyclic antidepressants (**TCAs**), are inhibitors of the P450 liver catabolic enzymes, thus potentially increasing each other's serum levels. *Chlorpromazine* increases **imipramine** serum levels. *Levomepromazine* can cause a significant increase in **clomipramine** serum levels. *Perphenazine* has been reported to increase the serum levels of **amitriptyline, desipramine, imipramine** and **nortriptyline**. *Thioridazine* has also been shown to increase **TCA** serum levels (mainly **desipramine**). Marked extrapyramidal side-effects (akathisia, dystonia, parkinsonism) have been reported (a few cases only) with *fluphenazine* or *perphenazine* when **fluoxetine** was added to the regimen. The mechanism is not known. A mutual increase in serum levels of both *thioridazine* and **paroxetine** is evident when these agents are combined (**paroxetine** inhibits P450IID6 which metabolizes *thioridazine*). Severe hypotension with a 30% fall in blood pressure was evident in few cases when **trazodone** was added to *chlorpromazine* or *trifuoperazine*.

Barbiturates. The serum levels of both **barbiturates** (reported predominantly with **phenobarbitone**) and *phenothiazines* (*chlorpromazine, thioridazine*) can be reduced by about 30%. presumably because **barbiturates** are potent hepatic catabolic enzyme inducers.

Cimetidine. No significant interactions, except for slight increase in *chlorpromazine* serum levels (without any clinical significance).

Disulfiram. There is an anecdotal report of a more than 50% decrease in *perphenazine* serum levels when **disulfiram** was added to the regimen (mechanism unknown).

Ethanol. An increased risk of emergence of acute dystonic reactions is described, mainly with *fluphenazine* and *trifluoperazine*, and is believed to be the consequence of an **alcohol**-induced lower neurological threshold or to be due to increased plasma levels of the antipsychotics. *Chlorpromazine* and to a lesser extent, *thioridazine* do not alter **alcohol** metabolism, but *haloperidol* can increase **alcohol** levels.

Guanethidine. *Chlorpromazine* was shown to reverse the antihypertensive effects of **guanethidine**. *Molindone* (a dihydroindole) apparently does not interact with **guanethidine** (data regarding other antipsychotic drugs are lacking).

Lithium. There are a few reports of rapid development of extrapyramidal side-effects (parkinsonism, tremor), or neurotoxicity (delirium, seizures) when co-administered with *thioridazine, fluphenazine, thiothixene, flupenthixol* and *haloperidol*. Some of these events were apparent while **lithium** serum levels were within normal range. *Chlorpromazine* serum levels are reduced in the presence of **lithium**. The mechanism is unclear, but could be related to the delayed gastric emptying induced by **lithium**, leading to a prolonged exposure of *chlorpromazine* to gastric-wall metabolic processing.

Naltrexone. There are anecdotal reports of prolonged and severe lethargy when co-administered with *thioridazine*.

Orphenadrine. This induces hepatic oxidizing enzymes, and reported to lower *chlorpromazine* serum levels. The clinical significance of this interaction is unclear.

Phenylpropanolamine. There are anecdotal data of fatal cardiac arrhythmia (ventricular fibrillation) while on a combined **phenylpropanolamine** and *thioridazine* regimen.

Pimozide. **Pimozide** and both *chlorpromazine* and *thioridazine* can prolong the QT interval, and isolated reports of additive effects were described.

Propranolol. Isolated data suggest that **propranolol** might reduce the elimination of *chlorpromazine* and *thioridazine* with a consequent increase in their serum levels/therapeutic effects.

Vitamin C. There are anecdotal data of a 25% decrease in serum levels of *fluphenazine* when vitamin C was added to the regimen (probably not of clinical significance).

> Note: Lack of stated interaction mean studies not reported, not that such combinations are safe.

12.2 Typical antipsychotics – haloperidol and miscellaneous drugs

Drug interactions

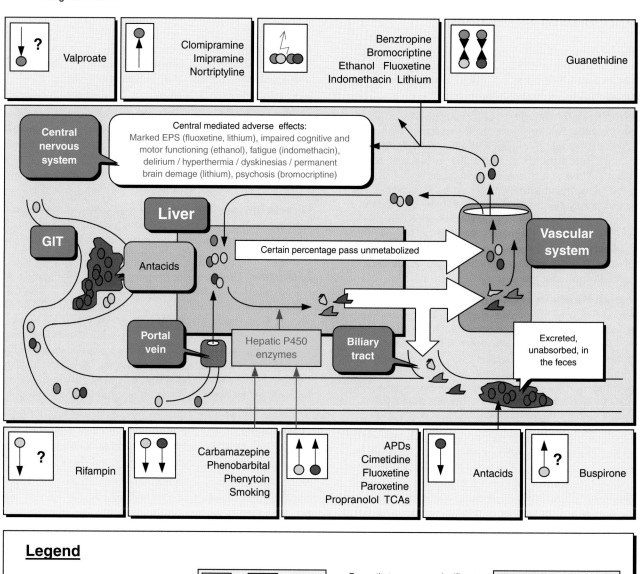

Valproate ?

Clomipramine / Imipramine / Nortriptyline

Benztropine / Bromocriptine / Ethanol Fluoxetine / Indomethacin Lithium

Guanethidine

Central nervous system

Central mediated adverse effects:
Marked EPS (fluoxetine, lithium), impaired cognitive and motor functioning (ethanol), fatigue (indomethacin), delirium / hyperthermia / dyskinesias / permanent brain demage (lithium), psychosis (bromocriptine)

Liver

GIT

Antacids

Certain percentage pass unmetabolized

Vascular system

Portal vein

Hepatic P450 enzymes

Biliary tract

Excreted, unabsorbed, in the feces

Rifampin ?

Carbamazepine / Phenobarbital / Phenytoin / Smoking

APDs / Cimetidine / Fluoxetine / Paroxetine / Propranolol TCAs

Antacids

Buspirone ?

Legend

Drugs that can increase the serum levels / effects of haloperidol or one of the other APDs — or — Name of drug

Drugs that can decrease the serum levels or effects of haloperidol or one of the other APDs — or — Name of drug

Drugs whose serum levels or effects can be increased by haloperidol or one of the other APDs — Name of drug

Drugs whose serum levels or effects can be decreased by haloperidol or one of the other APDs — Name of drug

The mechanism is unclear — ? Name of drug

Drugs that can cause significant and severe side-effects due to additive effects (not due to toxicity) — Name of drug

Drugs whose therapeutic effects were shown to be opposed by haloperidol or one of the other APDs (via receptor site interaction) — Name of drug

Stimulates →
Inhibits →
Haloperidol ○
Other APDs (not haloperidol) ●
Other agents (not APDs) ●
Metabolites of haloperidol / other agents ▸

APDs Antipsychotic drugs
EPS Extrapyramidal side-effects
TCAs Tricyclic antidepressants

Significant Drug Interactions

Butyrophenones (e.g. haloperidol) interactions

Antidepressants. An increase (about twice) in serum levels of tricyclic antidepressants *(TCAs)* is found in up to 10% of treated patients (mostly established with ***clomipramine*** and ***nortriptyline***). Such serum level abnormalities were not observed with ***desipramine***, although additive toxicity was reported (induction of seizure disorder). Marked extrapyramidal side-effects (akathisia, dystonia, parkinsonism) have been reported (a few cases only) with *haloperidol* when ***fluoxetine*** was added to the regimen. ***Fluoxetine*** and ***paroxetine*** were shown to increase *haloperidol* serum levels (by about 20%), presumably via inhibition of the P450 enzymes.

Anticonvulsants. ***Phenytoin*** and ***carbamazepine*** have been reported to decrease *haloperidol* serum levels by about 50% due to their hepatic P450-inducing properties. Preliminary data suggest that ***valproate*** has no effects on serum levels of *haloperidol*, while *haloperidol* itself can decrease the serum levels of ***valproate***.

Barbiturates. ***Phenobarbital*** can lower *haloperidol* serum levels via induction of hepatic enzymes.

Buspirone. A few uncontrolled studies showed an increase of about 50% in *haloperidol* serum levels.

Ethanol. Numerous reports suggest that combined antipsychotic drug–*alcohol* consumption further impairs driving abilities and cognitive or neuromotor functioning, and this effect is noted mostly with flupenthixol, chlorpromazine and, to a lesser extent, thioridazine, sulpiride and *haloperidol*. ***Alcohol*** serum levels could be elevated by concurrent use of *haloperidol*.

Guanethidine. The antihypertensive effects of ***guanethidine*** can be opposed by the concurrent use of *haloperidol*.

Indomethacin. Isolated cases of severe drowsiness and fatigue were reported when co-administered with *haloperidol*.

Lithium. There are anecdotal and rare reports of severe adverse effects induced by the combined *haloperidol*–***lithium*** regimen (extrapyramidal side-effects, delirium, hyperthermia, dyskinesia and some permanent brain damage). The effects are presumed to be mediated by additive effects of both agents on the basal striatal adenylate cyclase system or simply to be a manifestation of ***lithium*** toxicity. Some data suggest that old age and administration during an acute phase of a manic episode hold a greater risk for developing these effects. There is opposite and quite massive evidence that the concurrent use of these agents is safe.

Rifampin. Can increase *haloperidol* elimination, with a concomitant decrease in serum levels.

Smoking. Components of cigarettes/tobacco are hepatic enzyme inducers leading to a decrease in *haloperidol* serum levels, and established data suggest that the average serum levels of *haloperidol* are about halved.

Miscellaneous antipsychotics (non-phenothiazines or haloperidol) interactions

Antacids. ***Aluminum hydroxide*** can reduce the absorption of *sulpiride* and lower its serum levels.

Antidepressants. *Thiothixene* levels are usually increased by *TCAs* (***doxepin, nortriptyline***). Additive adverse effects were also reported when co-administered with ***clomipramine*** (rapid development of tardive dyskinesia). Marked extrapyramidal side-effects (akathisia, dystonia, parkinsonism) have been reported (a few cases only) with *thiothixene* or *sulpiride* when ***fluoxetine*** was added to the regimen. Unlike the established interactions between most phenothiazines and *TCAs*, in which serum levels of both agents could increase, no apparent interaction is evident to date, between *flupenthixol* and ***imipramine*** or any other *TCA*.

Benzodiazepines. Most data are consistent with relatively safe use of combined *antipsychotic drugs (APDs)* and ***benzodiazepines***.

Benztropine. There is an isolated case of reversible esophageal atonia and dilatation with *thiothixene*, due probably to additive anticholinergic effects. There is another isolated report of impaired esophageal contractility with increased upper esophageal sphincter pressure with *molindone*.

Bromocriptine. Most data are consistent with relatively safe use of combined *APDs* and ***bromocriptine***. There are anecdotal data about the emergence of psychotic symptoms when ***bromocriptine*** was added to *molindone*.

Carbamazepine. This increases the clearance of *thiothixene*, with a consequent decrease in its serum levels.

Cimetidine. This increases the serum levels of *thiothixene* via inhibition of hepatic microsomal enzymes.

Ethanol. See butyrophenones and ethanol, this page.

Guanethidine. *Chlorpromazine* can reverse the antihypertensive effects of ***guanethidine***. *Molindone* apparently does not.

Lithium. There are isolated cases of severe extrapyramidal adverse effects (parkinsonism, akathisia, dyskinesia) and neurotoxicity when *flupenthixol, sulpiride* or *thiothixene* was added to the regimen (or ***lithium*** added to the *APDs*). This effect might be mediated by the enhanced binding of these antipsychotics to dopaminergic receptors when ***lithium*** is co-administered. ***Lithium*** may also increase the half-life of *molindone* by 2–4 fold.

Propranolol. This increases the serum levels of *thiothixene* via inhibition of hepatic microsomal enzymes.

Note: Lack of stated interaction mean studies not reported, not that such combinations are safe.

12.3 Atypical antipsychotics – clozapine, olanzapine, risperidone and sertindole
Drug interactions

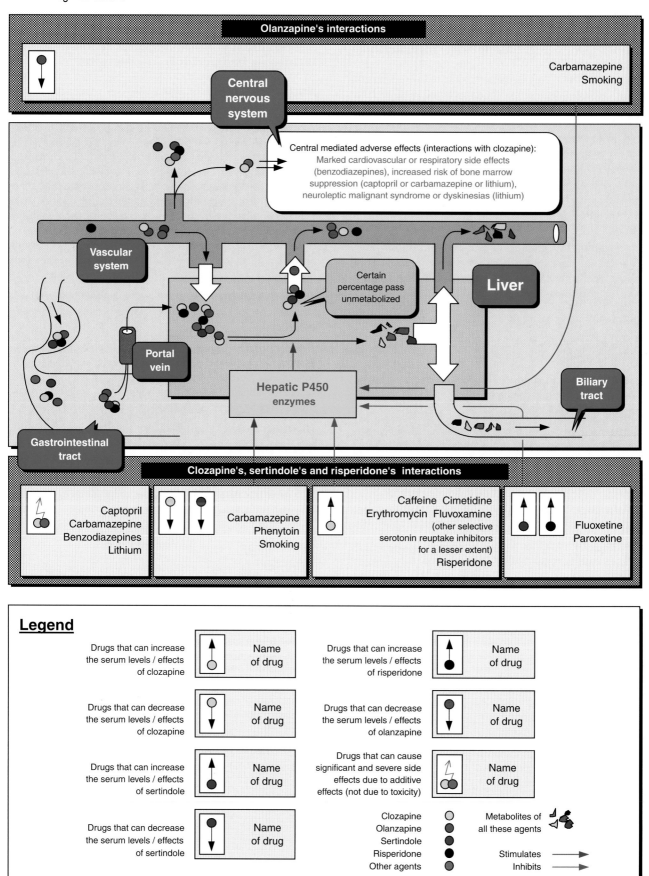

Significant Drug Interactions

Clozapine's interactions

Anticonvulsants. These can decrease *clozapine's* serum levels by about 60% (**carbamazepine**) and 85% (**phenytoin**) due to hepatic P450-inducing properties. There is no evidence for **valproate**–*clozapine* interactions, thus **valproate** is often used to decrease the risk for *clozapine*-induced seizures. **Carbamazepine** can potentially increase the risk for development of agranulocytosis when co-administered with *clozapine*, so should be avoided.

Antidepressants. *Clozapine* is metabolized by CYPIA2, and **fluvoxamine** is the predominant drug, among the major psychotropic agents, to inhibit CYP1A2's activities. Several reports have described a substantial increase in *clozapine* serum levels following the co-administration of **fluvoxamine**. **Fluoxetine, paroxetine** and **sertraline** were also found to increase *clozapine* serum levels, presumably by inhibiting a secondary metabolic step, distal to *clozapine* (since none of these agents affect CYP1A2). **Citalopram** has not been found, to date, to interact with *clozapine*.

Antipsychotic drugs (APDs). Anecdotal cases are described of a substantial (about 2-fold) increase in *clozapine* serum levels following the co-administration of **risperidone**. The mechanism is unclear but is speculated to involve a competitive inhibition of CYP2D6, which also metabolizes *clozapine* to some extent.

Benzodiazepines. Most data suggest that the combined regimen is safe and effective, although severe cardiovascular or respiratory adverse effects may occur with high doses of *clozapine* when combined with **diazepam**, **flurazepam** or **lorazepam. Clonazepam** and *clozapine* do not seem to interact.

Caffeine. Like *clozapine*, this is a substrate of the CYP1A2, so can increase *clozapine* serum levels.

Diuretics. There is an increased risk of bone marrow suppression with a combined **captopril**–*clozapine* regimen, since each agent alone has the capacity to induce this side-effect.

Erythromycin. Anecdotal data suggest it can (via CYP1A2 blockade) increase *clozapine* serum levels.

H₂ blockers. There is an anecdotal report of a 60% increase in serum levels of *clozapine* and the development of toxicity with **cimetidine** (a non-specific catabolic enzyme inhibitor). **Ranitidine** has no significant effects on this metabolic pathway.

Lithium. There are isolated reports of neuroleptic malignant syndrome, myoclonus and dyskinesias when co-administered with *clozapine*. A fatal agranulocytosis has been reported with this combination.

Smoking. Components of cigarettes are hepatic enzyme inducers (especially CYP1A2), leading to a decrease in *clozapine* serum levels or therapeutic/side-effects. Close monitoring is suggested, especially if **smoking** is stopped.

Olanzapine's interactions

Antidepressants. To date, in vivo studies with a combined *olanzapine–imipramine* regimen have not revealed any pharmacokinetic interactions.

Benzodiazepines. There are no reports of pharmacokinetic interactions between *olanzapine* and **benzodiazepines** (studied mainly with **diazepam**).

Carbamazepine. This was anecdotally reported to decrease *olanzapine* serum levels by about 50%. The clinical significance of this effect is unclear.

Smoking. Cigarette components induce CYP1A2, which metabolizes *olanzapine*, and combined *olanzapine–***cigarette smoking** have been reported to lower *olanzapine* serum levels (by up to 33%).

Warfarin. To date, in vivo studies with a combined *olanzapine-***warfarin** regimen have not revealed any pharmacokinetic interactions.

Sertindole's interactions

Anticonvulsants. Carbamazepine and **phenytoin** have been reported to decrease *sertindole* serum levels by about 2–3-fold. This is assumed to be via their hepatic CYP3A-inducing properties.

Antidepressants. Some data suggests that **fluoxetine** and **paroxetine** can increase *sertindole's* serum levels by about 2-fold (both inhibit CYP2D6 and 3A4). As *sertindole* can cause QTc elongation, this may be clinically relevant.

Smoking. Cigarette **smoking** has been shown to reduce *sertindole* serum levels by about 25%. This is presumably due to the CYP3A-inducing capacity of **smoking** components (although relatively weak compared with their CYP1A2-inducing abilities).

Risperidone's interactions

Antidepressants. Fluoxetine and **paroxetine** can increase *risperidone* serum levels in more than 50% of treated patients (both inhibit CYP2D6 which is the predominant enzyme metabolizing *risperidone*).

APDs. See under **Clozapine's** interactions (this page).

Note: Lack of stated interaction mean studies not reported, not that such combinations are safe.

13.1 Benzodiazepines/buspirone
Drug interactions

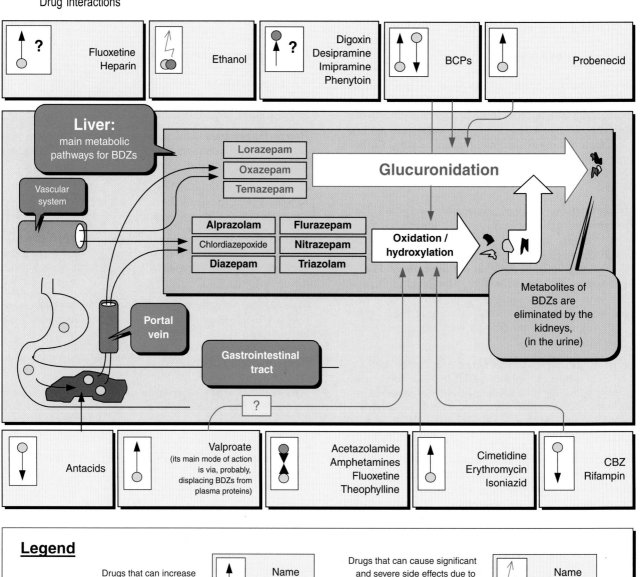

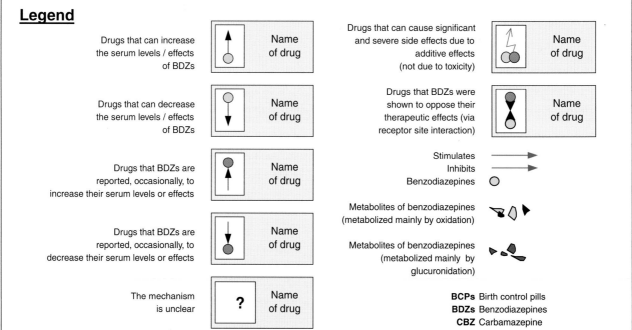

Significant Drug Interactions

Benzodiazepines interactions

Acetazolamide. This improves oxygenation at high altitudes. *Benzodiazepines (BDZs)* antagonize this effect due to impaired respiratory response to hypoxia. Concomitant use should be avoided in high altitudes.

Antacids. Few cases are reported of slight and insignificant delay in drug absorbtion (*chlordiazepoxide, diazepam*) and possibly more significant delay in absorption with *clorazepate* (activated by acid conditions).

Antibiotics/fungal preparations. For ***erythromycin*** there are many cases of increased serum levels of *midazolam* or *triazolam* when co-administered with ***erythromycin.*** The P450IIIA enzymes are speculated to be inhibited by ***erythromycin.*** **Isoniazid** reduces the clearance of *diazepam* or *triazolam* with a possible enhancement of their therapeutic or adverse effects. For ***ketoconazole***, there is an isolated report of about 40% reduction in the clearance of *chlordiazepoxide.* ***Rifampin*** is a potent catabolic enzyme inducer, thus enhancing the elimination of many agents, including *BDZs* such as *diazepam* and *nitrazepam* (half-life decreases to about 15–35% of baseline). *Temazepam (*an agent that undergoes metabolism via hepatic glucuronidation was found not affected).

Anticonvulsants. The co-administration of ***carbamazepine*** can infrequently cause significant decreases in serum levels of some *BDZs* (*clonazepam, alprazolam*). ***Valproate*** displaces *diazepam* from plasma protein binding and possibly inhibits its metabolism, leading to increased serum levels. A few studies suggest that *clonazepam, chlordiazepoxide* and *diazepam* may elevate serum levels of ***phenytoin.***

Birth control pills (BCPs). **BCPs** inhibit oxidative metabolism and at the same time enhance glucuronidation. Consequently, the half-life of *BDZs* such as *alprazolam, chlordiazepoxide, diazepam* and *triazolam* were found to be increased, and the half-life of *lorazepam,* and to a lesser extent *oxazepam,* can be significantly reduced.

Digoxin. *Diazepam* was noted, anecdotally, to increase ***digoxin's*** serum levels.

Disulfiram. This inhibits the metabolism of *diazepam* and *chlordiazepoxide* leading to enhancement of their therapeutic and/or adverse effects. The effects of *lorazepam* and *oxazepam* are practically unchanged. Isolated data suggest that ***disulfiram*** does not affect the metabolism of *alprazolam.*

Ethanol. **Ethanol** and *BDZs* produce synergistic central depression, probably via separate activity on the GABA$_A$ receptor.

H$_2$ blockers. **Cimetidine** inhibits the liver enzymes associated with oxidative metabolism. The serum levels of most *BDZs* affected by this metabolic pathway were found to be increased when ***cimetidine*** was co-administered (*alprazolam, diazepam, chlordiazepoxide, flurazepam, nitrazepam, triazolam*). *BDZs* metabolized by glucuronide conjugation (*lorazepam, oxazepam, temazepam*) are not affected by ***cimetidine. Ranitidine*** probably has no significant interaction with most *BDZs.*

Heparin. This increases the free fraction of *chlordiazepoxide, diazepam, lorazepam* and *oxazepam.* The mechanism is probably via *heparin's* induction of concomitant free fatty acid changes, which consequently alter *BDZs* pharmacokinetics.

Probenecid. This inhibits the hepatic glucuronidation metabolism and the renal excretion of many drugs, including *BDZs.* As a result, elimination half-lives of agents such as *lorazepam* were reported to increase (up to 2-fold).

Selective serotonin reuptake inhibitors (SSRIs).
Fluoxetine can raise the serum levels of *alprazolam* and *diazepam,* without any apparent effect on the pharmacokinetics of *clonazepam* or *triazolam.*

Theophylline. Can antagonize the sedative or the anxiolytic effects of *BDZs* (*diazepam*) probably via direct excitant action.

Tricyclic antidepressants. *Alprazolam* was found to increase ***imipramine*** and ***desipramine*** serum levels by about 25%. The mechanism is unknown.

Buspirone's interactions (not shown in the scheme)

Ethanol. *Buspirone* does not increase ***alcohol*** serum levels (as opposed to most other anxiolytics), and it does not potentiate ***alcohol's*** cognitive and motor dysfunctioning.

Haloperidol. *Buspirone* might increase ***haloperidol*** serum levels by about 25%.

> Note: Lack of stated interaction mean studies not reported, not that such combinations are safe.

13.2 Alcohol (ethanol)
Drug interactions

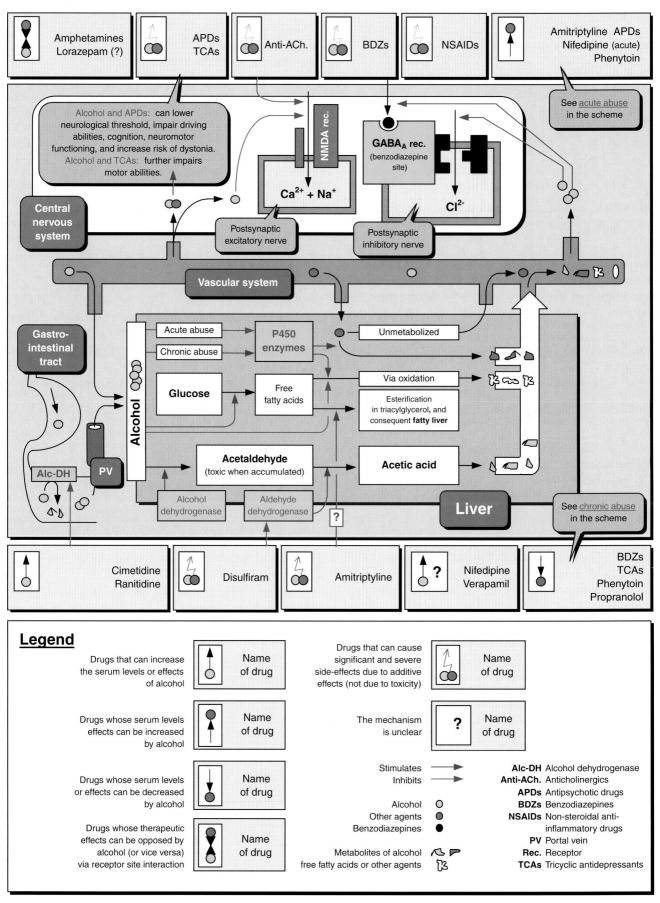

Significant Drug Interactions

Amphetamines. Can reduce some of the impairments attributed to *alcohol* abuse (memory, attention, recognition, reaction time and decision making).

Anticonvulsants. Acute *alcohol* consumption increases serum **phenytoin** levels while chronic *alcohol* abuse can decrease them.

Antidepressants. With tricyclic antidepressants (**TCAs**), chronic use of *alcohol* can enhance activity of the P450 liver catabolic enzymes with a consequent decrease in **TCAs** serum levels but few studies found *alcohol* to increase the serum levels of **amitriptyline** by up to 2-fold (due, possibly, to inhibition of **amitriptyline** metabolism). Some data suggest central receptor interactions between *alcohol* and **TCAs** that can cause impaired motor abilities (evident with **amitriptyline, clomipramine, doxepin,** and **nortriptyline**). **Mianserin** and **trazodone** can aggravate impaired driving skills caused by *alcohol* while no clinically significant interactions between **nefazodone** and *alcohol* are observed.

Selective serotonin reuptake inhibitors (**SSRIs**): **fluoxetine, paroxetine** and **fluvoxamine** do not interact significantly with *alcohol*, but isolated reports suggest that **fluvoxamine** and **paroxetine** can slightly augment the motor, attention and functioning impairments caused by *alcohol*.

Antipsychotic drugs (APDs). Numerous reports suggest that a combined **antipsychotic**–*alcohol* regimen further impairs driving abilities, cognitive, or neuromotor functioning and this effect is noted mostly with **flupenthixol** and **chlorpromazine** and, to a lesser extent, with **thioridazine, remoxipride, sulpiride** and **haloperidol**. An increased risk of emergence of acute dystonic reactions is described, mainly with **fluphenazine** and **trifluoperazine,** and is believed to be the consequence of *alcohol*-induced lower neurological threshold or to be due to the increased plasma levels of the antipsychotics.

Chlorpromazine and, to a lesser extent, **thioridazine** do not alter *alcohol* metabolism; **haloperidol**, can increase alcohol serum levels.

Anxiolytic agents. Benzodiazepines (**BDZs**): *Alcohol* and **BDZs** produce synergistic central nervous depression due to complimentary action on the GABA$_A$ receptor and glutamate block by *alcohol*. *Alcohol* can upregulate oxidative enzymes which leads to enhanced **BDZ** metabolism and a possible decrease in serum levels and therapeutic effects. **Buspirone** does not add to the impaired psychomotor skills when co-administered with *alcohol*.

Calcium-channel blockers (CCBs). These (**nifedipine, verapamil**) can increase *alcohol* serum levels by about 15–50%. The mechanism is speculated to be via the inhibition of hepatic alcohol metabolism. Some data suggest that *alcohol* might also inhibit the metabolism of **nifedipine**, thus raising its serum levels and consequent effects.

Disulfiram. This antagonizes aldehyde dehydrogenase (which metabolizes acetylaldehyde, the first metabolite of *alcohol*) leading to accumulation of acetaldehyde with a consequent antabuse reaction (flushing, weakness, vertigo, headaches, nausea, vomiting, dyspnea, hypotension, tachycardia), 10–30 minutes following the ingestion of *alcohol*.

H$_2$ blockers. Some but not all studies found that **cimetidine** or **ranitidine** can increase the serum *alcohol* levels by 10–300% perhaps as these drugs inhibit alcohol dehydrogenase in the gastric mucosa leading to enhanced *alcohol* absorption.

Non steroidal anti-inflammatory drugs (NSAIDs). *Alcohol* can stimulate the conversion of **paracetamol** to hepatotoxic derivatives, so worsening hepatic damage. Heavy drinkers, especially, are at a greater risk. **Ibuprofen** was found not to interact significantly with *alcohol* although an isolated report of acute renal failure with combined *alcohol*–**ibuprofen** use has been published. The risk of gastrointestinal bleeding is enhanced by concomitant use of *alcohol* and **NSAIDs** (and **aspirin**). The mechanism involves the damaging effects of both agents on gastric mucosal cells. Some **NSAIDs** might impair driving performance.

Propranolol. *Alcohol* impairs **propranolol** absorption, leading to possible impairments in **propranolol** effects.

> Note: Lack of stated interaction mean studies not reported, not that such combinations are safe.

SECTION D

TREATMENT STRATEGIES

14.1 Major depressive disorder (non-resistant) (1)
Treatment strategies (based on published data)

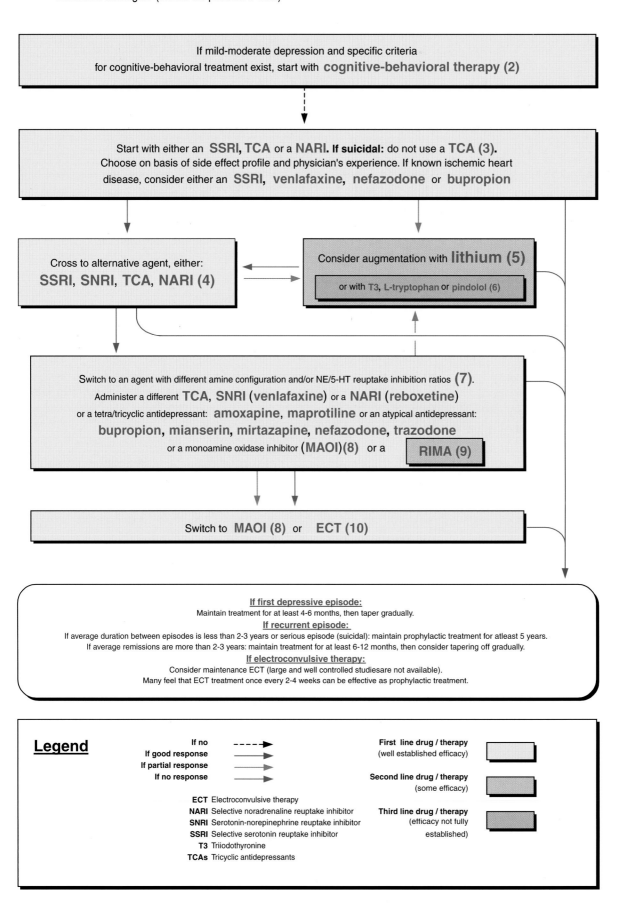

If mild-moderate depression and specific criteria
for cognitive-behavioral treatment exist, start with **cognitive-behavioral therapy (2)**

Start with either an **SSRI, TCA** or a **NARI**. **If suicidal:** do not use a **TCA (3).**
Choose on basis of side effect profile and physician's experience. If known ischemic heart
disease, consider either an **SSRI, venlafaxine, nefazodone** or **bupropion**

Cross to alternative agent, either:
SSRI, SNRI, TCA, NARI (4)

Consider augmentation with **lithium (5)**

or with T3, L-tryptophan or pindolol (6)

Switch to an agent with different amine configuration and/or NE/5-HT reuptake inhibition ratios (7).
Administer a different **TCA, SNRI (venlafaxine)** or a **NARI (reboxetine)**
or a tetra/tricyclic antidepressant: **amoxapine, maprotiline** or an atypical antidepressant:
bupropion, mianserin, mirtazapine, nefazodone, trazodone
or a monoamine oxidase inhibitor (MAOI)(8) or a   **RIMA (9)**

Switch to **MAOI (8)** or   **ECT (10)**

If first depressive episode:
Maintain treatment for at least 4-6 months, then taper gradually.
If recurrent episode:
If average duration between episodes is less than 2-3 years or serious episode (suicidal): maintain prophylactic treatment for atleast 5 years.
If average remissions are more than 2-3 years: maintain treatment for at least 6-12 months, then consider tapering off gradually.
If electroconvulsive therapy:
Consider maintenance ECT (large and well controlled studiesare not available).
Many feel that ECT treatment once every 2-4 weeks can be effective as prophylactic treatment.

Legend

If no	- - - - ▶
If good response	──────▶
If partial response	──────▶
If no response	──────▶

First line drug / therapy
(well established efficacy)

Second line drug / therapy
(some efficacy)

Third line drug / therapy
(efficacy not fully
established)

ECT Electroconvulsive therapy
NARI Selective noradrenaline reuptake inhibitor
SNRI Serotonin-norepinephrine reuptake inhibitor
SSRI Selective serotonin reuptake inhibitor
T3 Triiodothyronine
TCAs Tricyclic antidepressants

Notes about the numbered items in the scheme

Antidepressants

1. Antidepressant agents work in about 65–75% of patients. The selective serotonin reuptake inhibitors (**SSRIs**) are usually preferred as first line agents due to their high therapeutic index, relative benign side effect profile (especially cardiac and anticholinergic), safety and mild withdrawal symptoms. Symptoms that mostly respond to antidepressant therapy are depressed mood, feeling of hopelessness and helplessness, sleep difficulties, decreased appetite, guilt, interest in daily activities, and loss of energy. Patients with early insomnia can benefit from a sedative agent (**amitriptyline, clomipramine, nefazodone, mirtazapine, imipramine, doxepin, trazodone**) although these carry the risk of daytime carry over sedation. Patients who suffer mostly from lack of energy and hypersomnia could benefit more from agents with predominantly adrenergic stimulatory properties (**bupropion, desipramine, fluoxetine, nortriptyline** or **reboxetine**). Elderly patients should receive the least-anticholinergic agents (**bupropion, desipramine, nortriptyline, reboxetine, SSRIs** or **trazodone**). Patients with a seizure disorder should not be given agents that can significantly lower their seizure threshold (**amoxapine, bupropion, clomipramine** or **maprotiline**). Patients with manifest ischemic heart disease should be treated very cautiously, and those with pre-existing conduction disease should avoid tricyclic antidepressant (**TCAs**), due to their prolongation of intraventricular conduction (quinidine-like effect). There are some anecdotal reports of **SSRIs** (mainly **fluoxetine**) that can cause severe sinus bradycardia. **Nefazodone, reboxetine, venlafaxine** and **bupropion** (except in very rare cases) have not been shown, to date, to induce clinically relevant conduction disturbances. **Venlafaxine** and **bupropion** can raise the blood pressure by up to 10%.

2. The relative indications for **cognitive–behavioural therapy** are a person who cannot tolerate or has a relative contraindication for **TCAs** (recent myocardial infarction, manifest ischemic heart disease, asymptomatic arrhythmias) or **SSRIs** (sinus bradycardia or manifest ischemic heart disease – due to their potential vasoconstrictive effects on coronary arteries).

3. TCAs have a narrow therapeutic index and are lethal in overdose. Therefore start with small doses, raise gradually, and be aware of the danger in administrating these agents to suicidal patients. Note that unusual pharmacokinetic disposition can greatly alter the effective dose.

4. The selective noradrenaline (norepinephrine)-reuptake inhibitor (**NARI** – **reboxetine**) is a newly introduced agent, and accumulating data, including some large and well-controlled studies, suggest that it is as efficacious as the other antidepressant drugs in all forms of depression. In particular, it has been shown to have a rather special efficacy in improving social function in depression. **Reboxetine** has also been shown to be better-tolerated than **TCAs**.

5. Lithium, in combination with a **TCA**, **SSRI** or monoamine oxidase inhibitor (**MAOI**), exerts beneficial results in about 50% of patients previously unresponsive to these agents. The effect is usually observed within 2 weeks, and requires doses between 600 and 900 mg/day of **lithium**.

6. Triiodothyronine (**T3**) is administered in doses of about 25–50 μg/day. The mechanism of action is unclear but may be particularly beneficial in patients with a history of thyroid disease (or family history of thyroid disease). L-**Tryptophan** can be used as adjuvant to **TCAs** and **MAOIs**. As a precursor of serotonin, it increases the availability of serotonin to central nervous system. It is usually given just before bedtime because of its substantial sedative effects. The main side-effects attributed to L-**tryptophan** are nausea and possible impairments of liver functions. Eosinophilia–myalgia syndrome (myalgia, fatigue, rash, breathing difficulties, swelling of extremities, congestive heart failure and possible death), once believed to be a consequence of L-**tryptophan**, is now considered the result of contamination in the manufacturing process. **Pindolol** has the capacity to accelarate and augment the antidepressant effects of **SSRIs** (see Section 5.3).

7. Most antidepressants can be differentiated either by their different ratio of selectivity for blocking the reuptake of norepinephrine or serotonin or by their receptor and enzyme interactions. It is advisable to administer agents with a significantly different pharmacological profile compared with that of the previously used agent (in unresponsive patients).

8,9. MAOIs have equal efficacy in the treatment of major depressive disorder (MDD) as **TCAs** (if used in right doses) (**8**). **MAOIs** might have a better efficacy in improving symptoms of atypical depression (mood reactivity, hypersomnia, increased appetite and rejection sensitivity). The use of **MAOIs** was limited due to dietary restrictions and adverse side-effect profile (insomnia, sedation, postural hypotension, and sexual dysfunctions). With the marketing of the reversible inhibitor of monoamine oxidase type A (**RIMA**), **moclobemide,** many of these potential troublesome effects are absent. **Moclobemide** has shown similar efficacy to **TCAs** in agitated depression (**9**).

10. Electroconvulsive treatment (**ECT**) is especially effective for treatment of MDD with melancholic features (late insomnia, diurnal variation, decreased appetite/weight and psychomotor retardation). It is usually administered to non-responders to pharmacotherapy, severe psychotics and suicidal or aggressive patients, and for patients sensitive to relevant pharmacotherapies.

14.2 Major depressive disorder with psychotic features (1)

Treatment strategies (based on published data)

If patient agrees and there are no relative contraindications to electroconvulsive therapy, or if elderly or if there is any contraindication to pharmacotherapy

If the patient cannot tolerate anticholinergic effects or sedation, or if there is a need for a few tablets per day or a contraindication to high-potency antipsychotic agents

If suicidal

Start, if possible, with a
**high potency
antipsychotic agent (2)**

Consider starting with
amoxapine (3)

Following a few days
(to evaluate potential
adverse effects)

Following 4-6 weeks

Add an
**antidepressant
agent (4)**

After the acute episode, if fully remitted administer
'lower effective dose' (5)
The patient is probably within the 30-50% that respond solely to an antipsychotic regimen

After the acute episode, if fully remitted administer
'lower effective dose' (5)

Start, add or change to
electroconvulsive therapy (ECT) (6)

Legend

If yes	⟶	
If no	---⟶	
If good response	⟶	
If partial response	⟶	
If no response	⟶	

First-line drug / therapy
(well-established efficacy)

Second-line drug / therapy
(some efficacy)

Third-line drug / therapy
(efficacy not fully established)

Notes about the numbered items in the scheme

Antipsychotic Therapy

1. Major depressive disorder with psychotic features responds poorly to either antidepressants alone or to antipsychotics alone (in both cases the response rates are between 30–40%). The combined antipsychotic–antidepressant regimen has shown, in well controlled studies, to be efficient in about 70–80% of patients. There is no evidence that any specific antipsychotic or antidepressant agent is more efficacious for the treatment of a depressive disorder with psychotic features. Therefore practically any antipsychotic or antidepressant agent might be used. It is advisable to start with one agent (to properly monitor side-effects and response).

It is preferable to begin with an antipsychotic and not with an antidepressant. By doing so, one can achieve a number of goals:
- One can obtain faster and better compliance due to the diminishing psychosis.
- If the diagnosis should turn-up to be mistaken and the person has a psychotic disorder, one has addressed it correctly.
- Antidepressants might induce psychosis in some predisposed patients, although there are accumulating data that the combined **antipsychotic–antidepressant** regimen is not associated with the emergence of psychosis in the vast majority of cases.

2. It is recommended to use a **high-potency antipsychotic agent**, because most of these agents have less anticholinergic side-effects. The need for a weak anticholinergic capacity is due to the possible anticholinergic additive effects of combined antipsychotic and antidepressant agents (most of which have some anticholinergic properties).

The doses of the antipsychotic agents are usually lower than the doses used in the treatment of schizophrenia, and doses equivalent to 2–4 mg/day of **haloperidol** are usually sufficient.

3. **Amoxapine** is a tetracyclic antidepressant agent with a significant antagonism of the dopamine type 2 receptors. It is estimated that 100 mg of **amoxapine** is equivalent, approximately, to 0.5–1.0 mg of **haloperidol**. Besides its antidopaminergic properties, **amoxapine** exerts a significant norepinephrine-reuptake inhibition properties (it has also a very weak serotonin reuptake inhibition capacity). **Amoxapine** is usually effective at doses of 150–200 mg/day (up to 400 mg/day can be given). Tablets of 150 mg are available, so patients are quite often on a one tablet per day regimen, which consequently further improves their compliance.

Amoxapine's dual capacities of increasing adrenergic neurotransmission with a concomitant blockade of dopaminergic transmission is theoretically similar to a combined antidepressant–antipsychotic regimen. Some data support this assumption, since **amoxapine** was found in several cases to have a significant beneficial result in improving both the depressive state and the psychosis associated with major depressive disorder with psychotic features.

Antidepressant Therapy

4. No specific antidepressant has proven to have better efficacy in this disorder. The doses used should be as in the treatment of any other depressive disorder. The efficacy of the antidepressant agent should be monitored by addressing, mainly, such symptoms as guilt feelings, hopelessness, anhedonia, sleep parameters or the psychotic features. Other possible depressive symptoms (especially affect and motor ones) should be carefully evaluated, since the use of a concomitant antipsychotic regimen could affect and mask an apparent improvement.

5. This is a suggested practice that is not based on any established data. To date, no large and well-controlled trials on maintenance treatment of major depressive disorder with psychotic features have been made (neither with any antipsychotic–antidepressant regimen nor with **amoxapine**).

6. Electroconvulsive therapy (**ECT**) is considered more effective than the combined antipsychotic–antidepressant regimen in the treatment of major depressive disorder with psychotic features. For this entity, it has significant beneficial effects in 80–90% of patients. It was also shown to decrease the number and duration of future hospitalizations (especially if continued as maintenance therapy). **ECT** has also been shown to be better tolerated by the elderly, and in that population it might exert an even higher efficacy. Seizure induction is the most relevant and necessary event that has to take place in order to achieve the therapeutic effects of **ECT** (studied with depressive episodes, but presumed to be so with other clinical entities as well). The exact mechanism of action of **ECT** is unclear although much data are available regarding its intra- and intercellular effects (see Section 8.1). **ECT** should be the therapy of choice in most instances if possible. **ECT** is considered a very safe modality compared with most of the antidepressant or antipsychotic drugs. The mortality rate for **ECT** is estimated to be about 1:10 000 of treated patients, and it is almost always associated with pre-existing cardiac disorder. Both anterograde and retrograde amnesia might arise following **ECT**, but are usually transient, and cognitive capacity is usually fully restored within a few hours. In rare cases the cognitive impairments exist for a few months (usually between 6 and 8 months) but they are practically always transient. **ECT** should be a first option for pharmacotherapy-resistant patients or in cases where an immediate response is necessary (suicidal patient for example).

14.3 Treatment-resistant depression (1)

Treatment strategies (based on published data)

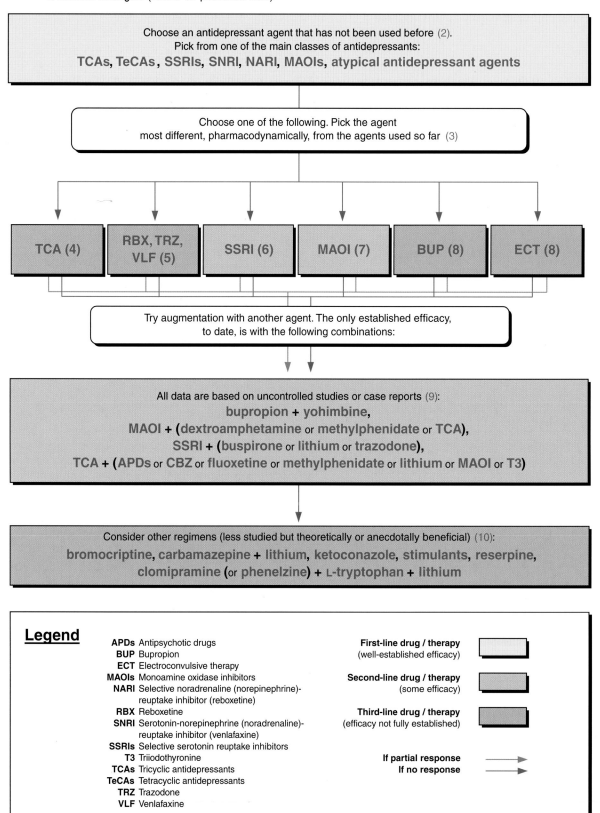

Choose an antidepressant agent that has not been used before (2).
Pick from one of the main classes of antidepressants:
TCAs, TeCAs, SSRIs, SNRI, NARI, MAOIs, atypical antidepressant agents

Choose one of the following. Pick the agent
most different, pharmacodynamically, from the agents used so far (3)

| TCA (4) | RBX, TRZ, VLF (5) | SSRI (6) | MAOI (7) | BUP (8) | ECT (8) |

Try augmentation with another agent. The only established efficacy,
to date, is with the following combinations:

All data are based on uncontrolled studies or case reports (9):
**bupropion + yohimbine,
MAOI + (dextroamphenidate or methylphenidate or TCA),
SSRI + (buspirone or lithium or trazodone),
TCA + (APDs or CBZ or fluoxetine or methylphenidate or lithium or MAOI or T3)**

Consider other regimens (less studied but theoretically or anecdotally beneficial) (10):
**bromocriptine, carbamazepine + lithium, ketoconazole, stimulants, reserpine,
clomipramine (or phenelzine) + L-tryptophan + lithium**

Legend

APDs	Antipsychotic drugs	
BUP	Bupropion	
ECT	Electroconvulsive therapy	
MAOIs	Monoamine oxidase inhibitors	
NARI	Selective noradrenaline (norepinephrine)-reuptake inhibitor (reboxetine)	
RBX	Reboxetine	
SNRI	Serotonin-norepinephrine (noradrenaline)-reuptake inhibitor (venlafaxine)	
SSRIs	Selective serotonin reuptake inhibitors	
T3	Triiodothyronine	
TCAs	Tricyclic antidepressants	
TeCAs	Tetracyclic antidepressants	
TRZ	Trazodone	
VLF	Venlafaxine	

First-line drug / therapy
(well-established efficacy)

Second-line drug / therapy
(some efficacy)

Third-line drug / therapy
(efficacy not fully established)

If partial response
If no response

Notes about the numbered items in the scheme

1. Treatment-resistant depression (**TRD**) is defined, in this case, as failure to achieve full remission after 3 adequate trials of antidepressant regimens. These regimens should include at least one tricyclic antidepressant (**TCA**) and one selective serotonin reuptake inhibitor (**SSRI**).

2. The major antidepressant classes are shown in Table 14.1.

3. Choose an agent that is different from previously used agents, in the following possible aspects:

- NE (norepinephrine)/5-HT (serotonin) reuptake inhibition ratio;
- affinity to specific receptors, besides the adrenergic or serotonergic (dopaminergic, muscarinic, histaminergic);
- different pharmacological class.

The mentioned steps are advised and they are based on common logic. No conclusive data are available on the role of these parameters in increasing the antidepressant response.

4,5. There is no sufficient data, via well-controlled trials, concerning the efficacy of these agents, although there is some data supporting the use of high dose **venlafaxine** in **TRD**.

6. Small uncontrolled studies and some case reports suggested the efficacy of **SSRIs** in **TRD**.

7. Some monoamine oxidase inhibitors (**MAOIs**) were tested in **TRD** with variable success rates. Most data suggest that **phenelzine** is efficacious in up to 65% of patients and **tranylcypromine** in about 50% of **TRD** patients. Since **MAOIs** possibly have an established efficacy in **TRD**, one might consider another **MAOI**, or, if the patient did not recieve an **MAOI** at all, a trial with **MAOI** should be made.

8. There are no well controlled trials on the efficacy of these agents (**bupropion, electroconvulsive therapy**) in **TRD**. However, accumulated clinical data indicate the efficacy of **electroconvulsive therapy** in **TRD**.

9. All the listed combinations have been reported to induce full remissions in **TRD**. Some of the data are based fully on anecdotal cases (e.g. **bupropion + yohimbine**), and the efficacy of the other regimens was suggested following case-series and small open-labeled trials. The data are incomplete and response rates are variable and range between 10% and 80%. No specific combination is currently recommended, or proved to be significantly more efficacious. The combined use of **clomipramine** (or **phenelzine**), L-tryptophan and **lithium** has also been reported in open trials to be beneficial in **TRD**.

10. **Ketoconazole** and **aminogluthetimide** inhibit the biosynthesis and the metabolism of steroids, including cortisol. A number of cases were reported of full remissions from **TRD** following treatment with these agents. The exact mechanism is unclear, and the significance of these regimens is questionable. **Bromocriptine, stimulants** (amphetamines), and **reserpine** have all been shown to improve depressive symptoms in patients suffering from major depressive disorder (not with atypical features). Their efficacy in **TRD** has not been established so far. Note that **reserpine**, an inhibitor of the vesicular monoamine transporter (see Section 1.11) is more widely accepted as an inducer of depression. The use of **stimulants** should usually be restricted to elderly patients with melancholic or anergic symptoms.

Table 14.1

TCAs	TeCAs	SSRIs	NARI	SNRI	MAOIs	Atypical
Amitriptyline	Amoxapine	Citalopram	Reboxetine	Venlafaxine	Isocarboxacid	Bupropion
Clomipramine	Maprotiline	Fluoxetine			Moclobemide*	Mianserin**
Desipramine	Mianserin**	Fluvoxamine			(reversible inhibitor of	Mirtazapine
Doxepin		Paroxetine			monoamine oxidase type A)	Nefazodone
Imipramine		Sertraline			Phenelzine	Trazodone
Nortriptyline					Tranylcypromine	

* **Moclobemide** belongs to a subclass of MAOIs termed reversible inhibitors of monoamine oxidase type A (RIMA).
** **Mianserin** is a tetracyclic antidepressant that is not a reuptake inhibitor, and many consider it to be an atypical agent (see Section 2.4).
TCAs tricyclic antidepressants; **TeCAs** tetracyclic antidepressants; **SSRIs** selective serotonin reuptake inhibitors; **NARI** selective noradrenaline (norepinephrine)-reuptake inhibitor; **SNRIs** serotonin–norepinephrine (noradrenaline)-reuptake inhibitors; **MAOIs** monoamine oxidase inhibitors.

14.4 Major depressive disorder with atypical features (1)
Treatment strategies (based on published data)

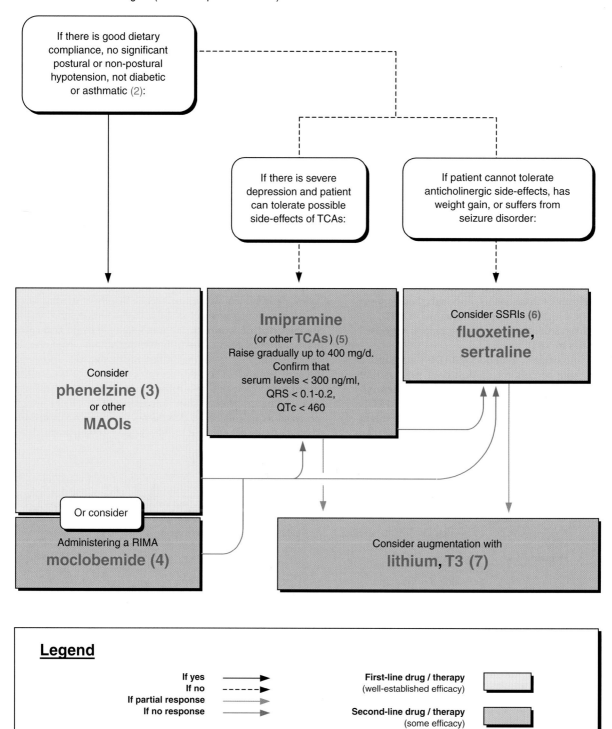

Notes about the numbered items in the scheme

Clinical Aspects

1a. The clinical picture is always characterized by mood reactivity (the patient has the capacity to be cheered-up, enjoy or respond favorably to positive experiences). The magnitude of the response is as much as 50% of that expected by a 'normal' non-depressed person.

b. Some of the other associated symptoms, most often seen with atypical depression, are as follows:

- *hypersomnia*. (Sleeping over 10 hours a day, at least 3 days per week and for a period of at least 3 months) is seen in about 35% of patients.
- *Hyperphagia*. Excessive eating or a weight gain of more than 3 kg in 3 months is seen in almost 50% of patients.
- *Leaden paralysis*. A physical feeling of heaviness mostly in the extremities. It should be present for at least 1 hour a day, 3 days a week, and last for at least 3 months.
- *Rejection sensitivity*. This is a pathological, over-sensitivity to interpersonal rejection.

c. Other, less often seen symptoms are as follows:

- Early insomnia without late insomnia.
- 'Reversed diurnal variation' – the patient's mood is better in the mornings.
- The classic symptoms of 'endogenous depression' are usually absent (guilt, weight loss, morning worsening).
- There is more severe motor retardation than is usually seen in major depressive disorder.
- Increased comorbidity with anxiety (panic disorder and social phobia), somatization disorders or substance abuse.

d. Onset is usually in the late teens or early twenties. More than 33% of patients have a family history of major depressive disorder.

Drug Treatment

2. The major or most often seen adverse side-effects of monoamine oxidase inhibitors (**MAOIs**) are as follows:

- *Postural hypotension*. This phenomenon is dose-dependent and can be worsened greatly if the patients is also receiving diuretics or antihypertensive agents.
- *Hyperadrenergic crisis*. **MAOIs** are not selective for the central nervous system only. They inhibit all monoamine oxidases, including the enzymes located in the gut and liver. These enzymes play an important role in catabolyzing sympathomimetic drugs and many foods containing pressor amines (tyramine, beef or chicken liver, some fish, overripe avocados, fava beans, and others). When a patient receives **MAOIs** and ingests pressor-amine-containing beverages, there is an increased risk that some of the pressors will not be metabolized quickly enough, leading to overstimulation of

the adrenergic system. The clinical picture can be characterized by severe headaches, mydriasis, diaphoresis, extreme hypertension, cardiac arrhythmias, myocardial infarctions and severe agitation.

- *Sexual dysfunction*, especially anorgasmia and impotence, is reported frequently. **Cyproheptadine** has been used to treat these sexual dysfunctions with some efficacy.
- Insomnia with possible, 'paradoxical' sedation during the daytime.
- **MAOIs** often alter serum glucose regulation, especially in patients receiving hypoglycemic agents.

3. Phenelzine (and other **MAOIs**) have been shown to exhibit superior efficacy over tricyclic antidepressants (**TCAs**) in atypical depression. Start with a dose of 15 mg/day every 3 days, and raise gradually to a total of 60–90 mg/day. Continue the therapy for at least 8–12 weeks for the best results, and before regarding the patient as non-responsive. **Tranylcypromine** has fewer anticholinergic side-effects, it causes less weight gain and sexual dysfunction, and its hepatotoxicity is relatively rare compared with **phenelzine**. **Tranylcypromine's** major side-effects are severe insomnia or agitation, and it is mostly effective in anergic depression.

4. Reversible inhibitors of monoamine oxidase type A (**RIMAs** e.g. **moclobemide**) are good candidates for the treatment of atypical depression due to their favorable side-effect profile (especially the absence of significant dietary restrictions and a shorter 'drug-free' interval needed between **MAOI** and **TCAs** administration, and vice versa: 1 day compared with 2 weeks). To date, no conclusive data is available for their efficacy in atypical depression.

5. Traditionally, patients with atypical depression are believed to respond poorly to **TCAs**. However, individual cases might respond well, and many case reports, and some open and double-blind studies, have reported about the beneficial effects of **TCAs** in atypical depressions. This was evident mainly with **imipramine**, and might be due to its sedative and anxiolytic effects.

6. Selective serotonin reuptake inhibitors (**SSRIs**) have been shown, in case reports and open-labeled trials, to exert beneficial responses in patients with atypical depression (60–80% remission rates with **fluoxetine**). Preliminary data suggest that **sertraline** might also be effective.

7. Lithium and **T3** (triiodothyronine) have proven efficacy as an augmenting agents in major depressive disorder. Their efficacy in atypical depression is not established, although some anecdotal data suggest the efficacy of the combined **fluoxetine–lithium–T3** regimen in this disorder.

14.5 Dysthymic disorder (1)
Treatment strategies (based on published data)

Consider treatment with a

MAOI (phenelzine) (2)

It probably has the highest efficacy in this disorder (30-70% beneficial results).
If there is a relative contraindication for an MAOI, consider administrating
an **SSRI (fluoxetine, sertraline)** or a **TCA (desipramine)**

Augment with
lithium or **T3 (3)**

Switch to:
imipramine, amitriptyline (4)

Consider treatment with one of the following (5):
amineptine, bupropion, reboxetine, RIMA, other **SSRIs.**
Note that these regimens are not studied in well-controlled
trials, but have shown beneficial effects
in case reports or small open-labeled studies

Legend

If partial response ⟶

If no response ⟶

MAOI Monoamine oxidase inhibitor
RIMA Reversible inhibitor of monoamine oxidase type A
SSRIs Selective serotonin reuptake inhibitors
T3 Triiodothyronine

First-line drug / therapy
(well-established efficacy)

Second-line drug / therapy
(some efficacy)

Third-line drug / therapy
(efficacy not fully established)

Notes about the numbered items in the scheme

Clinical Aspects

1a. The disorder is characterized by a less severe and more chronic course than major depressive disorder.

b. Lifetime prevalence is about 5%, and females are affected twice as often as males.

c. For the diagnosis of dysthymic disorder (by DSM-IV) along with depressed mood for more than 2 years, 2 out of the following 6 criteria are to be met: poor appetite/overeating, insomnia/hypersomnia; low energy/fatigue, low self esteem, poor concentration/difficulties in making decisions; hopelessness.

d. The illness may persist for 2–20 years with a median duration of about 5 years.

e. The prognosis worsens if the patient has coexisting major depressive episodes. Such patients suffer from the highest rates of relapses (also termed 'double depression').

f. Treatment of dysthymic disorder has not been studied in well controlled trials with the DSM-IV criteria. The main suggested treatment modalities are pharmacotherapy and cognitive–behavioral psychotherapy.

g. The prognosis of treated dysthymic disorder is variable. Data apparently suggest that only 10–20% of diagnosed patients attain complete remission a year following the diagnosis. About 25% of patients suffer from chronic, non-remitting course.

Drug Treatment

2. Few controlled trials have demonstrated the efficacy of **phenelzine** in ameliorating dysthymic symptoms. In some instances the reported efficacy was about 70%, compared with less than 50% with the tricyclic agent **desipramine** or some of the **selective serotonin reuptake inhibitors** (**SSRIs**; reported mainly with **fluoxetine** and **sertraline**). Generally, because the beneficial effects of these agents have not been established in large and well controlled studies, the validity of the presumed efficacy is questionable. It should be noted that the long-term outcome of these treatments has not been sufficiently studied, and anecdotal data suggest that these patients might suffer from severe depressive relapses, refractory to further treatment regimens.

3. The augmentation of **phenelzine** with **lithium** or **T3** has been proven efficacious in major depresive disorder, but has not been studied in dysthymic disorder.

4. A few case reports and open-labeled studies have demonstrated the efficacy of **imipramine** and **amitriptyline** in improving dysthymic symptoms in about 40–60% of patients. The symptoms most often responding to therapy were social and interpersonal functioning. **Imipramine** has been found to be less effective than **phenelzine** in some of these studies.

5. Anecdotal data about **amineptine** (a tricyclic agent) suggests its efficacy in up to 90% of patients diagnosed as suffering from dysthymic disorder. The relevance of this data is questionable due to the small study population and the lack of proper control. Further trials should be made to establish the suggested potential.

The efficacy of other **tricyclic antidepressants** and the other **SSRIs** and **bupropion** have been suggested in case reports and small open-labeled studies, but not in major well-controlled studies. **Reboxetine**, a newly introduced selective norepinephrine-reuptake inhibitor, has also been reported to exert beneficial antidepressive effects in dysthymic disorder. **Moclobemide**, a reversible inhibitor of monoamine oxidase type A (**RIMA**), has not shown, to date and in well-controlled studies, to be efficient in dysthymic disorder. However, the use of **moclobemide** is reasonable due to the established efficacy of **MAOIs** in this disorder.

14.6 Unipolar disorder – maintenance treatment

Treatment strategies (based on published data)

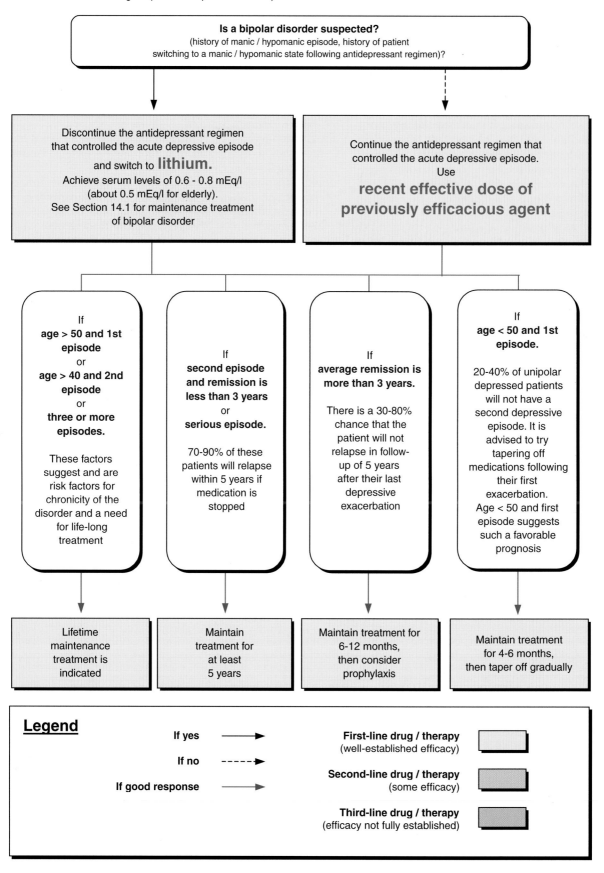

Is a bipolar disorder suspected?
(history of manic / hypomanic episode, history of patient
switching to a manic / hypomanic state following antidepressant regimen)?

Discontinue the antidepressant regimen
that controlled the acute depressive episode
and switch to **lithium.**
Achieve serum levels of 0.6 - 0.8 mEq/l
(about 0.5 mEq/l for elderly).
See Section 14.1 for maintenance treatment
of bipolar disorder

Continue the antidepressant regimen that
controlled the acute depressive episode.
Use
**recent effective dose of
previously efficacious agent**

If
**age > 50 and 1st
episode**
or
**age > 40 and 2nd
episode**
or
**three or more
episodes.**

These factors
suggest and are
risk factors for
chronicity of the
disorder and a need
for life-long
treatment

If
**second episode
and remission is
less than 3 years**
or
serious episode.

70-90% of these
patients will relapse
within 5 years if
medication is
stopped

If
**average remission is
more than 3 years.**

There is a 30-80%
chance that the
patient will not
relapse in follow-
up of 5 years
after their last
depressive
exacerbation

If
**age < 50 and 1st
episode.**

20-40% of unipolar
depressed patients
will not have a
second depressive
episode. It is
advised to try
tapering off
medications following
their first
exacerbation.
Age < 50 and first
episode suggests
such a favorable
prognosis

Lifetime
maintenance
treatment is
indicated

Maintain
treatment for
at least
5 years

Maintain treatment for
6-12 months,
then consider
prophylaxis

Maintain treatment
for 4-6 months,
then taper off gradually

Legend

If yes ⟶

If no ----▸

If good response ⟶

First-line drug / therapy
(well-established efficacy)

Second-line drug / therapy
(some efficacy)

Third-line drug / therapy
(efficacy not fully established)

14.7 Major depressive disorder with seasonal patterns (1)
Treatment strategies (based on published data)

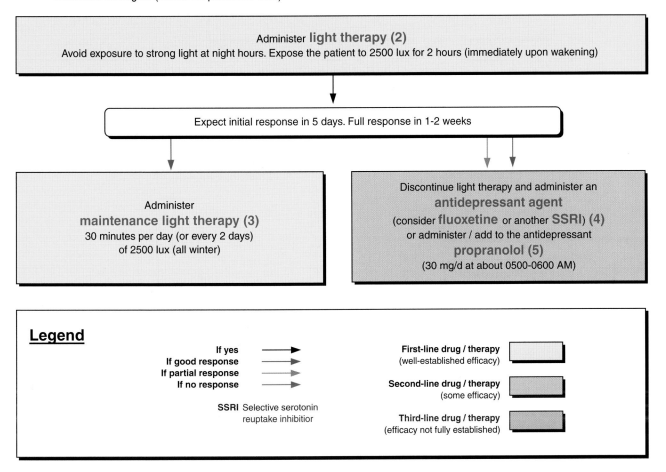

Notes about the numbered items in the scheme

Clinical Aspects

1. The major clinical characteristics of major depressive disorder with seasonal pattern (MDD-SP) are as follows:

- A depressive episode that occurs at the same time each year, virtually since first experienced. The worst time is around January and February (also termed 'winter depression').
- The mood change is characteristically modest and is manifested by low self-esteem, decreased social and occupational functioning, hypersomnia, fatigue, increased appetite, and weight gain.

Geographically, the incidence of major depressive disorder with seasonal pattern increases in areas further away from the equator. This is presumably related to the shortening of the day in these regions.

Melatonin is often speculated to be involved but there are no confirmed data to support this assumption.

Treatment

2. The mechanism of **light therapy** is reviewed in Section 8.2. Four essential parameters are considered:

a. Wave length. A wave length of about 509 nm (blue-green range) is the most efficient for suppressing melatonin production.

b. Intensity. The brighter the light, the better is the reponse. The most agreed upon value is an intensity of 2500 lux.

c. Duration. There is a linear relation between intensity and duration (2 hours of 2500 lux equals 1 hour of 5000 lux). Empirical data suggests the efficacy of 2 hours (of 2500 lux), or equivalent, for the best results.

d. Timing of administration. **Light therapy** immediately upon wakening is associated with the best results. This is in line with the 'phase-shift' hypothesis. Even so, recent data challenge the validity of the 'phase-delay' theory of MDD-SP since some recent studies have shown beneficial results with different timings of the exposure to light (including during the evenings).

3. Maintenance therapy should be administered all winter (30 minutes of 2500 lux every day or two).

4. There is no specific antidepressant agent with well-establised and increased efficacy in this disorder, although there are some data suggesting a better efficacy of serotonergic agents such as **fluoxetine**. If an antidepressant agent is administered, follow the treatment algorithm of major depressive disorder (without seasonal pattern).

5. Short-acting β-adrenergic antagonists (e.g. **propranolol**) have some efficacy in ameliorating the depressive symptoms of this disorder. The mechanism is presumably via suppression of melatonin secretion (findings are inconsistent).

14.8 Major depressive episode as part of bipolar I disorder (1)
Treatment strategies (based on published data)

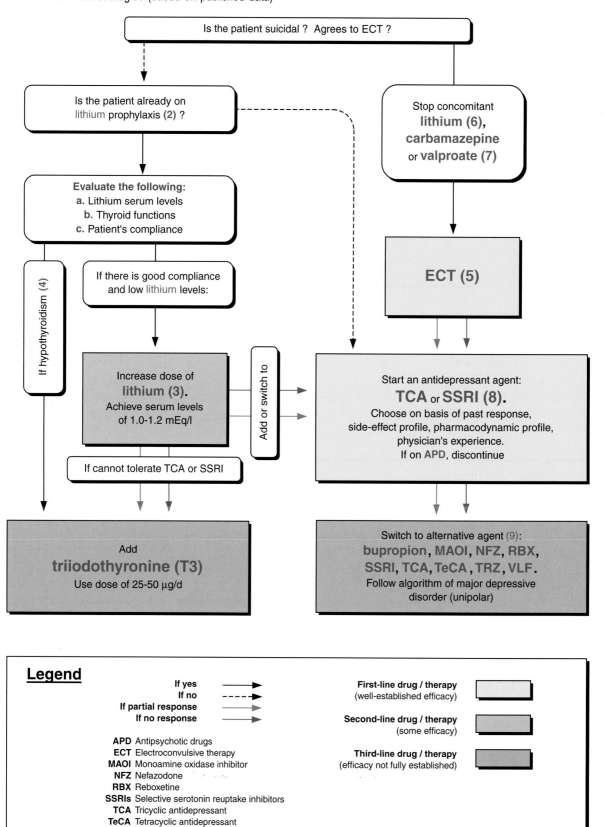

Is the patient suicidal ? Agrees to ECT ?

Is the patient already on
lithium prophylaxis (2) ?

Stop concomitant
lithium (6),
carbamazepine
or **valproate (7)**

Evaluate the following:
a. Lithium serum levels
b. Thyroid functions
c. Patient's compliance

If hypothyroidism (4)

If there is good compliance
and low lithium levels:

ECT (5)

Increase dose of
lithium (3).
Achieve serum levels
of 1.0-1.2 mEq/l

Add or switch to

Start an antidepressant agent:
TCA or **SSRI (8)**.
Choose on basis of past response,
side-effect profile, pharmacodynamic profile,
physician's experience.
If on APD, discontinue

If cannot tolerate TCA or SSRI

Add
triiodothyronine (T3)
Use dose of 25-50 µg/d

Switch to alternative agent (9):
**bupropion, MAOI, NFZ, RBX,
SSRI, TCA, TeCA, TRZ, VLF.**
Follow algorithm of major depressive
disorder (unipolar)

Legend

If yes →
If no ⇢
If partial response →
If no response →

First-line drug / therapy
(well-established efficacy)

Second-line drug / therapy
(some efficacy)

Third-line drug / therapy
(efficacy not fully established)

APD Antipsychotic drugs
ECT Electroconvulsive therapy
MAOI Monoamine oxidase inhibitor
NFZ Nefazodone
RBX Reboxetine
SSRIs Selective serotonin reuptake inhibitors
TCA Tricyclic antidepressant
TeCA Tetracyclic antidepressant
TRZ Trazodone
VLF Venlafaxine

Notes about the numbered items in the scheme

1. Systematic studies on major depressive episodes as part of bipolar I disorder, and on the role of pharmacotherapy while on **lithium** maintence therapy are absent. The main issue that needs to be addressed is whether or not the same treatment principles that hold for major depressive disorder (unipolar depression), are applicable for the treatment of depressive episodes as part of bipolar I disorder.

2–4. Many bipolar patients are on **lithium** maintenance treatment while exhibiting a breakthrough depressive episode (**2**). The therapist should address, firstly, the following:

- *Compliance with treatment.* If the compliance is good and **lithium** serum levels are lower than 0.8–1.0 mEq/l, an attempt to increase the **lithium** dose should be made in order to achieve serum levels between 1.0 and 1.2 mEq/l. Large and well controlled studies on the desired **lithium** serum levels in breakthrough depressive episodes are absent, but small open-labeled studies suggest the efficacy of such an increase in **lithium** serum levels (**3**).

- *Thyroid-function tests.* The role of enhancing thyroid function is relatively well established in major depressive disorders (unipolar depression), although patients who benefit from it usually have a normal baseline thyroid functions. In spite of the fact that there are no large or well controlled studies on **Triiodothyronine** (**T3**) augmentation to **lithium** in major depressive disorder (as part of bipolar I), a trial of **T3** augmentation to **lithium** is warranted, especially if baseline thyroid functions are decreased (**4**). **Lithium** augmentation should be given if the decreased thyroid functions are attributed to any cause (either **lithium** therapy or from any other etiology), or there is a contraindication to administer tricyclic antidepressants (**TCAs**).

5,6. If the patient is suicidal, and there are no clear contra-indications, try a course of electroconvulsive therapy (**ECT**) (**5**). The efficacy of **ECT** in major depressive disorder (unipolar depression) is well established, and it is similar to that of tricyclic antidepressants (**TCAs**). More research is needed in order to determine the efficacy of **ECT** in major depressive disorder as part of bipolar I disorder, although it seems promising.

Administration of **ECT** to patients receiving **lithium** has been reported to cause memory impairments, and to induce delirium and other neurological abnormalities. Therefore **lithium** should be discontinued before **ECT** is used (**6**).

7. Carbamazepine and **valproate** are anticonvulsants, and they oppose the desired convulsive activities of **ECT** (which is essential for its antidepressant activity), so they should also be withdrawn.

8. The standard treatment of breakthrough depression in bipolar I patients is either to add an antidepressant to an ongoing **lithium** therapy, or (if the patient is not receiving **lithium**) to administer an antidepressant as a sole agent. Since there are no large, well-controlled studies relevant to this entity, the common practice and logic should be to follow the treatment algorithm for major depressive disorder (unipolar depression). There is some inconsistent evidence that suggests that the co-administration of an antidepressant agent to **lithium** can precipitate a manic episode or induce cycling in bipolar I patients. However, this is not fully established, and the best reasonable alternative seems to be the administration of an antidepressant. If the patient is on an antipsychotic medication consider discontining it, especially if there are no psychotic features, and the patient does not need sedation (since antipsychotics might further impair functioning and/or cause adverse side-effects that might eventually worsen the depressive episode).

9. The efficacy of the non-**TCAs** in major depressive disorder (as part of bipolar I) has not been studied enough. A trial of **tetracyclic antidepressants, monamine oxidase inhibitors, trazodone, nefazodone, venlafaxine, reboxetine** or **bupropion** is warranted if the patient does not respond to **TCAs** or **selective serotonin reuptake inhibitors (SSRIs)**. The above-mentioned agents have proven efficacy in major depressive disorder (unipolar) and they seem to exert similar beneficial results in depressive disorder associated with bipolar I disorder. Inconsistent data suggest that the use of **SSRIs** is advisable due to their relatively low risk of inducing cycling.

14.9 Acute manic episode

Treatment strategies (based on published data)

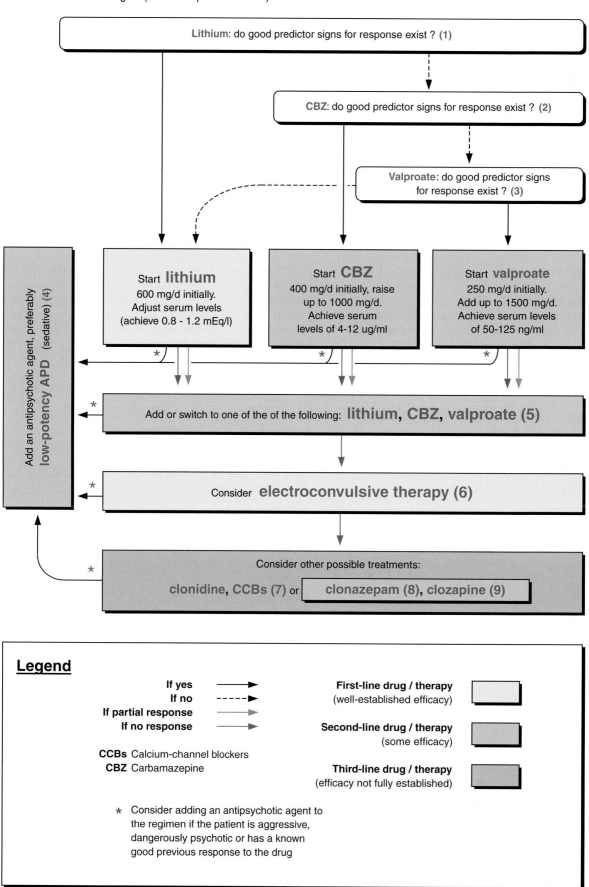

Lithium: do good predictor signs for response exist ? (1)

CBZ: do good predictor signs for response exist ? (2)

Valproate: do good predictor signs for response exist ? (3)

Add an antipsychotic agent, preferably **low-potency APD** (sedative) (4)

Start **lithium**
600 mg/d initially.
Adjust serum levels
(achieve 0.8 - 1.2 mEq/l)

Start **CBZ**
400 mg/d initially, raise
up to 1000 mg/d.
Achieve serum
levels of 4-12 ug/ml

Start **valproate**
250 mg/d initially.
Add up to 1500 mg/d.
Achieve serum levels
of 50-125 ng/ml

Add or switch to one of the of the following: **lithium, CBZ, valproate** (5)

Consider **electroconvulsive therapy** (6)

Consider other possible treatments:
clonidine, CCBs (7) or **clonazepam** (8), **clozapine** (9)

Legend

If yes ⟶
If no ⇢
If partial response ⟶
If no response ⟶

First-line drug / therapy
(well-established efficacy)

Second-line drug / therapy
(some efficacy)

Third-line drug / therapy
(efficacy not fully established)

CCBs Calcium-channel blockers
CBZ Carbamazepine

* Consider adding an antipsychotic agent to
the regimen if the patient is aggressive,
dangerously psychotic or has a known
good previous response to the drug

Notes about the numbered items in the scheme

1. Lithium. Possible good predictor signs or symptoms for the use of this agent:

a. First degree relatives with mood disorders.

b. Euphoric mania: 60–80% respond favorably to **lithium.** In dysphoric mania or mixed episode the response rate is only about 20%.

c. Good compliance to pharmcotherapy, and lack of suicidal behavior.

d. Less than 3 life-time manic episodes.

e. Absence of psychotic features.

f. Good response in previous exacerbations.

Lithium exerts beneficial effects in about 40–80% of acute manic episodes as part of bipolar I disorder. It was found more effective than placebo, antipsychotic agents or **carbamazepine** in the treatment of most manic episodes (in well controlled trials). The usual dose ranges between 1200 and 2100 mg/day.

2. Carbamazepine. Possible good predictor signs or symptoms which can direct at using this agent:

a. Secondary mania (due to pharmacotherapy, brain disorder, trauma).

b. Dysphoric mania.

c. Comorbidity of alcohol or other substance abuse.

d. Good response in previous exacerbations.

e. Absence of psychotic features.

f. Obesity.

g. Poor compliance to pharmacotherapy (due to its relatively wide therapeutic window).

h. Mixed episode.

i. Rapid cycling. Better efficacy, probably, than **lithium,** but less efficient than **valproate**. The data are based on small, uncontrolled trials in which **carbamazepine** was shown to reduce the number of recurrences (of manic or depressive episodes) to about 30% as compared with **lithium**.

j. Fertile or pregnant women who need an antimanic drug as a necessary regimen.

k. Acute manic episode as part of schizoaffective disorder.

Carbamazepine's efficacy in acute manic episodes is well established (over 15 double-blind studies have been published so far). It is more efficacious than placebo, and at least as effective as antipsychotics. There are no well-established data comparing **carbamazepine** directly with **lithium**. Beneficial effects are found in up to 60% of patients, and thus it is considered less effective than **lithium**.

3. Valproate. Possible good predictor signs or symptoms that indicate using this agent:

a. Rapid cycling mania.

e. No psychotic features.

b. Dysphoric mania.

f. Stable or decreasing frequency of manic exacerbations.

c. Mixed episode.

d. No response to **lithium** or **carbamazepine.**

g. Less-severe form of manic episode.

Valproate's efficacy in acute manic episodes is based mainly on open-labeled or small double-blind studies. It improves manic symptoms in up to 50% of patients. It was found less effective than **lithium** in small double-blind studies (60% versus 90% efficacy in certain populations).

4. Antipsychotic agents these are second line treatments for manic episode due to:

a. They have a worse side-effect profile than **lithium** or anticonvulsants (**carbamazepine** or **valproate**).

b. The efficacy of antipsychotics in ameliorating acute manic symptoms is not better than that of **lithium, carbamazepine** or **valproate** (possibly).

c. Some evidence suggests that antipsychotics lengthen or exacerbate the next depressive episode (if part of bipolar I/schizoaffective disorders).

d. The co-administration of **haloperidol** (and possibly other antipsychotics), with **lithium** might induce, in rare cases, severe extrapyramidal side-effects, delirium, dyskinesias, hyperthermia and some permanent brain damage. These effects are presumed to be mediated by their additive effects on the adenylate cyclase system.

5. Some data suggests that a combined regimen of **lithium** and another anticonvulsant (**carbamazepine** or **valproate**) might be more efficacious than the use of each agent alone. Well controlled studies are absent.

6. Electroconvulsive therapy (**ECT**) is an effective treatment for manic episodes. It has a response rate of up to 75%, especially if bilateral electrode placement is used. Poor responders to **lithium** might also benefit from **ECT**. **ECT** is also found efficient and is indicated for pregnant women and people with predisposition to develop neuroleptic malignant syndrome or severe extrapyramidal symptoms.

7. The beneficial effects of **clonidine** and **calcium-channel blockers** have been reported in a few case studies. The clinical significance of these findings is questionable.

8. Clonazepam is widely used to produce an acute calming effect, and a lot of data are accumulating about its efficacy in longer term usage.

9. Clozapine has shown to be effective in ameliorating acute manic symptoms (both treatment-resistant and as a first option regimen). Its use should be restricted due to its hematological and other potentially serious adverse side-effects. There is contraindication to administer **clozapine** with **carbamazepine** due to their synergistic effects on bone marrow suppression. The role of the other new-generation antipsychotics has not yet been established in this disorder, but should be considered due to their improved side-effect profile.

14.10 Bipolar I disorder with rapid cycling (1)

Treatment strategies (based on published data)

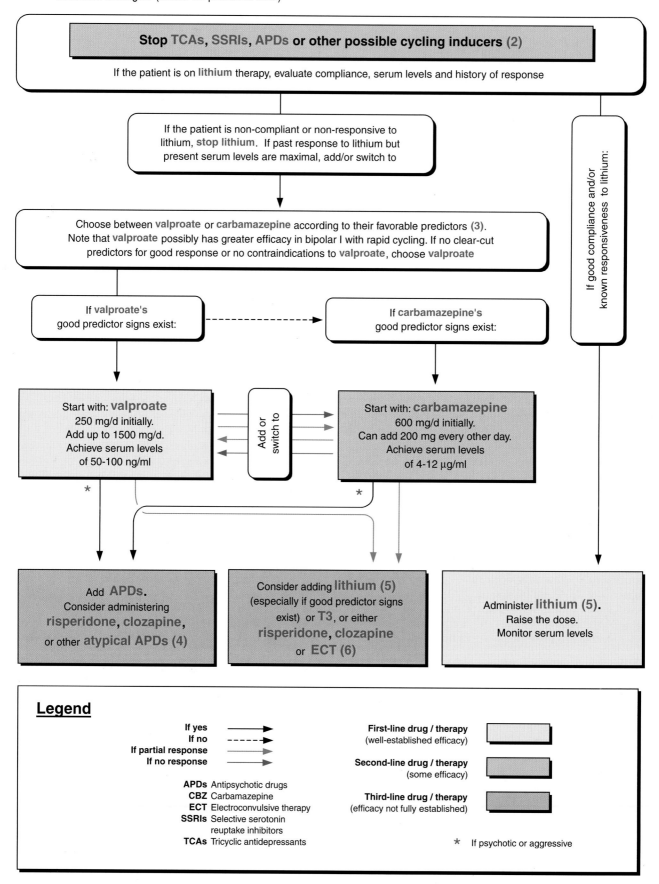

Stop TCAs, SSRIs, APDs **or other possible cycling inducers (2)**

If the patient is on **lithium** therapy, evaluate compliance, serum levels and history of response

If the patient is non-compliant or non-responsive to lithium, **stop lithium**. If past response to lithium but present serum levels are maximal, add/switch to

If good compliance and/or known responsiveness to lithium:

Choose between **valproate** or **carbamazepine** according to their favorable predictors **(3)**. Note that **valproate** possibly has greater efficacy in bipolar I with rapid cycling. If no clear-cut predictors for good response or no contraindications to **valproate**, choose **valproate**

If **valproate's** good predictor signs exist:

If **carbamazepine's** good predictor signs exist:

Start with: **valproate** 250 mg/d initially. Add up to 1500 mg/d. Achieve serum levels of 50-100 ng/ml

Add or switch to

Start with: **carbamazepine** 600 mg/d initially. Can add 200 mg every other day. Achieve serum levels of 4-12 µg/ml

Add **APDs.** Consider administering **risperidone, clozapine,** or other **atypical APDs (4)**

Consider adding **lithium (5)** (especially if good predictor signs exist) or **T3**, or either **risperidone, clozapine** or **ECT (6)**

Administer **lithium (5)**. Raise the dose. Monitor serum levels

Legend

If yes	⟶
If no	⤏
If partial response	⟶
If no response	⟶

APDs Antipsychotic drugs
CBZ Carbamazepine
ECT Electroconvulsive therapy
SSRIs Selective serotonin reuptake inhibitors
TCAs Tricyclic antidepressants

First-line drug / therapy (well-established efficacy)

Second-line drug / therapy (some efficacy)

Third-line drug / therapy (efficacy not fully established)

* If psychotic or aggressive

Notes about the numbered items in the scheme

Clinical Aspects

1a. Rapid cycling is a course specifier in the DSM-IV diagnostic criteria. For the diagnosis of rapid cycling, the person has to exhibit at least 4 episodes of mood disturbances in the last 12 months. These episodes should be separated by a partial or full remission of at least 2 months or by a switch to an episode of opposite polarity (major depressive episode to manic episode, or vice versa). Note that mood disturbances relevant for the diagnosis of rapid cycling can be major depressive disorder, manic episode, mixed episode or hypomanic episode.

b. Most affected individuals are females (about 70–90%).

c. About 90% begin with a depressive episode.

d. Most patients develop rapid cycling late in the course of their bipolar disorder.

g. Ultrafast cyclers (cycles of mood changes fluctuate in hours to days) are usually older men and the ultrafast cycling begins early in the course of their bipolar I disorder.

e. The course of 10–20% of bipolar I patients eventually acquires the characteristics of rapid cycling.

f. Rapid cyclers are relatively unresponsive to **lithium.**

g. Some of the associated factors with rapid cycling are:
- mental retardation.
- hormonal changes (in a few cases serum cortisol levels rise during the depressive episodes and decrease during the manic episodes).
- hypothyroidism.
- alcohol or other substance abuse.
- family history of bipolar I disorder.

Treatment

2. Some agents have the capacity to induce or exacerbate the cycling. The major ones are the tricyclic antidepressants (**TCAs**) (in as many of 50% of bipolar I patients), monoamine oxidase inhibitors (**MAOIs**), **tetracyclic agents** and selective serotonin reuptake inhibitors (**SSRIs**).

3A. Carbamazepine. Possible good predictor signs or symptoms that indicate using this agent:

a. Secondary mania (due to pharmacotherapy, electroconvulsive therapy, brain disorder, trauma).

b. Dysphoric mania.

c. Comorbidity of alcohol or other substance abuse.

d. Good response in previous exacerbations.

e. Absence of psychotic features.

f. Obesity.

g. Poor compliance to pharmacotherapy, due to a relatively wide therapeutic window.

h. Mixed episode.

i. Rapid cycling. There is probably better efficacy than **lithium**, but less than **valproate**. Data are based on small, uncontrolled trials in which **carbamazepine** was shown to reduce th number of recurrences (of manic or depressive episodes) to about 30% as compared with **lithium**.

j. Fertile or pregnant women who need an antimanic drug as a necessary regimen.

k. Acute manic episode as part of schizoaffective disorder.

B. Valproate. Possible good predictor signs or symptoms that indicate using this agent:

a. Rapid cycling mania. For this entity **valproate** should be considered the first line of therapy.

b. Dysphoric mania.

c. Mixed episode.

d. No response to **lithium** or **carbamazepine.**

e. No psychotic features.

f. Stable or decreasing frequency of manic exacerbations.

g. Less-severe form of manic episode.

4. Note that **antipsychotic drugs** (**APDs**) can actually induce or exacerbate the cycling. These agents should be administered with great care in rapid cyclers. The **typical APDs** (low-potency and sedative agents are usually preferred) should be reserved for severely agitated, psychotic or agressive patients and their duration of use should be limited.

5. Lithium. Possible good predictor signs or symptoms that indicate using this agent:

a. First-degree relatives with mood disorders.

b. Euphoric mania; 60–80% respond favorably to **lithium**. In dysphoric mania or mixed episode the response rate is only about 20%.

c. Good compliance with pharmacotherapy, and lack of suicidal behavior.

d. Less than 3 lifetime manic episodes.

e. Absence of psychotic features.

f. Good response in previous exacerbations.

The combined **lithium–carbamazepine** regimen was anecdotally reported to have beneficial effects in rapid cycling. There are also some other reports of the beneficial effects of combined **carbamazepine–triiodothyronine** in rapid cycling.

6. Clozapine, electroconvulsive therapy (ECT) and **risperidone** (less established at this point) have shown the capacity to control rapid cycling in case reports and small open-labeled studies. Other anticonvulsants, e.g. **gabapentin** and **vigabatrin** have been reported to work (case reports).

14.11 Bipolar I disorder – maintenance treatment (1)
Treatment strategies (based on published data)

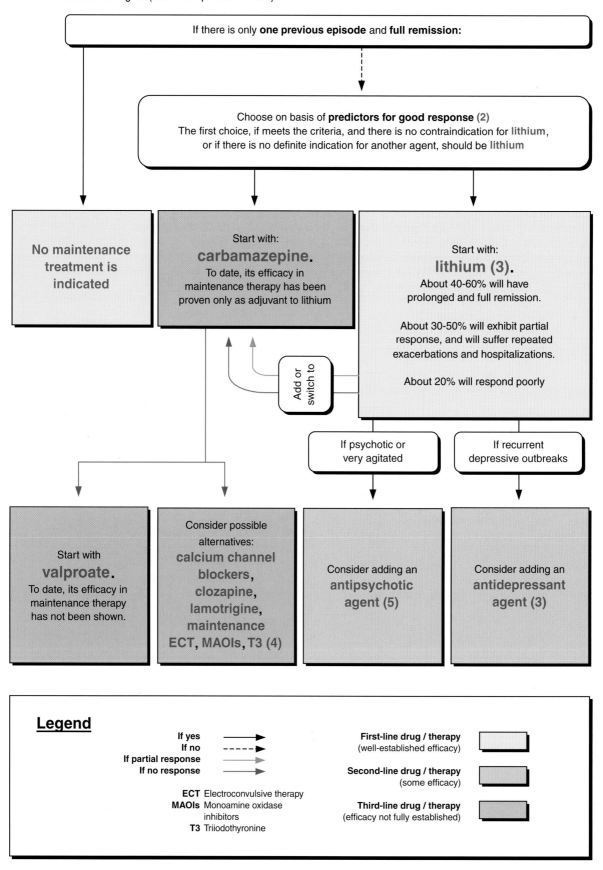

If there is only **one previous episode** and **full remission:**

Choose on basis of **predictors for good response (2)**
The first choice, if meets the criteria, and there is no contraindication for lithium,
or if there is no definite indication for another agent, should be lithium

No maintenance treatment is indicated

Start with:
carbamazepine.
To date, its efficacy in maintenance therapy has been proven only as adjuvant to lithium

Add or switch to

Start with:
lithium (3).
About 40-60% will have prolonged and full remission.

About 30-50% will exhibit partial response, and will suffer repeated exacerbations and hospitalizations.

About 20% will respond poorly

If psychotic or very agitated

If recurrent depressive outbreaks

Start with
valproate.
To date, its efficacy in maintenance therapy has not been shown.

Consider possible alternatives:
calcium channel blockers, clozapine, lamotrigine, maintenance ECT, MAOIs, T3 (4)

Consider adding an
antipsychotic agent (5)

Consider adding an
antidepressant agent (3)

Legend

If yes	→
If no	- - - →
If partial response	→
If no response	→

ECT Electroconvulsive therapy
MAOIs Monoamine oxidase inhibitors
T3 Triiodothyronine

First-line drug / therapy
(well-established efficacy)

Second-line drug / therapy
(some efficacy)

Third-line drug / therapy
(efficacy not fully established)

Notes about the numbered items in the scheme

1. The prophylactic treatment is related to periods following both depressive and manic episodes.

2. Lithium. Good predictor signs (factors that, if they exist, increase the possibility of good response) are as follows:

- 'Classic' bipolar disorder – a history of clear onset of symptoms followed by full remissions and no impairment in daily functioning between the mood episodes.
- 'Euphoric mania' – in such a case, the response rate to lithium is about 60–80%. Note that these statistics are related to acute manic episodes and not to prophylactic treatment.
- Low number of lifetime episodes (<3).
- Absence of psychotic features.
- First-degree relatives with mood disorders.

3. Several well-controlled studies have demonstrated the efficacy of **lithium** in the prophylactic treatment of bipolar I disorder. **Lithium**, in general, was found to decrease the number of relapses and the severity of the episodes, especially of the manic episodes (up to 80% response rates). There are conflicting data about the efficacy of **lithium**, as a sole agent, in the prophylactic treatment following a depressive episode compared with a combined **lithium–antidepressant** regimen. Current data suggest an almost similar efficacy, with a possible marginal improved efficacy for the combined regimen. Due to the capacity of antidepressants to induce or exacerbate manic episodes in bipolar I patients, the best practice is probably to administer **lithium** alone and to reserve the combined **lithium–antidepressant** regimen for those patients who suffer recurrent depressive episodes while on **lithium** therapy alone. **Lithium** serum levels should be kept within the ranges of 0.8–1.0 mEq/l. It is assumed that within this range, the relapse rates are decreased by 3-fold compared with serum levels of 0.4–0.6 mEq/l, along with a decreased severity of the episodes themselves (especially the manic episodes). Moreover, serum levels within the range of 0.8–1.0 mEq/l were found to reduce the risk of developing a rapid cycling course.

4. The role of these agents in the prophylactic treatment of bipolar I disorder is not established.

- **Calcium-channel blockers (verapamil).** This agent is primarily used to treat supraventricular tachyarrhythmias and angina pectoris. A few uncontrolled studies have shown some efficacy of **verapamil** in treating acute manic episodes (these findings have not been replicated so far), and some investigators have reported **verapamil's** efficacy in the prophylactic treatment of bipolar disorder.
- **Clozapine** has shown some mood-stabilizing properties, especially in rapid cyclers. Its efficacy in maintenance treatment of bipolar I disorder is not yet established.
- **Lamotrigine** is a new anticonvulsant suggested to be as efficacious as **lithium** in bipolar disorder.
- **Maintenance electroconvulsve therapy (ECT).** To date, not enough data are available about the role of maintenance **ECT** treatment in bipolar I disorder, although the beneficial role of **ECT** in acute manic or depressive exacerbations is very well established.
- **Monoamine oxidase inhibitors (MAOIs).** There are no established data concerning the efficacy of these agents. A reasonable practice would be to reserve **MAOI** treatment for those patients who switch to manic episodes while on antidepressant prophylactic treatment (the **MAOI** should be administered following the next depressive episode).
- **Triiodothyronine (T3)** - Since **T3** has some efficacy in improving depressive symptoms, it might be considered as maintenance therapy following a depressive episode. Controlled studies on the efficacy of **T3** in bipolar I disorder are not available.

5. The increased risk of developing serious adverse side-effects (mainly tardive dyskinesia, extrapyramidal side-effects, sexual dysfunctions and anticholinergic effects) and the capacity of the antipsychotic regimens to induce depressive episodes in bipolar I patients should alert the therapist not to administer antipsychotics unless the patient is very agitated or psychotic in such a way that impairs his or her daily functioning.

15.1 Acute exacerbation of schizophrenia

Treatment strategies (based on published data)

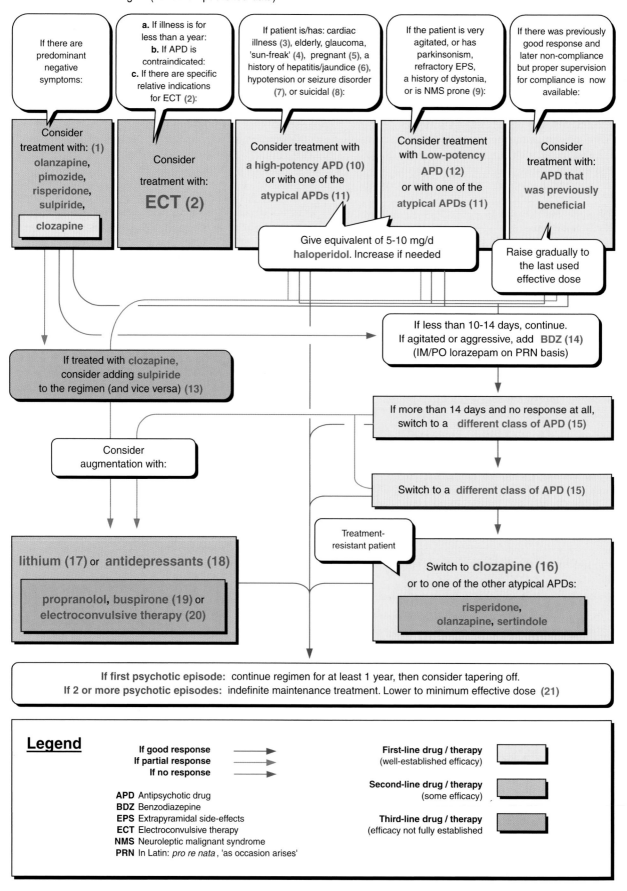

Notes about the numbered items in the scheme

1. Clozapine (and possibly **risperidone** and the other atypical antipsychotic drugs) have shown established efficacy in improving negative symptoms. Anecdotal reports suggest that **pimozide** and **sulpiride** also have some efficacy in ameliorating negative symtoms.

2. Electroconvulsive therapy (**ECT**) has some efficacy in acute exacerbations of schizophrenia. It is assumed that beneficial results can be achieved in 20–60% of patients (in reducing the acute symptomathology). **ECT** is much more beneficial if predominant affective symptoms are evident. **ECT** has no established role in the long-term management of schizophrenia.

3. Thioridazine, other **low-potency agents** and **pimozide** may cause a cardiac conduction block, ventricular tachycardia, prolonged PR, QT segments and ST depressions (in EKG recordings). These abnormalities are far more frequently reported with these agents than with high-potency antipsychotic drugs (**APDs**).

4. Low-potency drugs act as photosensitizers – leading to severe sunburn on prolonged exposure. It is especially observed with **chlorpromazine** and **thioridazine**.

5. There are insufficient data to prefer a specific antipsychotic regimen for a pregnant woman. **Haloperidol** perhaps causes less 'floppy baby syndrome'. Therefore it might be recommended to use if necessary, and especially in the third trimester. Try not to administer **APDs** in the first trimester. Some data suggest that **clozapine** has fewer teratogenic effects than other **APDs**.

6. All **APDs** can alter liver functions, especially **chlorpromazine,** which can cause cholestatic jaundice, secondary, probably, to hypersensitivity of predisposed individuals.

7. Noticed especially with the use of **low-potency APDs** and with **clozapine**.

8. Pimozide, thioridazine, chlorpromazine and other **low-potency agents** should be carefully administered to suicidal patients due to their narrow therapeutic index and lethality in overdoses.

9. The associated risk factors are organic brain disorder, dehydration, high dose and route of administration (depot more risky), use of concurrent lithium, high-potency antipsychotics, young adult male, alcoholic patient during delirium, malnutrition, exhaustion, concurrent medical illness or a prior history of neuroleptic malignant syndrome (NMS).

10. High-potency agents: **haloperidol, trifluoperazine, thiothixene**.

11. Clozapine, risperidone, olanzapine and **sertindole** have been shown in clinical and preclinical trials to have similar efficacy to **typical APDs** in non-resistant patients. This was accompanied by a diminished capacity to develop tardive dyskinesia and extrapyramidal adverse side-effects. The use of **clozapine** as a first drug agent should be avoided if possible due to its potential hazardous adverse effects.

12. Low potency agents: **chlorpromazine, thioridazine, levomepromazine, clothiapine**.

13. One controlled study and a few cases are reported concerning the beneficial effects of the combined **clozapine–sulpiride** regimen. The mechanism is unclear. It could be related to the enhanced D_2 dopaminergic blockade achieved with **sulpiride** (**clozapine** is a relatively weak D_2 antagonist).

14. Benzodiazepines (BDZs) are relatively safe (compared with antipsychotics) and reliable sedatives. Their use should be limited to controlling aggression, agitation, hyperactivity and dangerous behaviors related to the acute psychotic episode. **Lorazepam** 1–2 mg every 2 hours is usually sufficient on an as-needed basis and its use is recommended since it can be administered intra- muscularly. The co-administration of **clonazepam** with **haloperidol** significantly reduced psychotic excitement and the risk of developing extrapyramidal symptoms. In cases of schizophrenia with depressive and/or obsessive-compulsive symptoms a combined antipsychotic and selective serotonin reuptake inhibitor (**SSRI**; e.g. **citalopram**; **fluvoxamine**) may prove beneficial.

15. The main classes are **phenothiazines, butyrophenones, thioxanthenes, dibenzoxapines, benzamides, dihydroindoles** and **diphenylbutylpiperidines**.

16. The use of **clozapine** is usually restricted to treatment-resistant schizophrenic patients, where it is efficient in about 30% of patients. The more general use of **clozapine** is restricted because of its relatively high incidence of bone marrow suppression and other adverse effects, along with its present high cost. **Risperidone** and **olanzapine** have a much safer side-effect profile. Their efficacy in treatment-resistant patients is not yet well established. The role of other atypical antipsychotics such as **quetiapine, sertindole**, and **ziprazidone** in the treatment of neuroleptic-resistant schizoprenic patients is as yet unclear.

17. Some data, mostly uncontrolled, suggest that **lithium** can decrease violent behavior and improve both positive and negative symptoms when combined with an antipsychotic agent.

18. Antidepressants are traditionally believed to improve social withdrawal and depressive symptoms. Antidepressants with 5-HT$_2$ antagonism capacities (e.g. **mianserin**) might also improve psychotic symptoms. This assumption has not yet been established by well-controlled trials, and it is based on the similarities between the receptor antagonistic profile of the combined antipsychotic–antidepressant regimen and the atypical antipsychotics **clozapine, olanzapine,** and **risperidone**. Other fast acting BDZs (e.g. alprazolam) may also be effective in combination with antipsychotics for reducing agitation and dangerous behaviour.

19. Propranolol and **buspirone** may be specifically effective in improving assaultive behavior (but not as antipsychotic drugs).

20. ECT has only anecdotally been reported to sufficiently augment **APDs**. This was mainly for severly agitated, catatonic or patients with predominant affective symptoms.

21. Maintenance doses equivalent to 300 mg/day **chlorpromazine** or 2–4 mg/day of **haloperidol** are significantly more effective in lengthening the time between relapses and lowering the risk of a relapse (50% of patients not on **APDs** relapse in 6 months, and up to 80% in 12 months). The use of effective maintenance treatment can lower the relapse rates to around 10–15% and 25% respectively.

15.2 Schizoaffective disorder – depressive episode

Treatment strategies (based on published data)

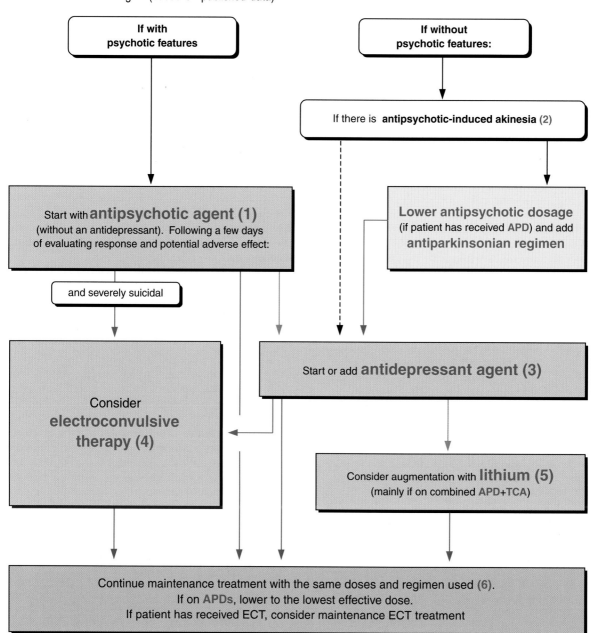

If with psychotic features

If without psychotic features:

If there is **antipsychotic-induced akinesia (2)**

Start with **antipsychotic agent (1)**
(without an antidepressant). Following a few days of evaluating response and potential adverse effect:

Lower antipsychotic dosage
(if patient has received APD) and add
antiparkinsonian regimen

and severely suicidal

Consider
electroconvulsive therapy (4)

Start or add **antidepressant agent (3)**

Consider augmentation with **lithium (5)**
(mainly if on combined APD+TCA)

Continue maintenance treatment with the same doses and regimen used (6).
If on **APDs**, lower to the lowest effective dose.
If patient has received ECT, consider maintenance ECT treatment

Legend

If yes	⟶
If no	----▶
If good response	⟶
If partial response	⟶
If no response	⟶

First-line drug / therapy
(well-established efficacy)

Second-line drug / therapy
(some efficacy)

Third-line drug / therapy
(efficacy not fully established)

APD Antipsychotic drug
ECT Electroconvulsive therapy
TCA Tricyclic antidepressant

Notes about the numbered items in the scheme

1. Some data suggest that the addition of an antidepressant agent might, in some cases, inhibit or delay recovery from the psychosis. Therefore, especially if the most predominant symptoms are psychotic, a trial with antipsychotics should be given first. It is almost always advisable to administer one regimen at a time (for side-effect evaluation and treatment response). The expected response rate when an antipsychotic regimen is given as a sole agent (and the patient has some depressive episodes) is about 30–40%. If affective symptoms are prominent, the addition of an antidepressant regimen should be considered (following a few days of evaluating potential adverse effects).

2. Consider the possibility of neuroleptic-induced akinesia. This side-effect can mimic any of the depressive symptoms. Therefore an attempt to lower neuroleptic doses and/or to add an antiparkinsonism regimen should be made. Another probable assumption is the emergence of so-called 'negative symptoms'. If so, lowering the neuroleptic dose might not be sufficient, and a switch to one of the atypical agents (e.g. **clozapine, risperidone, olanzapine**) should be considered.

3. A combined regimen of antidepressants and antipsychotics can be tried, although published data about such combinations in schizoaffective disorder–depressed type are lacking and often contradictory. A few studies found higher efficacy of this combination compared with each drug alone, but this effect was not always replicated. In major depressive disorder with psychotic features, the role of combined antipsychotic and antidepressant agents is more firmly established (this increases the response rates from about 40% for each regimen alone to around 70% with the combined therapy). For that reason, it is logical to assume (even though it is not established in schizoaffective disorder) that a combined regimen might exert better efficacy. If using a combined antipsychotic–antidepressant therapy, a trial of at least 9 weeks is needed for proper response.

4. The role of electroconvulsive therapy (**ECT**) in schizoaffective –depressed type is not proven, but should be considered. **ECT** has a proven efficacy in the treatment of affective disorders and is also beneficial in some of the psychotic disorders, especially if affective components are present (catatonia, psychotic mania, major depressive disorder with psychotic features). Therefore **ECT** might prove to be a beneficial tool for the treatment of depressive episodes as part of schizoaffective disorder.

5. Lithium has been found, to date, to be effective in reducing depressive symptoms in patients with schizoaffective disorder–depressed type only when added to a preexisting regimen of antipsychotics and antidepressants.

6. There are not enough or well-established data concerning the maintenance treatment of schizoaffective disorder–depressed type (especially with concomitant psychotic features). A logical practice, though not proven in well-controlled trials, is to continue with the same regimen that improved the acute depressive exacerbation. As in the maintenance treatment of other psychotic disorders, the long-term use of high-dose antipsychotic agents should be questioned. Therefore the present recommendation is to lower the antipsychotic doses to a lower effective dose (about a **chlorpromazine** equivalent of 300 mg/day or a **haloperidol** equivalent of 2–4 mg/day). These estimates were tested in maintenance treatment following schizophrenic exacerbations, and their validity for schizoaffective disorder should be challenged. In schizophrenic patients the above-mentioned doses were found to lengthen the time between exacerbations and to lower the risk of a relapse. Some data imply that recurrent depressive episodes (as part of schizoaffective disorder) might respond well to **lithium** or **carbamazepine** maintenance therapy.

15.3 Schizoaffective disorder – manic episode (1)

Treatment strategies (based on published data)

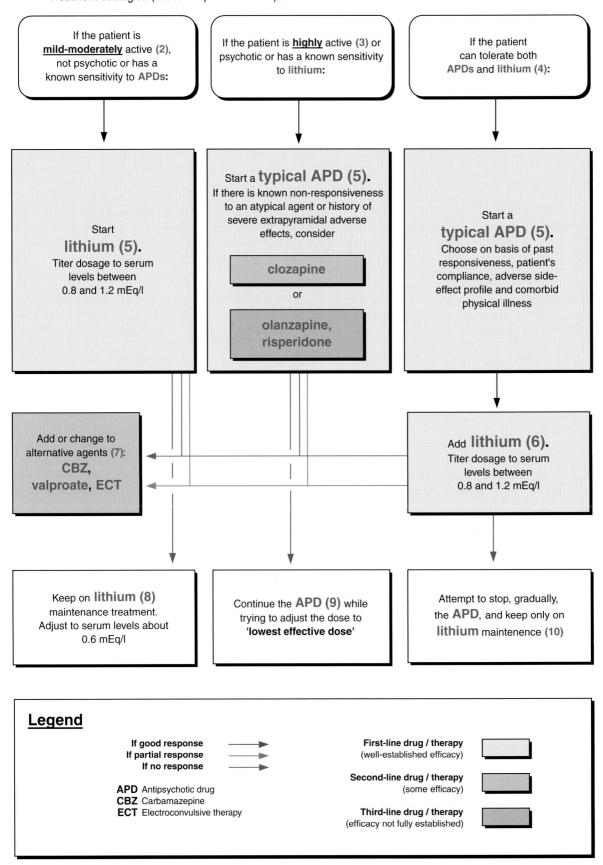

Notes about the numbered items in the scheme

Clinical Aspects

1a. The diagnosis of schizoaffective disorder is based on the present of a major depressive or manic episode along with DSM-IV criterion A for schizophrenia (at least once during the course of the disorder).

b. For the diagnosis, delusions or hallucinations must be present for a period of 2 weeks (or more) without a concomitant major depressive or manic episode.

c. There are 2 subtypes of schizoaffective disorder: manic type and depressed type. The manic type is characterized by criteria **1a** and **1b** with repeated mood episodes, at least one of which was a manic episode. The depressed type is characterized by the same criteria but all the mood episodes experienced by the patient were of the depressive type.

d. Schizoaffective – manic type has a high family history of bipolar disorder.

e. Schizoaffective – depressed type has a high family history of unipolar depressions and schizophrenia.

f. It is believed that schizoaffective disorder is a heterogenous cluster of disorders. Some patients probably have schizophrenia with prominent mood symptoms, others might have a mood disorder with prominent schizophrenic symptoms, while some have a distinct clinical syndrome.

h. The prevalence of schizoaffective disorder is between 0.5% and 0.8% of the general population. Women are at greater risk for developing the disorder.

Treatments

2. There is no significant correlation between the predominant symptomathology (psychotic versus affective) and the efficacy of different agents, especially antipsychotic drugs (**APDs**) or **lithium**. Most studies found a similar efficacy in treating an acute manic episode (as part of schizoaffective disorder) between **APDs** and **lithium**, and this is more significant when the patient is mild–moderately active.

3. In highly active patients **APDs** have a somewhat better efficacy than **lithium.**

4. A combined **APDs–lithium** regimen was found in several well-controlled studies to be more efficacious than each agent alone in the treatment of an acute manic episode of schizoaffective disorder.

5. The doses of **APDs** and **lithium** used for treating the manic episode of schizoaffective disorder are the same as for treating manic episode as part of bipolar I disorder or schizophrenia. **Clozapine** has been shown to be effective in ameliorating acute manic symptoms as part of bipolar I disorder (both treatment-resistant and as a first-option regimen). Its use should be restricted due to its hematological and other potentially serious adverse side-effects. The role of the other new-generation **antipsychotics** (**risperidone**, **olanzapine**, **sertindole**) has not yet been established in this disorder, but they should be considered as good candidates.

6. The combined **APD–lithium** regimen probably has superior efficacy in the treatment of the acute episode.

7. Carbamazepine, valproate and electroconvulsive therapy (**ECT**) have proven efficacy in the treatment of acute manic episode as part of bipolar I disorder. It is reasonable to assume similar efficacy in schizoaffective disorder–manic type, although large and controlled trials have not been done to date using the DSM-IV criteria for the disorder. The role of these agents as possible augmentors to **APDs** is not fully established in schizoaffective disorder. If used as augmentation, note that **carbamazepine** is contraindicated as adjuvant to **clozapine** due to their synergistic effects on bone marrow suppression.

8. Lithium was found to be an efficient modality for prophylactic treatment in schizoaffective disorder, especially when the following factors exist:

- Predominant mood symptoms.
- Serum levels above 0.6 mEq/l.
- Better efficacy (as prophylactic agent) in schizoaffective disorder – manic type as compared with depressed type.
- When a family history of mood disorder is evident.

9. If the patient cannot tolerate **lithium**, continue maintenance treatment with the **APD**. Doses should be gradually decreased, if possible, to a 'lower effective' dose (equivalent to **chlorpromazine** 300 mg/day or **haloperidol** 2–4 mg/day).

10. When the acute episode is controlled and the clinical state is stabilized, an attempt should be made to completely taper off the antipsychotic regimen and keep on **lithium** or **carbamazepine** maintenance treatment alone, because:

- **Lithium** alone is as efficient as antipsychotics in the prophylactic treatment of schizoaffective disorder. The role of **carbamazepine** as a prophylactic drug is not yet established, but there are accumulating data that it might prove to be quite efficacious.
- Long-term antipsychotic treatment should be avoided, if possible, due to possible serious adverse side-effects (for example, tardive dyskinesia).

15.4 Delusional disorder (1)

Treatment strategies (based on published data)

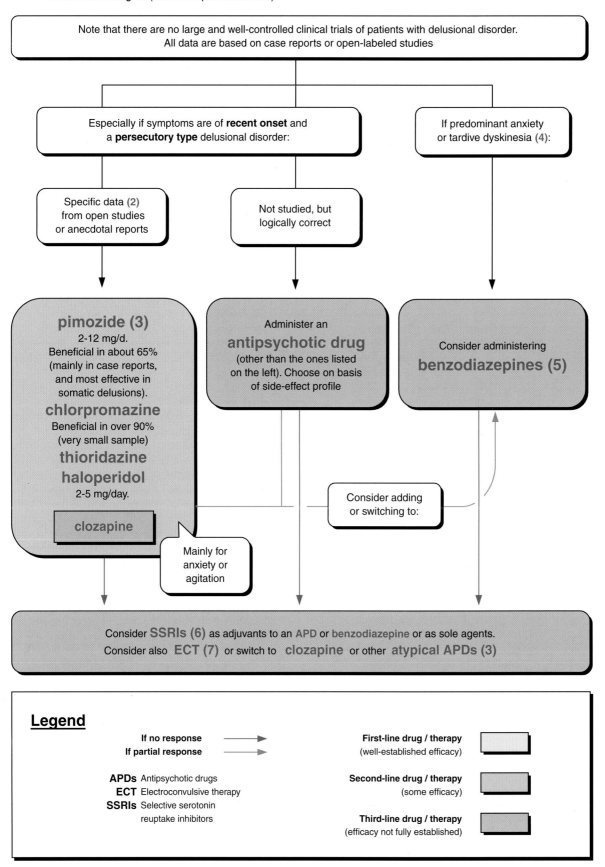

Note that there are no large and well-controlled clinical trials of patients with delusional disorder.
All data are based on case reports or open-labeled studies

Especially if symptoms are of **recent onset** and
a **persecutory type** delusional disorder:

If predominant anxiety
or tardive dyskinesia (4):

Specific data (2)
from open studies
or anecdotal reports

Not studied, but
logically correct

pimozide (3)
2-12 mg/d.
Beneficial in about 65%
(mainly in case reports,
and most effective in
somatic delusions).
chlorpromazine
Beneficial in over 90%
(very small sample)
thioridazine
haloperidol
2-5 mg/day.

clozapine

Administer an
antipsychotic drug
(other than the ones listed
on the left). Choose on basis
of side-effect profile

Consider administering
benzodiazepines (5)

Consider adding
or switching to:

Mainly for
anxiety or
agitation

Consider SSRIs (6) as adjuvants to an APD or benzodiazepine or as sole agents.
Consider also ECT (7) or switch to clozapine or other atypical APDs (3)

Legend

If no response

If partial response

APDs Antipsychotic drugs
ECT Electroconvulsive therapy
SSRIs Selective serotonin
reuptake inhibitors

First-line drug / therapy
(well-established efficacy)

Second-line drug / therapy
(some efficacy)

Third-line drug / therapy
(efficacy not fully established)

Notes about the numbered items in the scheme

Clinical Aspects

1a. Delusional disorder is believed to be a distinct entity, mainly due to specific genetics, course of illness and clinical features.

b. Core symptoms are persistent delusions, nonbizarre in their nature, along with the absence of prominent hallucinations, no thought disorder or mood disorder, or a significant flattening of the effect.

c. Most patients suffer from one main delusional theme.

d. There is a slight tendency for females to be affected by the disorder more than males.

e. Onset is usually between ages 40 and 49 years.

f. Prognosis is moderate, and data suggest that:
- About 50% of patients are employed.
- About 80% get married.
- Complete remmision and the elimination of the delusional themes are very rare.
- Recent onset symptoms and specific subtypes (mainly the persecutory type) may be more responsive to pharmacotherapy.

Treatment

2. All data are based on anecdotal reports or relatively small open-label studies. Pharmacotherapy should be administered for at least 8 weeks, and if no response is evident then consider stopping the antipsychotic medications (due to adverse side effects, either acute or chronic, which can further reduce the patients compliance). In such cases, **benzodiazepines (BDZs)**, especially if the patient is severely anxious, can have beneficial effects.

3. Pimozide exerts beneficial responses in up to 65% of patients, although data are based mainly on case reports. Some investigators believe that somatic delusions may be most responsive, and cases of erotomanic and jealous types were also reported to be responsive to **pimozide**. Other reports have shown the efficacy of antipsychotic drugs (**APDs**) such as **haloperidol**, **thioridazine** and **chlorpromazine** in reducing some of the symptoms, mainly the anxiety and agitation. All antipsychotics should be given in low doses (**haloperidol** equivalents of 2–5 mg/day usually), and if no response is observed within 6–8 weeks (with proper compliance) then the therapist should consider changing medications. **Clozapine** has been reported, anecdotally, to improve resistant delusional symptoms while the role of the other **atypical APDs** in delusional disorder is unclear as yet.

4. Since the delusional themes are relatively resistant to pharmacotherapy and patient's compliance is usually lacking, if the predominant clinical symptoms are agitation or anxiety, or if the patient is prone to experience acute adverse side-effects (dystonia, parkinsonism) or has a history of/ongoing tardive dykinesia, the best regimen might be **BDZs** for the relief of the acute symptoms and for a relative immediate response that could improve compliance.

5. Specific **BDZs** have not been studied, in well controlled studies. Their role should be the relief of acute anxiety and agitation, and to enhance compliance. The abuse potential of **BDZs** is usually not a major concern in these patients.

6. Selective serotonin reuptake inhibitors (**SSRIs**) are anecdotally reported to improve some of the symptoms associated with delusional disorder (especially affective parameters). The role of antidepressants has been suggested due to the incidence of affective disorders in families of delusional disorder patients. **SSRIs** or other antidepressants do not ameliorate the core psychotic themes.

7. The role of electroconvulsive therapy (**ECT**) in delusional disorder has not been studied. **ECT** has proven efficacy in psychotic disorders such as catatonia (as part of bipolar I disorder) or psychotic depression, and it is very efficacious in affective disorders (major depressive disorder, bipolar I). Since delusional disorder has psychotic and possibly affective components, **ECT** may be considered a good candidate in specific cases.

16.1 Panic disorder (1)

Treatment strategies (based on published data)

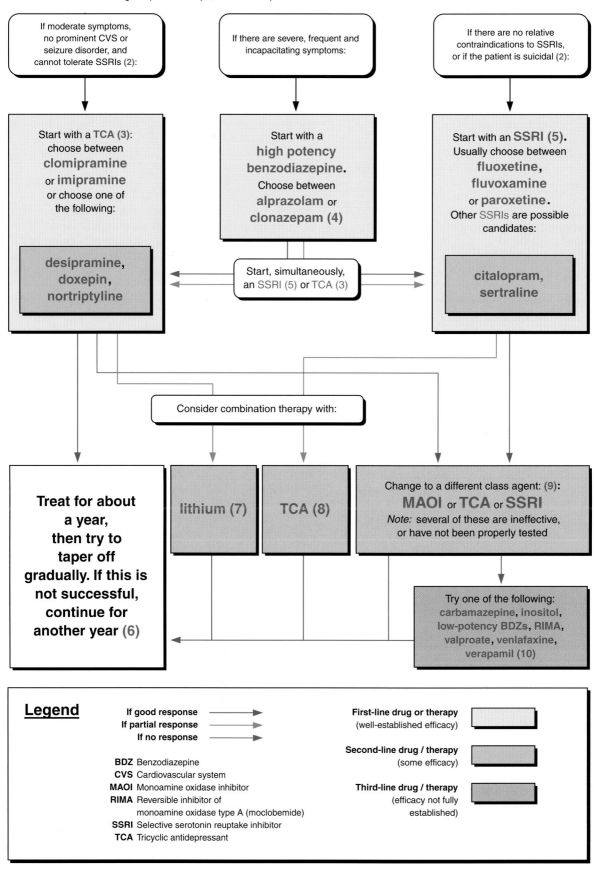

If moderate symptoms, no prominent CVS or seizure disorder, and cannot tolerate SSRIs (2):

If there are severe, frequent and incapacitating symptoms:

If there are no relative contraindications to SSRIs, or if the patient is suicidal (2):

Start with a TCA (3): choose between **clomipramine** or **imipramine** or choose one of the following:

desipramine, doxepin, nortriptyline

Start with a **high potency benzodiazepine.** Choose between **alprazolam** or **clonazepam (4)**

Start, simultaneously, an SSRI (5) or TCA (3)

Start with an **SSRI (5).** Usually choose between **fluoxetine, fluvoxamine** or **paroxetine.** Other SSRIs are possible candidates:

citalopram, sertraline

Consider combination therapy with:

Treat for about a year, then try to taper off gradually. If this is not successful, continue for another year (6)

lithium (7)

TCA (8)

Change to a different class agent: (9): **MAOI** or **TCA** or **SSRI** *Note:* several of these are ineffective, or have not been properly tested

Try one of the following: **carbamazepine, inositol, low-potency BDZs, RIMA, valproate, venlafaxine, verapamil (10)**

Legend

If good response	⟶
If partial response	⟶
If no response	⟶

BDZ Benzodiazepine
CVS Cardiovascular system
MAOI Monoamine oxidase inhibitor
RIMA Reversible inhibitor of monoamine oxidase type A (moclobemide)
SSRI Selective serotonin reuptake inhibitor
TCA Tricyclic antidepressant

First-line drug or therapy (well-established efficacy)

Second-line drug / therapy (some efficacy)

Third-line drug / therapy (efficacy not fully established)

Notes about the numbered items in the scheme

Clinical Aspects

1a. About 50% of panic attacks, part of panic disorder (PD), begin with attacks consisting of 3 or less symptoms out of the 13 possible symptom criteria eligible for the diagnosis of PD by the DSM-IV. Four out of 13 are required for the diagnosis of PD.
b. About 20% of all panic attacks appear without any sense of anxiety.
c. Lifetime prevalence of PD is about 1.5–3%. The women to men ratio is about 4:1.
d. Mean age of onset is about 23 years. Onset at ages older than 40 or younger than 15 is rare.
e. First-degree relatives of patients with PD have a 25% lifetime risk of developing the disorder.

Treatment

2. Relative contraindications for administering a selective serotonin reuptake inhibitor (**SSRI**) are severe gastrointestinal discomfort, specific sexual dysfunctions such as decreased libido or impotence, or a suspected sensitivity to these drugs. Moderate symptoms are diagnosed if only a few attacks are present and the patient can tolerate the disorder without a marked impairment in his/her daily functioning. **Clomipramine** and **imipramine** are tricyclic antidepressants (**TCAs**) which have significant anticholinergic capacity and can cause numerous adverse cardiac side-effects. Patients with known seizure disorder should not receive these agents due to their ability to reduce the seizure threshold. They can also provoke panic attacks early in therapy.

3. TCAs, high potency benzodiazepines (clonazepam, alprazolam) and most **monoamine oxidase inhibitors** (**MAOIs**) exert similar efficacy as antipanic agents (estimated to be around 70–80%). **Clomipramine** was traditionally believed to be the most efficacious antipanic agent. This has not been established in large, well-controlled studies. **Imipramine** is the most-studied medication in PD. There is no convincing evidence that it has superior efficacy over most other **TCAs**, except for a few agents that were found to be practically ineffective in treating PD (**trazodone, bupropion** and **maprotiline**). It is estimated that their possible impaired ability to downregulate the α_2-adrenergic receptors might play a role in their lack of antipanic properties. **Buspirone** has shown some efficacy in augmenting the antipanic effects of cognitive–behavioral therapy. **Desipramine, doxepin** and **nortriptyline** were all shown also to possess antipanic capabilities.

4. Use **benzodiazepines (BDZs)**, **alprazolam** and **clonazepam** with caution due to their abuse potential, dependence, possible cognitive impairments and rebound effects on abrupt stoppage. There is no tolerance to the antipanic effects of the **BDZs**. The use of **BDZs** is relevant when there is a contraindication to use **TCAs** or **SSRIs**, or when the disorder is incapacitating and a need for immediate anxiolytic relief is indicated.

5. SSRIs are most effective in panic disorder. Meta-analysis of most double-blind placebo-controlled trials of panic disorder patients suggested the superior efficacy of **SSRIs** (mainly reported with **fluoxetine, fluvoxamine,** and **paroxetine**) over other agents, including **TCAs** and **alprazolam**. **SSRIs** have a wider therapeutic window, they are usually better tolerated, and are considered, relative to the **TCAs** or **tetracyclic** agents, safer in overdose. Therefore **SSRIs** are recommended as the drug of choice in panic disorder or for suicidal patients who have access to the drugs and lack proper supervision. Other **SSRIs** (**sertraline** and **citalopram**) have not yet been studied in large and well-controlled trials of PD, but they are assumed to exert similar effects.

6. Panic disorder is a chronic disorder and about 50-70% of patients who stop their pharmacotherapy experience a renewed exacerbation of the disorder. For this reason it is recommended to continue the treatment for at least a year, following with a tapering-off attempt.

7,8. Lithium and **TCAs** could, in some cases, improve the antipanic response of certain individuals already receiving a **TCAs** or a **SSRI**.

9. MAOIs, especially **phenelzine**, might have superior efficacy over **TCAs** (tested versus **imipramine**) in more severe and chronic patients, and in patients unresponsive to **imipramine**. It seems evident that patients receiving **MAOIs** are less prone to develop the 'overstimulation' phenomena that is apparently more associated with **TCAs**. The role of **moclobemide**, a reversible inhibitor of **monoamine oxidase type A (RIMA)**, has not been established, to date, in panic disorder.

10. Anecdotal reports have shown that **anticonvulsants (carbamazepine, valproate)** have some antipanic properties. **Venlafaxine** can be beneficial, but the data are based on small open-label trials. Preliminary data with **inositol**, a potential antidepressant agent, have shown beneficial results in reducing the frequency and severity of panic attacks in PD patients, without inducing any major adverse side-effects. A **Low-potency BDZ** (**diazepam**) was found in a few cases and in predisposed patients to have antipanic properties when given in very high doses.

16.2 Simple phobia
Treatment strategies (based on published data)

16.3 Social phobia
Treatment strategies (based on published data)

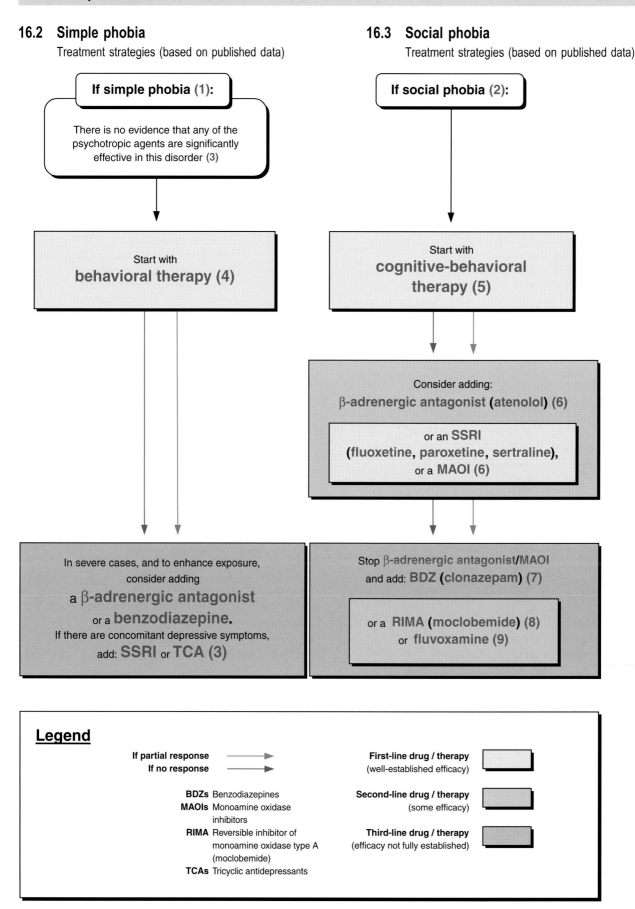

If simple phobia (1):

There is no evidence that any of the psychotropic agents are significantly effective in this disorder (3)

Start with
behavioral therapy (4)

In severe cases, and to enhance exposure, consider adding
a **β-adrenergic antagonist**
or a **benzodiazepine.**
If there are concomitant depressive symptoms, add: **SSRI** or **TCA** (3)

If social phobia (2):

Start with
cognitive-behavioral therapy (5)

Consider adding:
β-adrenergic antagonist **(atenolol)** (6)

or an **SSRI**
(fluoxetine, paroxetine, sertraline),
or a **MAOI (6)**

Stop β-adrenergic antagonist/MAOI
and add: BDZ **(clonazepam)** (7)

or a **RIMA (moclobemide)** (8)
or **fluvoxamine (9)**

Legend

If partial response ⟶

If no response ⟶

BDZs Benzodiazepines
MAOIs Monoamine oxidase inhibitors
RIMA Reversible inhibitor of monoamine oxidase type A (moclobemide)
TCAs Tricyclic antidepressants

First-line drug / therapy
(well-established efficacy)

Second-line drug / therapy
(some efficacy)

Third-line drug / therapy
(efficacy not fully established)

Notes about the numbered items in the scheme

Clinical Aspects

Simple phobia

1. The rule of thumb for diagnosing simple phobia is when the patient's fear is of circumscribed stimulus, object or situation. One needs to exclude, mostly, the following:

- panic disorder (a fear of having another panic attack);
- social phobia (a fear of social humiliation or embarrassment);
- hypochondriasis (fear of having a serious illness);
- Obsessive–compulsive disorder (feared avoidance of an object or a situation due to obsessions).

Social phobia

2. The major aspect is the patients fear of getting into a social situation in which he or she could feel humiliated or embarrassed when acting in front of others.

Treatment

Simple phobic treatment

3. A few regimens have been studied, without any definite success, in the treatment of simple phobia:

Benzodiazepines (mostly **diazepam**) reduce the fear-induced avoidance, but have no effect on anxiety or autonomic symptoms. The use of these agents in simple phobia is usually aimed at helping patients to engage in exposure program.

No significant efficacy was evident in the few studies with **imipramine**, other tricyclic antidepressants (**TCAs**) or selective serotonin reuptake inhibitors (**SSRIs**) and simple phobia (in ameliorating phobic themes). Depressive symptoms associated with simple phobia have been shown to benefit from these medications.

β**-adrenergic antagonists** were not found efficacious in augmenting behavioral treatments. In some cases, a symptomatic relief was observed, but was not sustained.

4. The main goal is to provide a fear-reduction behavioral therapy, usually via systematic desensitization and controlled exposure. Cognitive and behavioral coping skills might be integrated in the sessions.

Social phobia treatment

5. The major aspect of cognitive–behavioral therapy is the integration of cognitive and exposure components. Exposure is efficient, mainly, on short-term behavioral changes, while the cognitive approach aids more in long-term maintenance effects and prevention of relapse. Social-skill training could be very beneficial in people who lack those skills, and much of the person's discomfort is due to this deficiency. Relaxation training is usually effective in people whose predominant symptoms are autonomic arousal. Exposure therapy as a sole modality of treatment is probably less effective, since it aids mainly in the short-term relief of symptoms.

6. β**-adrenergic antagonists** (best studied with **atenolol**) and **monoamine oxidase inhibitors** (**MAOIs**) were found to be effective in the treatment of social phobias. β**-adrenergic antagonists** seem to reduce the autonomic symptoms (and so are viewed as agents for treatment of 'specific social phobia'). **MAOIs** affect both the autonomic arousal related to social phobia and the cognitive dysfunction associated with the disorder. **MAOIs** (especially **phenelzine**) are considered to be better agents, compared with β**-adrenergic antagonists**, when compared on large populations. The role of **selective serotonin reuptake inhibitors** (**SSRIs**) in social phobia is quite established. **SSRIs** seem to be as effective as **MAOIs** or cognitive–behavioral therapy and the efficacy of **fluoxetine, paroxetine** and **sertraline** was demonstrated in several well controlled studies. Information about most other **SSRIs** is still lacking.

7. One controlled study showed good efficacy of **clonazepam** in improving anxiety, avoidance and social phobic symptoms. Other anecdotal reports about different **benzodiazepines** are contradictory.

8. Recent studies have demonstrated the efficacy of the **reversible inhibitor of monoamine oxidase type A, moclobemide**, in social phobia. It was found to be as effective as several of the **SSRIs**, while producing fewer adverse side-effects.

9. Fluvoxamine demonstrated some efficacy in social phobia, but to date it seems to be beneficial in fewer cases than the other **SSRIs**.

16.4 Generalized anxiety disorder (GAD) (1)
Treatment strategies (based on published data)

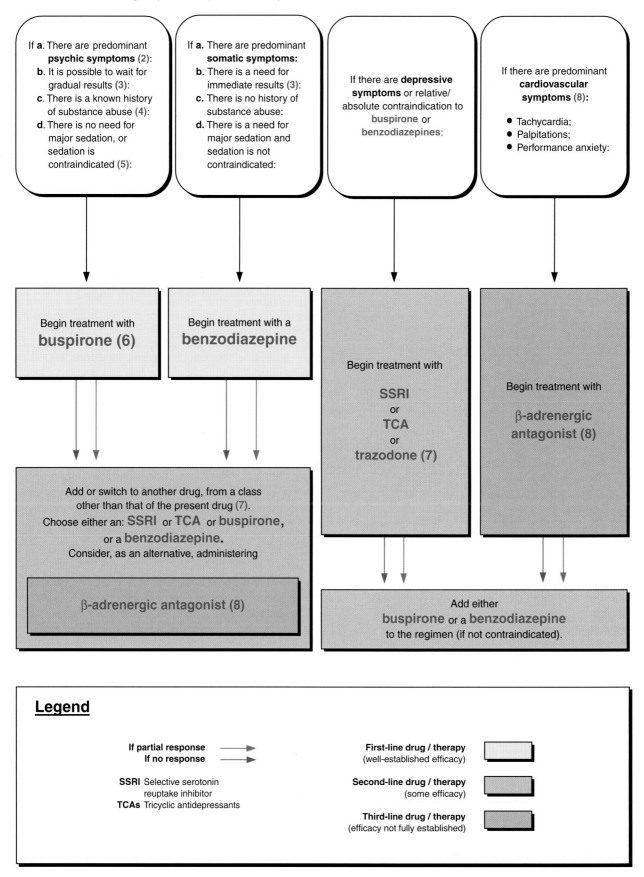

If **a**. There are predominant **psychic symptoms (2)**:
b. It is possible to wait for gradual results (3):
c. There is a known history of substance abuse (4):
d. There is no need for major sedation, or sedation is contraindicated (5):

If **a**. There are predominant **somatic symptoms:**
b. There is a need for immediate results (3):
c. There is no history of substance abuse:
d. There is a need for major sedation and sedation is not contraindicated:

If there are **depressive symptoms** or relative/absolute contraindication to **buspirone** or **benzodiazepines**:

If there are predominant **cardiovascular symptoms (8)**:
- Tachycardia;
- Palpitations;
- Performance anxiety:

Begin treatment with **buspirone (6)**

Begin treatment with a **benzodiazepine**

Begin treatment with **SSRI** or **TCA** or **trazodone (7)**

Begin treatment with **β-adrenergic antagonist (8)**

Add or switch to another drug, from a class other than that of the present drug (7).
Choose either an: **SSRI** or **TCA** or **buspirone**, or a **benzodiazepine**.
Consider, as an alternative, administering

β-adrenergic antagonist (8)

Add either **buspirone** or a **benzodiazepine** to the regimen (if not contraindicated).

Legend

If partial response →
If no response →

SSRI Selective serotonin reuptake inhibitor
TCAs Tricyclic antidepressants

First-line drug / therapy (well-established efficacy)

Second-line drug / therapy (some efficacy)

Third-line drug / therapy (efficacy not fully established)

Notes about the numbered items in the scheme

Clinical Aspects

1. In DSM-IV, the diagnosis is based on several elements:

a. The experienced anxiety is not a manifestation of another major psychiatric disorder (mainly psychotic/mood disorders or posttraumatic stress disorder).

b. Patients suffer from at least 3 out of 6 symptoms of motor tension: restlessness; being easily fatigued; impaired concentration; irritability; muscle tension and impaired sleep.

c. The anxiety has a duration of at least 6 months, and is not focused on one subject only.

d. The diagnosis and the differential diagnosis are based on the quantity of the anxiety. The anxiety in generalized anxiety disorder (GAD) is not of:

- having a panic attack (panic disorder with anticipatory anxiety);
- being embarrassed in public (social phobia);
- being contaminated (obsessive compulsive disorder);
- having multiple physical symptoms / complaints (somatization disorder);
- gaining weight (anorexia nervosa);
- having serious illness (hypochondriasis).

Treatment

2. Buspirone has better efficacy, compared with **benzodiazepines** (**BDZs**), in reducing psychic anxiety, while **BDZs** (studied mostly with **diazepam**) are better in eliminating somatic anxiety.

3. The acute effects of **buspirone** tend to build up gradually in 2–4 weeks. **BDZs** exhibit their effects more rapidly. Do not confuse this rapid effect of **BDZs**, which is targeted at diminishing somatic anxiety, from **buspirone's** quicker and better efficacy in ameliorating psychic anxiety.

4. To date, **buspirone** (unlike **BDZs**) has not been shown to possess significant adverse effects such as abuse potential, tolerance, withdrawal symptoms, rebound anxiety, sedation, significant psychomotor impairments or increasing the effects of other central nervous system depressants.

5. Buspirone is particularly attractive in individuals who cannot tolerate the sedative effects of **BDZs** (pilots, cab and truck drivers, students) or in patients on central nervous system depressants, or in those with a history of drug or alcohol abuse.

6. Buspirone is superior to placebo in improving both anxiety and depressive symptoms associated with GAD. It was also found to be as effective as several **benzodiazepines** (studied mostly with **lorazepam**) in reducing anxiety symptoms (while producing fewer side-effects).

7. Accumulating data suggest that **tricyclic antidepressants** (**TCAs**) and some of the **atypical antidepressants** are also beneficial in GAD, although probably less so than **buspirone** or **benzodiazepines**. It is well established that **TCAs** can reduce anxiety in several disorders (panic disorder, anxiety symptoms as part of a major mood disorder, anxiety related to posttraumatic stress disorder). **Imipramine**, **clomipramine** and **trazodone** have shown some capacity to reduce anxiety related to GAD. The **selective serotonin reuptake inhibitors** (**SSRIs**) have not been studied in well-controlled studies in GAD, though anecdotal and preliminary reports suggest that they might have beneficial effects.

8. β-**adrenergic antagonists** are effective in reducing nonspecific anxiety that is predominantly manifested by cardiovascular complaints: palpitations, tachycardia, tremor and other peripheral manifestations of anxiety. They also possibly have a beneficial effect in reducing performance anxiety. The β-**adrenergic antagonists** do not exert beneficial results in GAD patients as a group.

16.5 Obsessive–compulsive disorder (1)
Treatment strategies (based on published data)

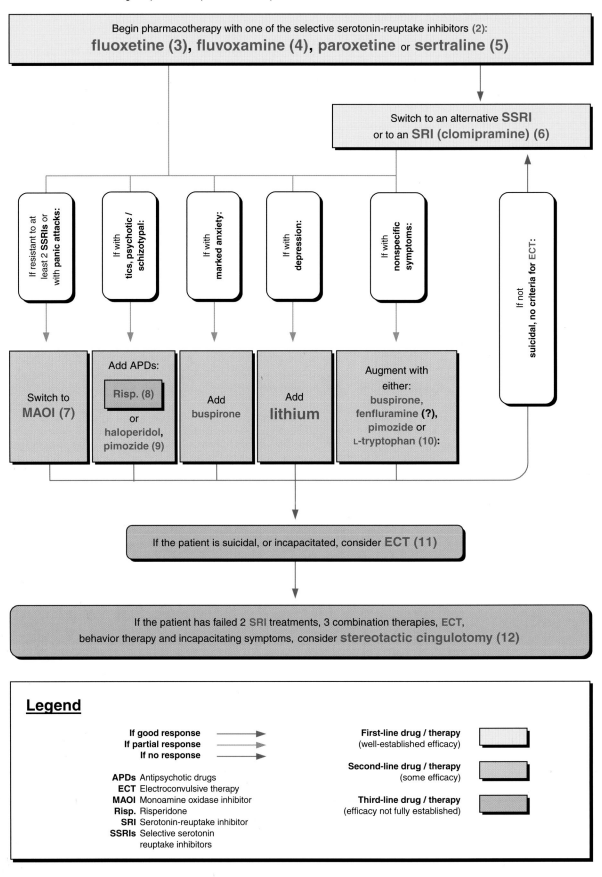

Begin pharmacotherapy with one of the selective serotonin-reuptake inhibitors (2):
fluoxetine (3), fluvoxamine (4), paroxetine or **sertraline (5)**

Switch to an alternative **SSRI**
or to an **SRI (clomipramine) (6)**

If resistant to at least 2 **SSRIs** or with **panic attacks:**

If with **tics, psychotic / schizotypal:**

If with **marked anxiety:**

If with **depression:**

If with **nonspecific symptoms:**

If not suicidal, no criteria for ECT:

Switch to **MAOI (7)**

Add APDs:
Risp. (8)
or
haloperidol, pimozide (9)

Add buspirone

Add **lithium**

Augment with either:
buspirone, fenfluramine **(?)**, pimozide or L-**tryptophan (10):**

If the patient is suicidal, or incapacitated, consider **ECT (11)**

If the patient has failed 2 **SRI** treatments, 3 combination therapies, **ECT**, behavior therapy and incapacitating symptoms, consider **stereotactic cingulotomy (12)**

Legend

If good response
If partial response
If no response

First-line drug / therapy
(well-established efficacy)

Second-line drug / therapy
(some efficacy)

Third-line drug / therapy
(efficacy not fully established)

APDs Antipsychotic drugs
ECT Electroconvulsive therapy
MAOI Monoamine oxidase inhibitor
Risp. Risperidone
SRI Serotonin-reuptake inhibitor
SSRIs Selective serotonin reuptake inhibitors

Notes about the numbered items in the scheme

Clinical Aspects

1. Obsessive–compulsive disorder (OCD) is the 4th most common psychiatric disorder. The mean age of onset is 20 years. About 70% have their onset before the age of 25 years, while only 15% have their onset after the age of 35.

The etiology of the disorder is not known. It is hypothesized that dysregulation of the serotonergic system plays a major role in the pathogenesis of the disorder. This theory is based on the efficacy of serotonin reuptake inhibitors, on 5-HIAA abnormalities found in CSF analysis of some OCD patients, and the reduction in 5-HT transporter in platelets of OCD patients (inconsistent).

About 35% of first-degree relatives of OCD patients are also afflicted by the disorder.

Between 5% and 7% of OCD patients also meet the criteria for Tourette's disorder (TD). About 50–70% of TD patients meet the criteria for OCD.

The most frequent personality disorders associated with OCD are avoidant, dependent and histrionic (more than 40% of all cases). Only 5% of OCD had an obsessive–compulsive personality disorder/traits prior to the onset of the disorder.

About 50–70% of OCD patients suffer, sometime throughout their disorder, from concomitant major depressive disorder.

Treatment

2. Meta-analysis of all the well controlled studies over the last 20 years suggested that only selective serotonin reuptake inhibitors (**SSRIs**) such as **fluoxetine, fluvoxamine, sertraline,** or **paroxetine** and the tricyclic antidepressants with marked serotonin reuptake inhibition (**SRI**) properties (**clomipramine**) have shown any efficacy in eliminating OCD symptoms. Direct comparison, in well controlled studies, did not show any significant differences between **clomipramine** and **fluoxetine** or **fluvoxamine**.

When a patient is given an anti-OCD regimen, one should expect the following:

a. There is usually only a partial reduction in the quality and/or quantity of the obsessions or compulsions (usually about 30–50% decrease in various parameters).

b. The response to treatment is usually evident in 4–12 weeks. For that reason responsiveness should be properly monitored and evaluated only following at least 12 weeks of treatment.

c. The improvement in OCD parameters is independent of mood changes.

3. Fluoxetine is considered equal in its efficacy for OCD to **clomipramine**, and it is usually better tolerated due to its much more favorable side-effect profile.

4. Fluvoxamine was shown to have superior efficacy over placebo in OCD. Some reports have claimed superior efficacy over tricyclic antidepressants (**TCAs**) that have no significant **SRI** properties.

5. Paroxetine and **sertraline** were shown to exhibit anti-OCD properties in well-controlled studies, and their efficacy is believed to be similar to that of the other **SSRIs**.

6. Clomipramine is the most-studied agent and it is probably more efficient than **imipramine, amitriptyline** or **desipramine. Clomipramine** is recommended at a maximal dose of about 250–300 mg/day. **Nortriptyline** and **buspirone** might have some efficacy for the treatment of OCD.

7. Phenelzine and **tranylcypromine** (to a lesser extent) are considered effective in OCD, and **phenelzine** might be as efficacious as **clomipramine**.

8. Risperidone was reported in a small open-label trial to be effective as an adjuvant to **fluvoxamine** in resistant OCD patients. The role of other atypical antipsychotics is yet to be ascertained.

9. The addition of **antipsychotics** can help in some cases, especially in patients with coexisting chronic tic disorders, schizotypal personality disorder or psychosis. The addition of low-dose **haloperidol** or **pimozide** to an **SSRI** can be beneficial in up to 65% of cases with comorbid tic disorder.

10. Some data suggest beneficial effects with the coadministration of **fluvoxamine** and either **buspirone** or **pimozide** with **fenfluramine** or **haloperidol**. The use of **fenfluramine** is controversial, and is not usually recommended due to its potential serious cardiac adverse effects. There are some reports on the beneficial effects of augmenting anti-OCD agents (especially **clomipramine**) with L-**tryptophan** (a precursor of serotonin), or **fenfluramine** (a serotonin releaser), or **buspirone** (a serotonergic transmission modulator) or **pimozide** (a adopaminergic antagonist).

11. Electroconvulsive therapy (ECT) is effective in only 20% of nonresponders to pharmacotherapy, and most of these patients had concomitant depressive symptoms.

12. The long-term prognosis is relatively poor, with only 35% of patients achieving full or substantial remission. Current data suggest that **cingulotomy** does not significantly alter cognitive or motor functioning and may help 50% of drug resistant patients. It is well accepted that some patients respond better to pharmacotherapy following surgery.

16.6 Posttraumatic stress disorder (PTSD) (1)

Treatment strategies (based on published data)

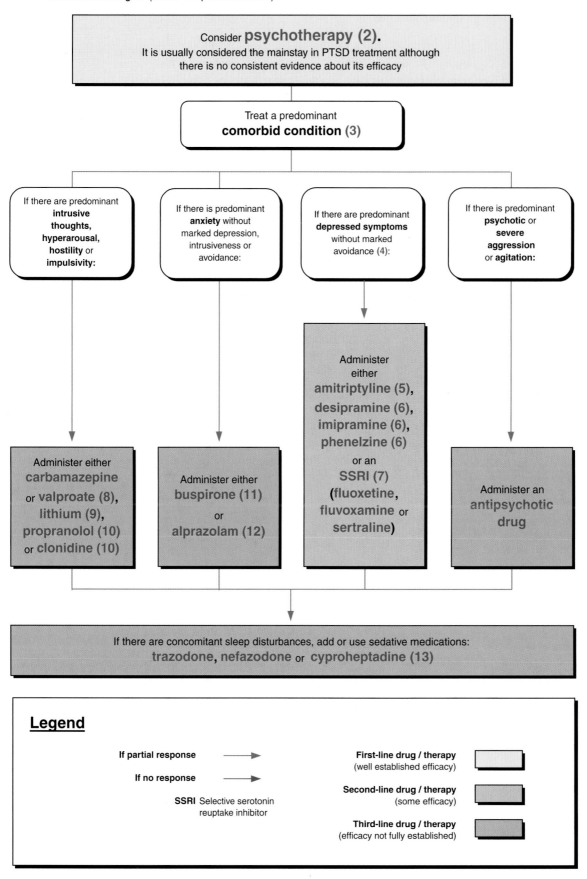

Consider **psychotherapy (2).**
It is usually considered the mainstay in PTSD treatment although there is no consistent evidence about its efficacy

Treat a predominant **comorbid condition (3)**

If there are predominant **intrusive thoughts, hyperarousal, hostility** or **impulsivity:**

If there is predominant **anxiety** without marked depression, intrusiveness or avoidance:

If there are predominant **depressed symptoms** without marked avoidance (4):

If there is predominant **psychotic** or **severe aggression** or **agitation:**

Administer either **carbamazepine** or **valproate (8),** **lithium (9),** **propranolol (10)** or **clonidine (10)**

Administer either **buspirone (11)** or **alprazolam (12)**

Administer either **amitriptyline (5),** **desipramine (6),** **imipramine (6),** **phenelzine (6)** or an **SSRI (7)** (**fluoxetine,** **fluvoxamine** or **sertraline)**

Administer an **antipsychotic drug**

If there are concomitant sleep disturbances, add or use sedative medications: **trazodone, nefazodone** or **cyproheptadine (13)**

Legend

If partial response ⟶

If no response ⟶

SSRI Selective serotonin reuptake inhibitor

First-line drug / therapy (well established efficacy)

Second-line drug / therapy (some efficacy)

Third-line drug / therapy (efficacy not fully established)

Notes about the numbered items in the scheme

Clinical Aspects

1. The diagnosis of the disorder is based on several main findings:

a. Exposure to a significant stressor that is a threat to the physical integrity of self or others.

b. The trauma is reexperienced by means of recurrent dreams, perceptions, thoughts, illusions, hallucinations, dissociative flashbacks, and an intense physiological response when exposed to either internal or external stimuli.

c. Persistent avoidance of stimuli that remind the patient of the trauma.

d. Persistent symptoms of increased arousal: insomnia, irritability, impaired concentration, alertness, exaggerated startle response.

The disorder may develop months or even years following the trauma. The prognosis is variable: 30% recover almost completely, 40% continue to suffer from mild symptoms and reduced daily functioning. About 20% exhibit moderate symptoms and up to 10% suffer from chronic, disabling condition. Lifetime prevalence is about 1% (1.3% for women and 0.5% for men). The prevalence increases in populations exposed to long-term and severe trauma. More than 50% of cases of posttraumatic stress disorder (PTSD) due to combat trauma do not remmit in 3 years. Most other cases of PTSD tend to remit in 6–8 months.

Treatment

2,3. Psychotherapy is aimed at helping the patient to absorb and understand the trauma, and it is the most effective modality for the treatment of PTSD symptoms (**2**). Psychotropic agents are given only to help in the symptomatic relief of certain comorbid conditions, especially when other major psychiatric disorders (from axis I) exist (**3**). These drugs lack the capacity to greatly reduce PTSD symptoms such as avoidance, isolation and emotional numbness.

4. The avoidance is considered unresponsive to pharmacotherapy and much more responsive to psychotherapy.

5. Amitriptyline, in doses of up to 300 mg/day, was found to reduce PTSD symptoms in about 40% of patients. The drug reduces mainly the depressive symptoms, but it also has a significant effect on anxiety, intrusiveness and, to a much lesser extent, avoidance.

6. Desipramine, imipramine and **phenelzine** are more effective than placebo in antidepressant activity (related to PTSD symptoms), but have a lesser capacity to reduce intrusiveness, arousal and avoidance than **amitriptyline**.

7. A few controlled studies are available concerning the efficacy of selective serotonin reuptake inhibitors (**SSRIs**) in PTSD. It is assumed that **SSRIs** have a beneficial potential via similar mechanisms by which tricyclic antidepressants (**TCAs**) induce their beneficial effect. **Fluoxetine** was shown to exert beneficial effects on arousal and numbing, particularly in patients without chronic treatment histories. **Fluvoxamine** was found to be beneficial for intrusive thoughts, avoidance, and arousal as part of combat-related PTSD. An open trial suggests the efficacy of **sertraline** in PTSD. Not enough data are currently available concerning the efficacy of **clomipramine** in PTSD.

8. Preliminary studies suggested the beneficial effect of **carbamazepine** in improving intrusion, hostility and impulsivity in up to 70% of PTSD patients, and a few anecdotal reports found **valproate** to be effective in reducing impulsive and arousal related to PTSD.

9. Lithium has some potential for improving intrusion and arousal in PTSD patients.

10. Some data support an hyperadrenergic state as a major associated factor with PTSD. **Propranolol** and **clonidine** reduce the total adrenergic tone, and a few reports describe the beneficial effects of these agents in reducing the autonomic hyperstimulation observed in PTSD patients.

11. Buspirone may help in PTSD, mainly by reducing the associated anxiety. **Buspirone** is known to be an effective augmentor in obsessive–compulsive disorder (OCD), and since OCD and PTSD share some overlap features, it is possible that **buspirone** exerts its effects in PTSD by similar mechanisms to its activity in OCD.

12. Alprazolam is effective in the treatment of non-specific anxiety and is not specific for symptoms associated with PTSD. It should be administered with caution, since it has a significant dependence potential.

13. The use of sedative antidepressants with anxiolytic features is mostly recommended for patients with predominant sleep disturbances. Drugs such as **trazodone** and **nefazodone** are anecdotally reported to be efficient for such indications. **Cyproheptadine** is a 5-HT$_2$ serotonergic and H$_1$ histaminergic antagonist with prominent sedative effects, and its beneficial effects in reducing sleep disturbances in PTSD has also been reported.

17.1 Paranoid personality disorder (1)

Treatment strategies (based on published data)

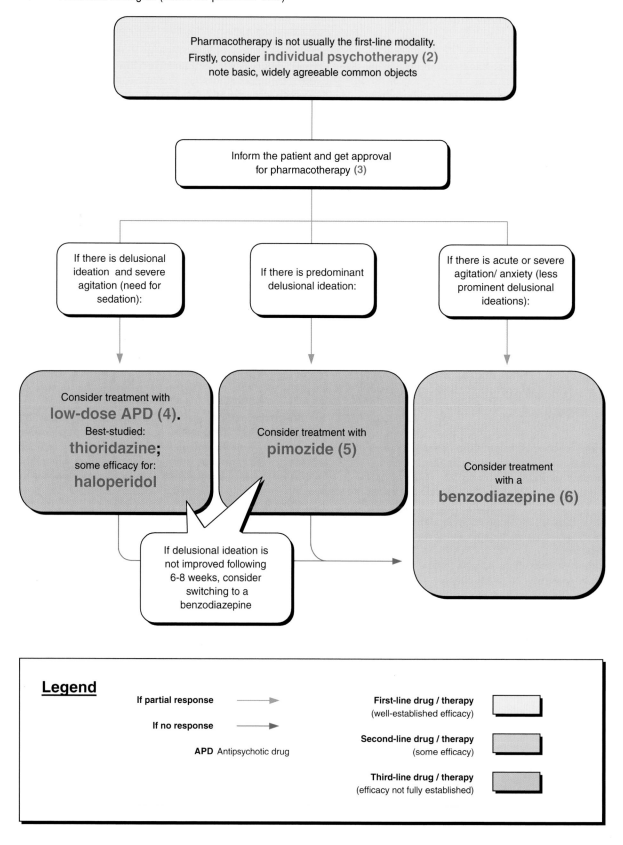

Pharmacotherapy is not usually the first-line modality.
Firstly, consider **individual psychotherapy (2)**
note basic, widely agreeable common objects

Inform the patient and get approval
for pharmacotherapy (3)

If there is delusional
ideation and severe
agitation (need for
sedation):

If there is predominant
delusional ideation:

If there is acute or severe
agitation/ anxiety (less
prominent delusional
ideations):

Consider treatment with
low-dose APD (4).
Best-studied:
thioridazine;
some efficacy for:
haloperidol

Consider treatment with
pimozide (5)

Consider treatment
with a
benzodiazepine (6)

If delusional ideation is
not improved following
6-8 weeks, consider
switching to a
benzodiazepine

Legend

If partial response ⟶

If no response ⟶

APD Antipsychotic drug

First-line drug / therapy
(well-established efficacy)

Second-line drug / therapy
(some efficacy)

Third-line drug / therapy
(efficacy not fully established)

Notes about the numbered items in the scheme

Clinical Aspects

1a. Paranoid personality disorder (PPD) is diagnosed, mainly, when there is a lifelong suspiciousness, hypersensitivity to criticism and a tendency to ascribe malicious intents to the action of others.

b. The patients tend to question without reasonable justification, and to see hidden meanings in others intentions.

c. The prevalence of PPD is estimated to be between 1% and 3% of the general population.

d. Several risk factors (men, elderly, impaired hearing, and being a prisoner) are associated with developing the disorder, although none of them have been found to date, to be statistically significant.

e. PPD tends to run in families. A family history of schizophrenia is not a characteristic feature in PPD patients.

f. About 75% of PPD patients meet the criteria for another psychiatric disorder.

Treatment

2. Psychotherapy is the main effective modality for the treatment of PPD. The therapy is quite difficult due to the patient's basic mistrust and frequent denial of having any mental disorder. The most basic approach to psychotherapy should include the following:

- Trust should be experienecd and learned.
- The therapist should introduce the patient to cognitive and behavioral techniques that will encourage the patient and make it easier for him or her to interact with the surroundings.
- Some of the paranoid ideations could be tested by the patient with the proper supervision and assurance of the therapist.

3. The patients, as a result of their basic mistrust and denial of illness, are usually noncompliant. It is advisable to build up a trusting relation and to try improve compliance. This might be done if medications are offered as a way to cope with such symptoms as anxiety and insomnia and as a tool that gives the patient a better coping mechanism with the 'hostile' surroundings. The need to inform the patient and get approval for the treatment is essential due to the possible side-effects related to antipsychotic drug (**APD**) treatment: mainly parkinsonism, anticholinergic effects and tardive dyskinesia.

4. Antipsychotic agents might have a beneficial effect in PPD, but to date there are very few established data about their actual efficacy. Some uncontrolled studies showed the efficacy of **APDs** such as **haloperidol** and **thioridazine** in improving delusional ideation, especially in agitated patients suffering from PPD. The doses used are usually low (less than 5 mg/day of **haloperidol** or the equivalent). Even though there are no conclusive data about other **APDs**, it is a reasonable assumption that they would exhibit similar effects. No apparent clinical guidelines are available concerning PPD treatment. Most clinicians do not administer **APDs** at doses of more than 10 mg/day equivalent of **haloperidol**. The **APDs** are usually given for brief periods only, and they are aimed at relieving some of the acute symptoms and not the chronic personality characteristics.

5. Pimozide was shown in several studies to have significant beneficial effects in improving paranoid ideation in PPD patients. More trials need to be done since these data are based on a few cases and small uncontrolled studies.

6. Benzodiazepines could be beneficial in the treatment of acute anxiety states related to PPD. PPD patients tend much less than cluster B personality disorder patients (borderline, narcissistic, histrionic and antisocial personality disorders) to abuse **benzodiazepines**, and their prompt effects can aid in building a trusting relation with the therapist. The use of **benzodiazepines** is especially prompted in cases of an acute stress-related anxiety, in which event the patient's compliance is usually improved. There is no evidence about the superior efficacy of a specific **benzodiazepine** in such circumstances.

17.2 Schizoid personality disorder (1)

Treatment strategies (based on published data)

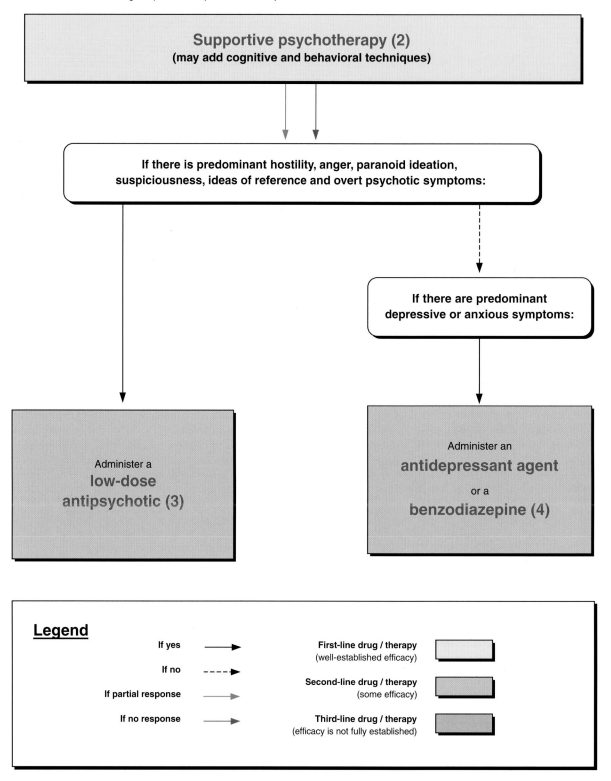

Notes about the numbered items in the scheme

Clinical Aspects

1. Schizoid personality disorder (SPD) is characterized, mainly, by indifference to social and familial relationships and a restricted range of emotions. DSM-IV specifies 7 criteria, of which at least 4 should be present in order to make the diagnosis of SPD. The criteria are as follows:

a. The individual neither desires nor enjoys close relationships, including being a part of a family.

b. SPD people almost always engage in solitary activities.

c. SPD people take pleasure in few, if any, activities.

d. There is diminished desire to have sexual experience with a partner.

e. There is indifference to praise or criticism by others.

f. The person has no close friends.

g. Constricted affect.

The prevalence of the disorder is not known, but is estimated to be between 1% and 16%, and males are probably more prone to be affected. The etiology of the disorder is unclear, and current data suggest the influence of both genetic and psychological factors in the evolvement of the disorder. Patients with SPD are at no greater risk of developing schizophrenia, but if they do get a diagnosis of schizophrenia at a later stage, their prognosis is poorer. This is consistent with some of the other axis I disorders, which have worse prognosis if there is a concomitant comorbidity with other personality disorders.

Treatment

2. There are very few controlled studies on the treatment of SPD. Current data prompts the use of **supportive psychotherapy** as the main treatment modality in SPD. The aim of the psychotherapy is to enable the patient to tolerate shifts in life circumstances, and to engage in some social behaviors, using the relationship between the patient and the therapist as the role model for relationships outside the therapy. The therapist might make use of some cognitive and behavioral techniques in order to reduce isolation and to strengthen social behaviors.

The use of classical psychoanalysis is virtually contraindicated, since the patient with SPD cannot, usually tolerate the intensity of such a treatment. The prognosis of SPD is relatively poor, and the observed symptoms are not usually responsive to therapy. However, when the patient, through psychotherapy, becomes involved in more social activities, the surrounding people respond better to the patient, and the overall effect could be beneficial both for the patient and society.

3. The use of pharmacotherapy in SPD is limited to the relief of acute symptoms. These are usually the symptoms that prompt the patient to receive medical assistance, and often include depressive or anxious states. In such a case the patient often agrees to become involved in psychotherapy. Symptoms such as agitation, hostility, anger, assaultiveness, suspiciousness or overt psychotic symptoms do not usually bring the patient to ask for medical help, and in those cases the patient is usually persuaded by family members to engage in the therapy. In such a case it is quite difficult for the patient to relate favorably to psychotherapy. Some data suggest the efficacy of **low-dose antipsychotics** in relieving symptoms such as hostility, suspiciousness, anger and psychotic-like features associated with SPD. In some of these cases, the use of **antipsychotics** leads to an improvement in social functioning and willingness to tolerate psychotherapy. There are no specific agents that proved to be more efficacious in this disorder, and at this stage, it is up to the clinician's personal judgment and experience to choose an antipsychotic agent.

4. There are no large and well-controlled studies of **antidepressants** or **anxiolytic** pharmacotherapy in SPD. A trial of **antidepressants** or **benzodiazepines** might be warranted for SPD patients with concomitant depressive or anxious symptoms. Current data suggest the use of these agents for symptom relief and for a relatively short duration, and the use of psychotherapy as the main modality for improving overall social and personal functioning.

17.3 Schizotypal personality disorder (1)

Treatment strategies (based on published data)

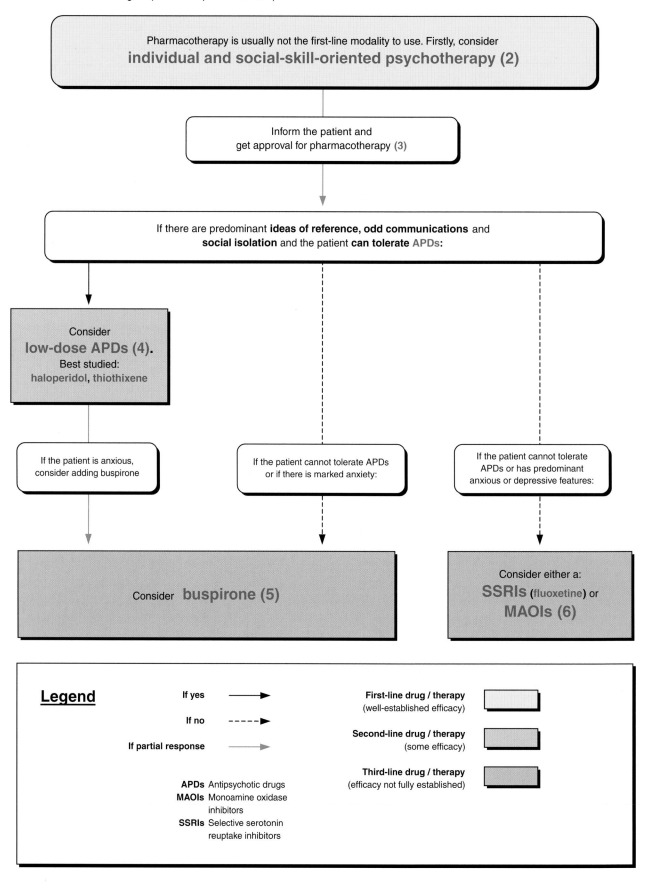

Pharmacotherapy is usually not the first-line modality to use. Firstly, consider
individual and social-skill-oriented psychotherapy (2)

Inform the patient and
get approval for pharmacotherapy (3)

If there are predominant **ideas of reference, odd communications** and
social isolation and the patient **can tolerate APDs:**

Consider
low-dose APDs (4).
Best studied:
haloperidol, thiothixene

If the patient is anxious,
consider adding buspirone

If the patient cannot tolerate APDs
or if there is marked anxiety:

If the patient cannot tolerate
APDs or has predominant
anxious or depressive features:

Consider **buspirone (5)**

Consider either a:
SSRIs (fluoxetine) or
MAOIs (6)

Legend

If yes	⟶
If no	----➤
If partial response	⟶

First-line drug / therapy
(well-established efficacy)

Second-line drug / therapy
(some efficacy)

Third-line drug / therapy
(efficacy not fully established)

APDs Antipsychotic drugs
MAOIs Monoamine oxidase inhibitors
SSRIs Selective serotonin reuptake inhibitors

Notes about the numbered items in the scheme

Clinical Aspects

1a. The diagnosis of schizotypal personality disorder (PD) is based mainly on pervasive deficits in interpersonal relatedness and peculiarities of ideas, appearance and behaviors.

b. There is an increased prevalence of schizotypal PD in relatives of schizophrenic patients. The prevalence of the disorder in the general population in not known.

c. Up to 25% of the people diagnosed as having schizotypal PD eventually (following a couple of years) get the diagnosis of schizophrenia.

d. There are some similarities between the abnormal physiological parameters that are found in schizotypal PD and those found in schizophrenia. The main ones are eye movement dysfunctions and a decreased serum amine oxidase levels.

e. The main characteristics of schizotypal PD are represented by the following diagnostic criteria, at least 5 of which must be present in order to make the diagnosis (by DSM-IV):

- Ideas of reference (delusions of reference are not included).
- Odd beliefs or magical thinking that are not consistent with cultural norms.
- Unusual perceptual experiences (bodily illusions are included).
- Odd thinking or speech (vague, metaphoric, stereotyped, circumstantial).
- Paranoid ideation or suspiciousness.
- Inappropriate or constricted affect.
- Odd, eccentric or peculiar behaviors or appearance.
- Lack of close interpersonal relations except with first-degree relatives.
- Excessive social anxiety, related mostly to paranoid themes.

Treatment

2. Schizotypal PD patients do not usually seek psychiatric help. When they finally do so, this is mostly when suffering from an acute crisis, so their main target is to get some symptom relief and not to engage in therapy aimed at changing their chronic psychopathology. Therefore the most relevant and beneficial measure is to provide the patient an **individual and skill oriented psychotherapy**. Supportive measures with an emphasis on the reduction of social isolation and concomitant behavioral techniques aimed at acquiring better adaptive behaviors might be added.

3. The patients, as a result of their basic mistrust and denial of illness, are usually noncompliant. It is advisable to build up a trusting relation and to try to improve compliance. This might be done if medications are offered as a way of coping with such symptoms as anxiety and insomnia, and as a tool that gives the patient a better coping mechanism with the 'hostile' surroundings. The need to inform the patient and get approval for the treatment is essential due to the possible side-effects related to antipsychotic drug (**APD**) treatment: mainly parkinsonism, anticholinergic effects and tardive dyskinesia.

4. Many studies have shown the efficacy of **APDs** in reducing some of the basic features of schizotypal PD. **APDs** were given in relatively low doses (best studied with **haloperidol** at doses of between 2 and 12 mg/day). and the symptoms that had some response to therapy were the following:

- ideas of reference;
- odd communication patterns;
- social isolation.

It should be noted that the total gain of schizotypal PD patients from pharmacotherapy is modest, and inconsistant at best.

5. Anecdotal data suggest the efficacy of **buspirone** in reducing both anxiety and 'soft' psychotic symptoms associated with schizotypal PD. The clinical significance of these effects in the treatment of schizotypal PD is unclear, and well-controlled studies should be made in order to further establish the efficacy of **buspirone**.

6. There are a few open-label studies and anecdotal reports that demonstrated the beneficial effects of **high-dose fluoxetine** or monoamine oxidase inhibitors (mostly reported with **phenelzine**) in reducing anxiety or depressive features associated with schizotypal PD, along with some of the core features of the disorder itself.

17.4 Borderline personality disorder (1)

Treatment strategies (based on published data)

Pharmacotherapy is usually not the first-line modality to use.
Consider **long-term individual psychotherapy (2)**.
Note basic, widely agreeable common objects

Consider pharmacotherapy.
A. Avoid **benzodiazepines (3)**.
B. Note that **tricyclic antidepressants** were found in many cases to have similar efficacy, compared with placebo, in borderline personality disorder patients with depressive symptoms (not major depressive disorder), and are capable, in some cases, of exacerbating symptoms such as irritability, impulsivity and aggressiveness

---

If there is atypical depression (4), a depressed or labile mood, or an impaired self-image:

If there is predominant behavioral dyscontrol:

If there is a predominant combination of impulsivity, assaultiveness and mild psychotic symptoms:

Consider either
MAOIs, RIMAs (5)
or
SSRIs
(fluoxetine) (6)

Consider either
carbamazepine (7)
or

lithium
or
valproate (8)

Consider
low-dose APDs (9).
Best-studied are
flupenthixol,
haloperidol,
thiothixene,
or consider either

clozapine (10),
risperidone, olanzapine

Legend

If partial response   ⟶

APDs   Antipsychotic drugs
MAOIs Monoamine oxidase
       inhibitors
RIMAs Reversibile inhibitors of
       monoamine oxidase type A
SSRIs Selective serotonin reuptake
       inhibitors

First-line drug / therapy
(well-established efficacy)

Second-line drug / therapy
(some efficacy)

Third-line drug / therapy
(efficacy not fully established)

Notes about the numbered items in the scheme

Clinical Aspects

1a. Borderline personality disorder (BPD) belongs to cluster B – the 'dramatic cluster' – which consists of narcissistic, borderline, histrionic and antisocial personality disorders. There is no pharmacotherapy of choice for any of the personality disorders associated with this cluster. Most of the treatments to be discussed were found effective in the short-term outcome only, and are based on small, open-label studies.

b. The disorder is characterized by stormy interpersonal relations, unstable affect and behavioral dyscontrol. The prevalence of BPD is about 2% of the general population and up to 20% of psychiatric inpatients.

c. Comorbidity with other axis I or II disorders is frequent:
- 25–75% suffer, sometimes during the disorder, from major depressive disorders.
- 5–20% suffer from coexisting bipolar mood disorder.
- There are many overlaps with other cluster B personality disorders.
- About 50–70% meet the criteria for one or more of the substance abuse disorders.

d. The prognosis is mostly invariable: many of the patients exhibit persistent morbidity, impaired occupational achievements, unstable interpersonal life and multiple hospitalizations. About 65% of BPD patients tend to improve somewhat with age in parameters such as working performance and interpersonal relations.

e. Some biological abnormalities are assumed to be related to BPD characteristic symptoms:
- Serotonergic dysregulation is often correlated with impulsivity, suicidality and aggression.
- An abnormal dexamethasone suppression test (DST) is seen in up to 60% of BPDs.
- An increased frequency, compared with controls, of non specific EEG abnormalities (especially slow-wave activities and spike phenomena).

Treatment

2. Some basic sommon objects are accepted as part of individual psychotherapy in BPD:
- Create a stable framework and address any deviations from it.
- Confront and direct patient's behaviors during sessions to minimize transference distortions.
- The therapist must tolerate negative transference without retaliation/withdrawing.
- Make the patient aware that he/she communicates affect via behaviors.
- Set limits to behaviors that endanger the therapeutic process.
- Focus on clarifications and interpretations of transference in the here and now basis. Developmental reconstructions, especially early in the therapy are not likely to yield beneficial results.

3. Benzodiazepines are beneficial in reducing anxiety in many psychiatric disorders. The use of **benzodiazepines**, especially **alprazolam**, should be avoided as much as possible in BPD patients due to their abuse potential. A couple of major studies even found **alprazolam** to worsen the clinical status of BPD patients by aggravating suicidality, behavioral dyscontrol and assaultiveness.

4. Atypical depression is characterizaed mainly by hypersomnia, hyperphagia, anxiety and absence of autonomic symptoms. This form of depressive state is often less severe than major depressive disorder and, in few cases at least, resembles the depressive states experienced by BPD patients.

5. A few, uncontrolled studies and case reports demonstrated the efficacy of monoamine oxidase inhibitors (**MAOIs**) in reducing the impulsivity, chronic emptiness, loneliness and mood lability of BPD patients. **Phenelzine** was found to be better, in these aspects, compared with **tricyclic antidepressants** such as **amitriptyline**. **Tranylcypromine** was also reported to be beneficial in improving depression, anxiety, rage, impulsivity, rejection sensitivity and suicidality in BPD patients. The reversible inhibitors of monoamine oxidase type A (**RIMAs**) (e.g. **moclobemide**) might also be efficacious, although well controlled studies have not, as yet, been published.

6. Some BPD patients have responded well to the selective serotonin reuptake inhibitors (**SSRIs**; mostly studied with **fluoxetine**) in parameters such as depressed mood, aggressiveness and impulsivity. The role of **SSRIs** is promising due to their enhanced stimulation of the serotonergic system (serotonergic dysregulation is often correlated with impulsivity, suicidality and aggression). There are practically no significant studies concerning the efficacy of other **SSRIs** in BPD.

7. Small uncontrolled studies, some anecdotal reports and small double-blind placebo-controlled studies found **carbamazepine** to be effective in improving dyscontrolled behaviors of nonpsychotic BPD patients. In these studies, at least some beneficial results were reported in up to 90% of patients. The main behavioral dyscontrol symptoms that responded to **carbamazepine** were impulsivity and aggressiveness.

8. There are no reports about the efficacy of other mood stabilizers (**lithium** or **valproate**) for this entity.

9. Low-dose antipsychotic agents, especially **flupenthixol**, **haloperidol** and **thiothixene**, were found to be effective in improving specific symptom combination (minor psychotic symptoms, somatic complaints, impulsivity and depressive symptoms). The minor psychotic features that can respond relatively well to these agents are impulsivity, ideas of reference, odd thinking/communications, social withdrawal and suspiciousness.

10. Clozapine has been shown to reduce total brief psychiatric rating scale (BPRS) scores in BPD paients in a small open-label trial. Its use in BPD should be carefully weighed due to its potential hazardous adverse effects and the lack of confirmed substantial efficacy. The other atypical antpsychotic drugs have not yet been studied in BPD.

17.5 Histrionic personality disorder (1)
Treatment strategies (based on published data)

Psychoanalytically oriented psychotherapy (2):
Aimed at bringing the patients to become consciously aware of their unrealistic gratification of dependency needs.

If there is predominant attention-seeking behavior, rejection sensitivity, constant need for approval from others to maintain self-esteem and mood, and the patient is predisposed to atypical depressive episodes following frustration:

If there are acute depressive or anxious symptoms:

Consider adminstering a
monoamine oxidase inhibitor (3)

Consider administering
antidepressants
or
benzodiazepines (4)

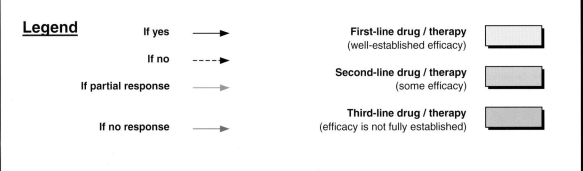

Legend

If yes	⟶
If no	----▶
If partial response	⟶
If no response	⟶

First-line drug / therapy
(well-established efficacy)

Second-line drug / therapy
(some efficacy)

Third-line drug / therapy
(efficacy is not fully established)

Notes about the numbered items in the scheme

Clinical Aspects

1. Histrionic PD (personality disorder) is characterized mainly by colorful and dramatic appearance, self-centeredness, seductiveness, and labile emotional expressions. DSM-IV specifies 8 criteria, at least 5 of which should be present in order to make the diagnosis of histrionic PD. The criteria are as follows:

   a. The person feels uncomfortable if not at the center of attention.

   b. The person is sexually seductive and/or provocative.

   c. The person displays labile and shallow expressions of emotions.

   d. The person uses physical appearance to draw attention to self.

   e. There is an impressive and detail-lacking style of speaking.

   f. There is self-dramatization, theatricality and exaggerated expression of emotions.

   g. The person is easily influenced by others.

   h. The person conceives relationships to be more intimate than they are.

The prevalence of the disorder is between 2% and 6%, and women are more prone to be affected. The etiology of the disorder is unknown, and there are no data regarding the genetic or neurobiological basis of the disorder. Many histrionic PD patients also meet the criteria for other personality disorders, especially from clusters B and C (antisocial, borderline, narcissistic, avoidant and dependent).

Treatment

2. There are very few controlled studies on the treatment of histrionic PD. The present data prompts the use of **psychoanalytically oriented psychotherapy** as the main treatment modality in histrionic PD. The aim of psychotherapy is to bring the patient to consciously be aware of his/her needs for constant gratification through interpretations of transference. Some believe that the right approach should focus on a balanced fulfillment and withholding of gratification as the correct route to achieve the best results in this disorder (to diminish the risk of severe acting-outs with a possible termination of the therapy).

3. Studies on the use of pharmacotherapy in histrionic PD are limited, and currently the only relevant data are the beneficial results achieved with monoamine oxidase inhibitors (**MAOIs**) for the treatment of hysteroid dysphoria. Hysteroid dysphoria is characterized by recurrent depressive episodes triggered by interpersonal rejections, which are often romantic in nature. The person is often seductive, self-centered and very demanding, and makes a great effort to draw attention to themselves. The depressed episodes resemble DSM-IV's entity of major depressive disorder with atypical features, and is characterized by hyperphagia, hypersomnia and mood reactivity. Alcohol abuse is associated with these patients.

4. For depressive or anxious symptoms, a trial with (respectively) **antidepressants** or **benzodiazepines** might be warranted, although there are no large or well controlled studies about their efficacy in histrionic PD. Current data suggest the use of these agents for symptom relief and for a relatively short duration, and to use psychotherapy as the main modality for improving the overall social and personal functioning.

17.6 Avoidant personality disorder (1)
Treatment strategies (based on published data)

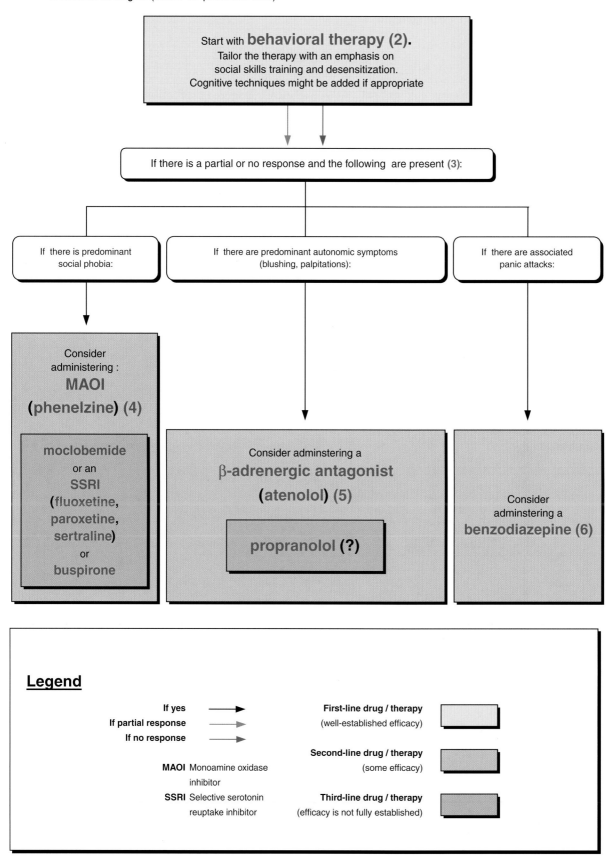

Start with behavioral therapy (2).
Tailor the therapy with an emphasis on
social skills training and desensitization.
Cognitive techniques might be added if appropriate

If there is a partial or no response and the following are present (3):

If there is predominant
social phobia:

If there are predominant autonomic symptoms
(blushing, palpitations):

If there are associated
panic attacks:

Consider
administering :
MAOI
(phenelzine) (4)

moclobemide
or an
SSRI
(fluoxetine,
paroxetine,
sertraline)
or
buspirone

Consider adminstering a
β-adrenergic antagonist
(atenolol) (5)

propranolol (?)

Consider
adminstering a
benzodiazepine (6)

Legend

If yes   ⟶

If partial response   ⟶

If no response   ⟶

MAOI Monoamine oxidase
inhibitor

SSRI Selective serotonin
reuptake inhibitor

First-line drug / therapy
(well-established efficacy)

Second-line drug / therapy
(some efficacy)

Third-line drug / therapy
(efficacy is not fully established)

Notes about the numbered items in the scheme

Clinical Aspects

1. The core features of avoidant personality disorder (avoidant PD) are the avoidance of activities that require interpersonal contacts, and an exaggerated hypersensitivity to rejections by others. DSM-IV specifies 7 main criteria, at least 4 of which should be present in order to make the diagnosis of avoidant PD. The main aspects pointed out by the DSM-IV criteria are as follows:

    a. There is avoidance of occupational activities that involve significant contacts with other people. This is due to fear from rejection, disapproval or criticism.

    b. There is an unwillingness to get involved with other people unless there is a certainty of being liked.

    c. Intimate relationships are characterized by numerous restraints due to the fear of being conceived of as ridiculous.

    d. There is a preoccupation with being rejected or criticized in social situations.

    e. The person is inhibited in new interpersonal situations because of feeling inadequate.

    f. The person views self as socially unfitted, unappealing, and inferior to others.

    g. The person is usually reluctant to engage in new activities due to the fear of being embarrassed in front of others.

The prevalence of avoidant PD is not known but is estimated to be between 1% and 10%. Avoidant PD is often associated with axis I disorders such as social phobia, and, to a lesser extent, obsessive–compulsive disorder (OCD). Patients with avoidant PD often exhibit trait symptoms from other cluster C disorders, namely dependent and obsessive-compulsive. The genetic component of avoidant PD is unclear. The environmental influence might be, in certain instances, a key etiological factor, especially when early childhood traumas such as incest, parental cruelty or sexual abuse are evident. The prognosis is variable, and many avoidant PD patients are able to function properly, provided they are in an appropriate familial and environmental setting.

Treatment

2. Behavioral therapy is the most commonly practiced modality in avoidant PD. It is aimed at encouraging the patient to get involved in tasks that are perceived, firstly, as potentially humiliating or embarrassing. The therapy should be specifically tailored for the patient, while focusing on social skill training, desensitization and cognitive techniques.

3. Avoidant PD is frequently associated with social phobia, autonomic symptoms such as palpitations, tachycardia, sweating and panic attacks. When these symptoms are incapacitating, and cause a significant or an acute distress, a trial of certain pharmacological agents might be warranted.

4. Monoamine oxidase inhibitors (**MAOIs**) have a proven efficacy in ameliorating both the autonomic arousal related to avoidant PD and also the cognitive dysfunction associated with the disorder. **Phenelzine** is the best-studied, but other **MAOIs**, as well as the reversible inhibitors of monoamine oxidase type A (**RIMA**) such as **moclobemide**, might prove to be beneficial. Some data suggest the efficacy of certain selective serotonin reuptake inhibitors (**SSRIs**, especially **fluoxetine**, **paroxetine** and **sertraline**), in ameliorating predominant phobic symptoms associated with avoidant PD. One study even demonstrated the efficacy of **SSRIs** in reducing the core cognitive misinterpretation of reality.

5. Atenolol, a relative selective β_1-adrenergic antagonist has an established efficacy in reducing the autonomic arousal associated with avoidant PD that is manifested by symptoms such as blushing, palpitations or increased heart rate. Other β-antagonists, such as **propranolol** might also prove to be beneficial, although systematic studies of these agents in avoidant PD are lacking.

6. Brief episodes of panic attacks are relatively common in avoidant PD, and **benzodiazepines** often exert beneficial results in reducing the frequency and intensity of these attacks. The role of tricyclic antidepressants (**TCAs**) in avoidant PD has not been studied systematically, and currently there are no reports of **TCAs'** efficacy in ameliorating panic or anxious states related to avoidant PD.

17.7 Obsessive–compulsive personality disorder (1)

Treatment strategies (based on published data)

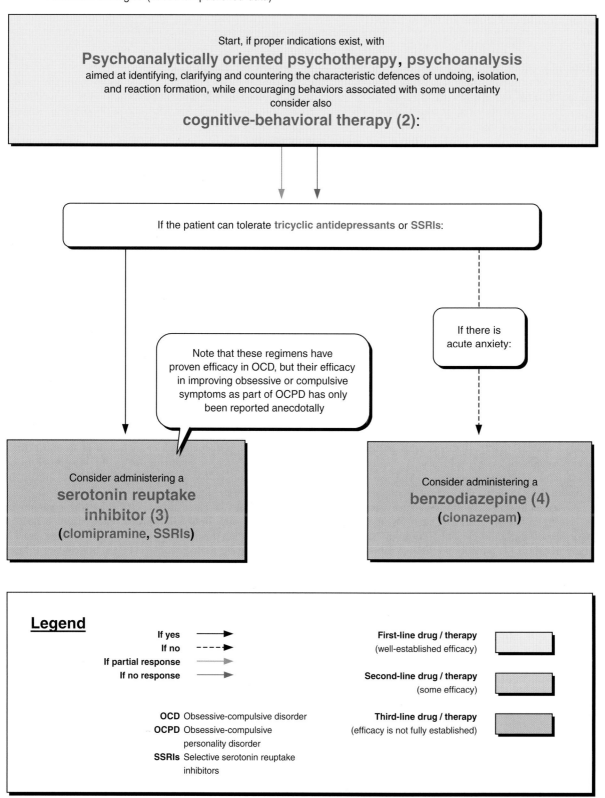

Notes about the numbered items in the scheme:

Clinical Aspects

1. Obsessive–compulsive personality disorder (OCPD) is characterized by multiple impairments in main aspects of psychiatric functioning: behavior, thought and mood. The behavioral component includes compulsive preoccupation with details, rules, orderliness, indecisiveness and overemphasis on work. The cognitive component is usually associated with moral rigidity, intrusive worries and overconsciousness. The abnormal mood related to OCPD is the inability of the patient to adequately express emotions. DSM-IV specifies 8 criteria, at least 4 of which should be present in order to make the diagnosis of OCPD:

> **a.** The person is preoccupied with details, lists and rules to the extent that the main point of the activity is not achieved.
>
> **b.** This is perfectionism that interferes with task formation and efficiency.
>
> **c.** There is overworking accompanied by withdrawing from leisure activities and friendships.
>
> **d.** There is moral rigidity.
>
> **e.** The person retains worn-out objects (even if they do not have sentimental value), and is unable to get rid of them.
>
> **f.** The person is unwilling to work with others unless they comply exactly to his/her way of doing things.
>
> **g.** The person adopts a close-fisted spending style with money.
>
> **h.** There is obstinacy.

The prevalence of OCPD is estimated to be between 1% and 2%, and males are affected 1.5–2 times more than females. There is a possible genetic component to the disorder, as reflected by the increased occurrence of OCPD in first-degree relatives of people with the disorder and the higher concordance rate for OCPD found in monozygotic twins compared with dizygotic twins. Some of the psychoanalytic schools refer to OCPD and OCD (obsessive–compulsive disorder) as a continuum of entities. However, current data, based on very few controlled studies, do not support this assumption. People with OCD might have a number of underlying personality disorders, including OCPD, but the latter is not considered as a risk factor for developing OCD. Only 4–6% of OCD patients have the diagnosis of OCPD. In fact, avoidant, dependent and histrionic personality disorders are the most frequently associated with OCD. The prognosis of OCPD is variable and unpredictable (significant statistical data are lacking).

Treatment

2. People with OCPD often seek psychiatric treatment because of their intact reality testing, the awareness of their pleasureless behaviors and interactions, and the emergence of social or occupational problems that they conceive as necessitating acute interventions. Such psychotherapies are indicated if the patient exhibits intact reality testing, and relatively good and mature ego functions. **Cognitive psychotherapy** has also been used with favorable results. The therapist should establish priorities as to which of the patient's problems should be dealt with first, focusing on the patient's emotions and feelings, encouraging behaviors associated with an uncertain outcome, and advocating changes in daily life circumstances.

3. There are no well-controlled studies about the efficacy of **clomipramine** (a non-selective serotonin reuptake inhibitor) or selective serotonin reuptake inhibitors (**SSRIs**) in OCPD. The efficacy of these agents in obsessive–compulsive disorder (OCD) is well established, and they have also been shown to exert beneficial results by ameliorating obsessive or compulsive behaviors associated with schizophrenia. These agents were also reported, anecdotally, to reduce obsessional thinking or compulsive behavior in various other psychiatric disorders (e.g. in impulse-control disorders such as kleptomania and trichotillomania) although rarely in OCPD. Therefore a trial with **SSRIs** (e.g. **fluoxetine, fluvoxamine**) or **clomipramine** is warranted, especially if the patient's symptoms become acutely worse and incapacitating.

4. Anecdotal data suggest the efficacy of **benzodiazepines** in reducing obsessive and compulsive symptoms besides their anxiolytic effects. The use of such **benzodiazepines** (reported with **clonazepam**) is especially recommended if the patient suffers from overwhelming anxiety related to a specific stressogenic event.

18.1 Anorexia nervosa (1)
Treatment strategies (based on published data)

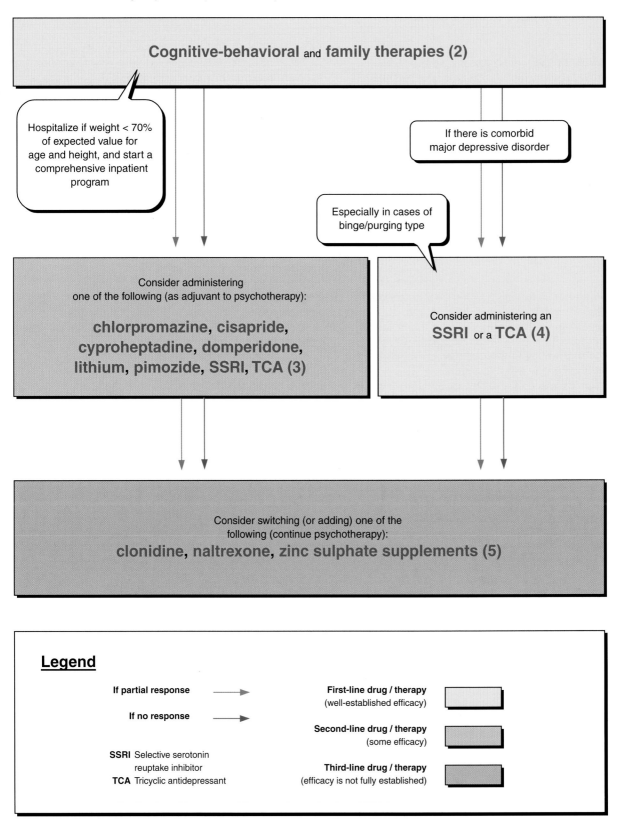

Cognitive-behavioral and family therapies (2)

Hospitalize if weight < 70% of expected value for age and height, and start a comprehensive inpatient program

If there is comorbid major depressive disorder

Especially in cases of binge/purging type

Consider administering
one of the following (as adjuvant to psychotherapy):

chlorpromazine, cisapride, cyproheptadine, domperidone, lithium, pimozide, SSRI, TCA (3)

Consider administering an
SSRI or a TCA (4)

Consider switching (or adding) one of the
following (continue psychotherapy):
clonidine, naltrexone, zinc sulphate supplements (5)

Legend

If partial response ⟶

If no response ⟶

SSRI Selective serotonin reuptake inhibitor
TCA Tricyclic antidepressant

First-line drug / therapy
(well-established efficacy)

Second-line drug / therapy
(some efficacy)

Third-line drug / therapy
(efficacy is not fully established)

Notes about the numbered items in the scheme

Clinical Aspects

1. Anorexia nervosa (AN) is characterized by a disturbance in body image, accompanied by an intense fear of becoming fat, affecting, primarily, young females. The prevalence is 0.5–1% of girls aged 12–18 years. The prognosis is variable: some exhibit spontaneous recovery, some respond favorably to psychotherapy and/or pharmacotherapy, but a relatively major subgroup exhibits a chronic deteriorating course that often leads to starvation and death. Mortality rates are estimated to be about 5–20%. Anorectic patients often take compensatory measures to loose weight (self-induced vomiting, laxative or diuretic abuse, engaging in excessive exercising). Many patients often have symptoms of bulimia nervosa (BN), especially binge eating. DSM-IV points out two types of AN: restricting and binge eating/purging type (see Table 18.1), and it specifies 4 main criteria needed for the diagnosis. The main aspects (DSM-IV criteria) are as follows:

a. Significant weight loss (body weight <85% of that expected for height and age).

b. Intense fear of gaining weight.

c. Distorted body image (impaired perception of one's body weight or shape) plus denial of the potential hazardous consequences of AN.

d. Amenorrhea.

Treatment

2. Cognitive–behavioral psychotherapy is considered the most effective treatment of AN, although large and well-controlled studies are lacking. **Family therapy** is often indicated to support, to reduce anxiety, and to evaluate specific familial interactions that might promote the disorder. If the patient's weight is reduced to under 70% of the expected weight, an inpatient program is required. A target weight and the rate of weight gain are set. If these are not met, nasogastric feeding can be used to save life. Anorectic patients are denied the use of the bathroom for 1–2 hours following their meals to decrease self-induced vomiting. Daily weighing, and recording of food intake and urine output, while administering a preprogrammed diet (about 500 calories over that required for age and height) is used.

3. Pharmacotherapy of AN has limited value. Some beneficial effects – usually demonstrated via small open-labeled studies or case reports – are seen with **chlorpromazine** and **pimozide** (antipsychotics that induce weight gain), **lithium**, **cyroheptadine** (an antihistaminergic and antiserotonergic agent that suppresses the inhibitory effects of the serotonergic transmission on appetite), **cisapride** or **domperidone** (gastric prokinetic agents that reverse the delayed gastric emptying observed in AN) and selective serotonin reuptake inhibitors (**SSRIs**) or **tricyclic antidepressants** (especially the binge/purging type), and where there is comorbid depression.

4. These agents have been proven to be effective in BN and thus might be beneficial in the treatment of AN (especially the binge/purging type).

5. Early reports of beneficial results with **clonidine**, **naltrexone**, or **zinc sulphate** supplements have not yet been confirmed in well-controlled studies.

Table 18.1 Parameters characteristic of the two types of AN

	Binge/purging type	Restricting type
Obsessive–compulsive features	☐	■
Comorbidity with other personality disorders	■	☐
Decreased sexual interest	■	■
Depressive symptoms and fear of obesity	■	■
Patient or familial history	■	☐
Impaired impulse control	■	☐
Social isolation	■	■
Substance abuse	■	☐
Suicidality	■	☐

■ seen more often; ☐ seen less often.

18.2 Bulimia nervosa (1)
Treatment strategies (based on published data)

Cognitive-behavioral therapy (2)
A focus on some or all of the following is required:
education, self-monitoring, trigger-response control, and addressing irrational beliefs, including body image

Regardless of past or
current depressive disorders

Consider adding to psychotherapy one of the following:
MAOI, SSRI (high dose fluoxetine), **TCAs** or **TeCAs (3)**.
Best-studied: **amitriptyline, desipramine, fluoxetine, imipramine,
isocarboxazide, phenelzine, trazodone**

Discontinue former pharmacological agent and consider adding to
the psychotherapeutic process one of the
anticonvulsants (4).
Some efficacy with
carbamazepine, phenytoin
Less-established efficacy with

valproate

Discontinue former pharmacological agent and consider adding to the psychotherapeutic
process one of the following:
**fenfluramine, fluvoxamine, lithium,
L-tryptophan (5), light therapy (6), naltrexone**

Legend

If partial response	→
If no response	→

MAOI Monoamine oxidase inhibitor
SSRIs Selective serotonin reuptake inhibitors
TCAs Tricyclic antidepressants
TeCAs Tetracyclic antidepressants

First-line drug / therapy
(well-established efficacy)

Second-line drug / therapy
(some efficacy)

Third-line drug / therapy
(efficacy is not fully established)

Notes about the numbered items in the scheme

Clinical Aspects

1. The core features of bulimia nervosa (BN) are recurrent episodes of binge eating accompanied by the feeling of being out of control. Binge eating is overly excessive eating, usually during short periods of time, that is accompanied by an inability to stop once started. Even so, and mainly due to compensatory measures to reduce weight, about 70% of affected persons remain within the normal range of body weight. The prevalence of BN is estimated to be between 1% and 2%, and it almost exclusively affects females. There are few axis I and II disorders associated with BN. The lifetime prevalence of a concomitant major depressive disorder is about 60%. Cluster B personality disorders (borderline and histrionic) are common among BN patients, while some other personality disorders from cluster C (obsessive–compulsive or avoidant) are also associated with BN but to a much lesser extent. There is an increased risk of alcohol abuse and some data suggest a familial relationship between these two disorders.

The prognosis of BN is variable and it is usually regarded as a chronic disorder with a waxing and waning course. About 33% of BN patients are functioning well after a 3-year follow-up period, and 33% exhibit some improvement in symptoms, while the remainders have a poor outcome. DSM-IV specifies the following 6 main criteria for the diagnosis of BN:

a. Eating large amounts of food in a discrete period of time (usually within 2 hours). The amount of food is disproportionate compared with what other people consume in similar time frames or circumstances.

b. Lack of control over the binge eating (cannot stop eating or control the amount or kind of food eaten).

c. Recurrent compensatory behaviors to prevent weight gain (laxative or diuretic abuse, self-induced vomiting, excessive exercising, enemas or fasting).

d. The binge eating and the associated compensatory behaviors occur at least twice a week for 3 months.

e. Self-evaluation is strongly influenced by body shape and weight.

f. The above-mentioned clinical characteristics do not occur exclusively during episodes of anorexia nervosa (AN).

Treatment

2. Many psychotherapeutic approaches have been successfully employed in BN. **Cognitive–behavioral techniques** are most frequently employed. They emphasize education, self-monitoring of eating behaviors and associated thoughts, relating between specific triggering events and the induction of binge eating (and learning to avoid these events), and addressing and challenging the irrational beliefs, including the patient's distorted body image.

3. Many well-controlled studies have shown efficacy of antidepressants in BN, regardless of past depressive disorder, or major depressive disorders in the family. The selective serotonin

Table 18.2 Parameters to help in differentiating between BN and AN:

	Bulimia nervosa	Anorexia nervosa
Affective lability	■	☐
Alcohol abuse	■	☐
Ego dystonic	■	☐
Hypothyroidism	☐	■
Impulsivity	■	☐
Menstrual abnormalities	☐	■
Normal body weight	■	☐
Seeks for help	■	☐
Sexual desire	■	☐
Shoplifting	■	☐

■ seen more often; ☐ seen less often.

reuptake inhibitor **fluoxetine** and tricyclic agents such as **amitriptyline**, **imipramine** and **desipramine** have been efficacious in reducing the frequency of the bulimic episodes, and the intensity of some of the associated symptoms. Other agents, such as **trazodone**, **phenelzine** and **isocarboxazide**, probably have similar efficacy. The doses used are approximately the same as for treating depressive episodes, and some response is usually observed within 2–4 weeks. As there is evidence of reduced serotonergic transmission in BN (especially of subsensitive postsynaptic 5-HT receptors in the hypothalamus), antidepressants exert their antibulimic effects presumably via the enhancement of serotonergic transmission.

4. Anticonvulsants such as **carbamazepine** and **phenytoin** have shown, in some case reports or small open-labeled studies, slight efficacy in reducing symptoms of BN. The use of these agents is theoretically warranted following anecdotal data that suggest non-specific electroencephalographic (EEG) abnormalities in BN. To date, **valproate** has not been shown to have significant efficacy in BN.

5. Fenfluramine, **lithium**, **fluvoxamine** and **L-tryptophan** have been anecdotally reported to exert some beneficial results in BN. **Naltrexone** was studied because of its opiate-antagonism capacity. The opiate system is presumed to be involved in stress-mediated feeding behaviors. However, **naltrexone** was found to be efficient only if administered in very high doses, which greatly increase the risk of developing hepatotoxicity.

6. An anecdotal report suggests the efficacy of **light therapy** (10 000 lux in the early morning for 2 weeks). The BN was not associated with any seasonal patterns but the subgroup of patients who did suffer from such seasonal fluctuations benefited more from this therapy.

19.1 Attention-deficit hyperactivity disorder (ADHD) - adult type (1)

Treatment strategies (based on published data)

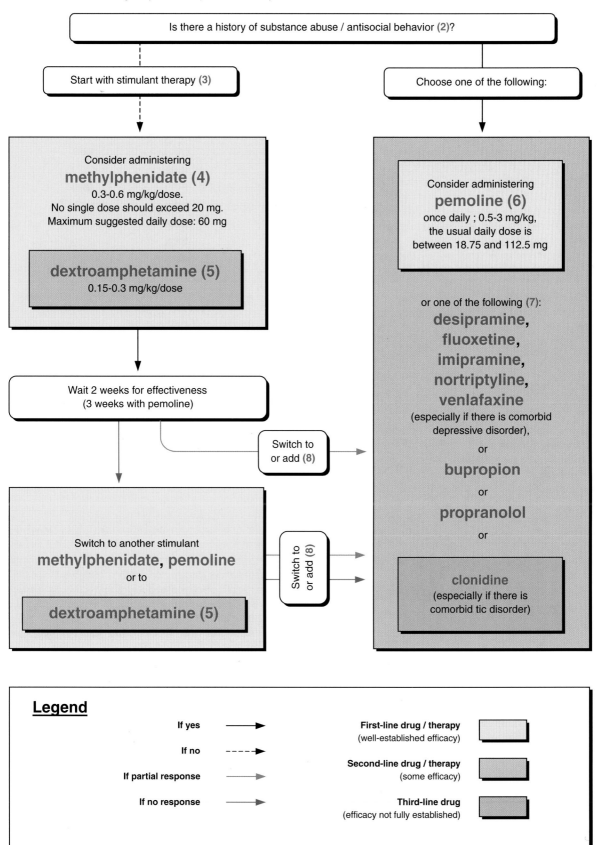

Is there a history of substance abuse / antisocial behavior (2)?

Start with stimulant therapy (3)

Choose one of the following:

Consider administering
methylphenidate (4)
0.3-0.6 mg/kg/dose.
No single dose should exceed 20 mg.
Maximum suggested daily dose: 60 mg

dextroamphetamine (5)
0.15-0.3 mg/kg/dose

Consider administering
pemoline (6)
once daily ; 0.5-3 mg/kg,
the usual daily dose is
between 18.75 and 112.5 mg

or one of the following (7):
**desipramine,
fluoxetine,
imipramine,
nortriptyline,
venlafaxine**
(especially if there is comorbid
depressive disorder),
or
bupropion
or
propranolol
or

Wait 2 weeks for effectiveness
(3 weeks with pemoline)

Switch to
or add (8)

Switch to another stimulant
methylphenidate, pemoline
or to

dextroamphetamine (5)

Switch to
or add (8)

clonidine
(especially if there is
comorbid tic disorder)

Legend

If yes	⟶	
If no	----▶	
If partial response	⟶	
If no response	⟶	

First-line drug / therapy
(well-established efficacy)

Second-line drug / therapy
(some efficacy)

Third-line drug
(efficacy not fully established)

Notes about the numbered items in the scheme:

Clinical Aspects

1. Attention-deficit hyperactivity disorder (ADHD) was believed until recently, to affect mainly children and adolescents. However, several prospective long-term follow-up studies have shown that the disorder continues into adulthood in about 10–60% of previously ADHD-diagnosed children. Thus the incidence of the disorder in adults is estimated to be between 1% and 3%. The core features of ADHD are the development of inappropriate poor attention span or age-related inappropriate hyperactivity or impulsivity, or both. It has to begin before the age of 7 years and last at least 6 months while causing a significant impairment in daily functioning.

Three subtypes are recognized by DSM-IV: inattentive, impulsive–hyperactive and combined. The symptoms must be evident in at least two different situations (home, school/academic, occupational, social). The disorder affects about 3–5% of prepubertal schoolage children, and males are affected 3–5 times more than females (mostly first-born boys).

The etiology of ADHD is unknown. Some genetic factors are associated with the disorder: there is a greater concordance rate in monozygotic twins, and siblings have an increased risk of developing ADHD. The genetic correlates between children and adults with ADHD are quite similar. Some soft neurological signs are observed more often in ADHD children: ambidexterity, right–left discrimination and reflex asymmetries. Socioeconomic status was not found to be a factor associated with the development of ADHD.

The most common clinical symptoms observed in adults with ADHD are inattention, impulsivity, intrusiveness, distractibility, low frustration tolerance, impatience, daydreaming, forgetfulness, and frequent shifts in activities. High divorce rates and poor academic or occupational functioning are commonly seen. Adults with ADHD have, like children, a high incidence of comorbid substance abuse, and depressive or anxiety disorders. Adults with ADHD respond less to pharmacotherapy (e.g. stimulants) than children do. The response rate for adults is estimated to be about 50%, as compared with around 70–80% in children and adolescents. The long-term adverse effects and efficacy of stimulants in adults with ADHD has not been studied in well controlled trials.

Treatment

2–6. Psychostimulants (mainly **methylphenidate, dextroamphetamine** and **pemoline**) that are used for treatment of ADHD are 'indirectly acting' amines. They act by increasing the release of biogenic amines (norepinephrine, serotonin and dopamine) from presynaptic nerve terminals into the synaptic cleft. Some of them also exhibit a capacity to block the reuptake of biogenic amines into presynaptic nerves. These stimulants, especially **methylphenidate** and **dextroamphetamine** have an abuse potential, so patients with a known history of substance abuse should, if possible, not receive these agents (**2**). A few open-label and some controlled studies with **methylphenidate** have shown beneficial results in about 25–75% of adult ADHD patients. It should be noted that to date no cases of stimulant abuse have been reported in well-controlled studies on adult patients with ADHD. **Methylphenidate** presumably has a linear dose–response curve, and incremental improvements have been reported using doses of 0.5, 0.75 and 1 mg/kg/day. Currently, there are no data about **dextroamphetamine** in adults with ADHD. Thus, in cases where there are no significant abuse potential (**3**), and no comorbid tic disorder is apparent, **methylphenidate** (**4**) should be considered firstly due to its relatively well-established efficacy in adults with ADHD. The use of **dextroamphetamine** in adults might be warranted based on its well-established efficacy in children (**5**). **Dextroamphetamine** has a significantly higher incidence of cardiac adverse effects (mostly tachycardia and hypertension) compared with the other stimulants. A few controlled studies have found **pemoline** (**6**) to be as efficacious as **methylphenidate** in adults with ADHD. The reported response rate is about 50%. **Pemoline** has a long half-life, thus enabling once-a-day dosing, and it has much less abuse potential than the other stimulants. It takes at least 3 weeks to reach full therapeutic effect, compared with about 2 weeks with the other stimulants. However, **pemoline** can cause fatal hepatic necrosis and so should be reserved for patients who have failed other treatments.

Psychostimulants have been found (in both children and adults) to improve attention and decrease hyperactivity and impulsiveness. They have not been shown to have beneficial effects in improving the specific learning disabilities (e.g. dyslexia) that are often associated with ADHD.

7. A number of non-stimulant agents have been reported to have some beneficial effects in adults with ADHD. The data are based mainly on case reports or small open-label studies. Some antidepressant agents (**desipramine, fluoxetine, imipramine, nortriptyline, venlafaxine**) were reported to exert beneficial effects in adults, but exact data on dosing strategies or efficacy rates are currently not established. The rationale for using these agents is based on their ability to increase the availability of biogenic amines to the synaptic cleft – a similar capacity to that of stimulants. **Bupropion**, a norepinephrine- and dopamine-reuptake inhibitor, was reported to be effective in about 75% of treated adults with ADHD (in an open-label study), but a high dropout rate (about 35%) limits the clinical significance of these findings. **Propranolol** has also been found to be beneficial in adults with ADHD (in small open-label studies). **Clonidine** might have some efficacy in children with ADHD (especially if there is concomitant tic disorder), but its efficacy in adults has not yet been studied. When used at night it can reduce the insomnia that stimulants sometimes produce.

8. The efficacy and safety of polypharmacotherapy in ADHD has not been studied systematically in adults. Combination treatment should be considered if there is an inadequate response to a single agent, or when there is a comorbid psychiatric disorder (e.g. depressive states, tics). Data in adults are lacking, but several successful combination therapies have been reported in children or adolescents (**methylphenidate** and **desipramine**, **methylphenidate** and **propranolol**).

20.1 Neuroleptic malignant syndrome (NMS) (1)

Treatment strategies (based on published data)

If suspected NMS, rule out major causes of NMS-like syndromes (2):
**malignant hyperthermia, lethal catatonia,
viral encephalitis, heat stroke**

a. **Withdraw the offending agent** (e.g. an antipsychotic) **immediately**
b. Institute **supportive measures**: cooling blankets, ice-water enema, oxygen
c. **Monitor** serum electrolytes, renal, hepatic and cardiac functions
d. Consider administering **low-dose heparin** (due to the patient's immobilization)
e. Continue the **antiparkinsonian** agent (if the patient receives one)

Start with the following regimens; choose either one or a combination of these:

dantrolene (4)
Initiate with
IV 0.8-2.5 mg/kg x 4/d.
or PO 50-100 mg x 2/d
and/or
benzodiazepine
(lorazepam) (up to 5 mg)

and/or

bromocriptine (5):
initiate with PO 2.5-10 mg
three times per day;
increase up to a
maximum of 60 mg/day

and/or

amantadine (5)
initiate with PO
100-200 mg
two times per day

Consider **electroconvulsive therapy (6)** or add **nifedipine (7)**

When fully remitted (wait at least 2 weeks) consider the following:
a. If the diagnosis is **bipolar disorder**, use **lithium, valproate** or **carbamazepine**
   If psychotic, add low-dose **antipsychotics**
b. If there is psychosis as part of **schizophrenia** (or other psychotic disorder),
   use **low-potency antipsychotics** and a **different class** of agents;
   if possible, use an atypical antipsychotic drug: **clozapine, olanzapine, risperidone,**
c. Consider prophylactic treatment with **bromocriptine** for several weeks

Legend

If good response   ⟶

If partial response   ⟶

If no response   ⟶

First-line drug / therapy
(well-established efficacy)

Second-line drug / therapy
(some efficacy)

Third-line drug / therapy
(efficacy not fully established)

Notes about the numbered items in the scheme

Clinical Aspects

1. The diagnosis of neuroleptic malignant syndrome (NMS) is problematic as many diagnostic criteria have been proposed but no single set of criteria has been adopted for general use. The etiology of NMS is unknown although two main theories (not necessarily contradictory) are proposed. One assumes a neuroleptic-induced alteration in dopamine-mediated hypothalamic thermoregulation. The antagonized dopamine receptors in the hypothalamus lead, probably, to impaired heat dissipation, while increased muscle rigidity accompanied by enhanced generation of heat is mediated by the blockage of dopamine receptors in the striatum. The second theory assumes an abnormal reaction of predisposed skeletal muscles and it suggests that **antipsychotic drugs** (**APDs**) alter calcium mobilization in muscle cells (for example, impaired calcium ion transport across the sarcoplasmic reticulum) with a consequent impairment in contractility. The characteristic features of neuroleptic malignant syndrome (NMS) are as follows:

a. It usually appears early in the course of neuroleptic treatment (in 80% of cases NMS appears within the first 2 weeks of treatment). All classes of **APDs** can cause NMS (including atypical drugs). Other drugs (**tetrabenazine, tricyclic antidepressants** and **selective serotonin reuptake inhibitors**) have also been shown to cause NMS (although very rarely). The incidence is between 0.7–2.2%, and more than 40% of NMS patients are diagnosed as a having mood disorder. The male-to-female ratio is about 3:2.

b. The associated risk factors are organic brain disorder, dehydration, high dose and route of administration (depot more risky), use of concurrent **lithium**, **high-potency antipsychotics**, young adult male, alcoholic patient during delirium, malnutrition, exhaustion, concurrent medical illness or a prior history of NMS.

c. Death is usually associated with rhabdomyolysis and acute renal failure. Mortality, without treatment is estimated to be around 20%.

d. High fever, usually between 38.5–40°C

e. Severe muscle rigidity, usually lead pipe and not cogwheel.

f. Altered consciousness.

g. Autonomic instability (diaphoresis, hypertension).

h. Laboratory abnormalities: elevated CK (creatine phosphokinase), usually between 2000 and 15 000; leukocytosis,

usually between 15 000 and 30 000; elevated liver enzymes (AST, ALT, LDH).

2. Malignant hyperthermia is a disorder associated with exposure to inhalation anesthetic agents and succinylcholine only. The increase in temperature progresses very rapidly – up to 1°C every 5 minutes. The disorder has a strong herediatery component related to chromosome 19. About 80% of family members are also susceptible to the disorder. The pathogenesis is assumed to be related to a muscle membrane defect that leads to increased intracellular calcium and a consequent severe muscle contractions.

Treatment

3. Antiparkinsonian agents, anticholinergics and/or dopaminergic drugs might have suppressing, beneficial effects on the evolvement of NMS.

4. Dantrolene is a muscle relaxant which inhibits calcium release from the sarcoplasmic reticulum with a subsequent decreased availability of calcium for muscle contracture. Do not administer more than 10 mg/kg/day due to possible hepatotoxicity. Follow the I.V. treatment with PO doses of 50–100 mg twice daily. It can be increased to a total of 700 mg/day.

5. Bromocriptine and **amantadine** are dopamine agonists that oppose the action of neuroleptics at the dopaminergic receptor site. They can be administered along with **dantrolene**. Their efficacy is not well established and only anecdotal case reports have been published concerning their beneficial effects.

6. Electroconvulsive therapy (**ECT**) is effective for treating catatonic states – mainly those related to bipolar mood disorder and schizophrenia. Its efficacy in NMS is not proven, and it is quite controversial. There are small studies that suggest its overwhelming superior effects in NMS (compared with supportive measures alone) but other reports point out the increased chance of developing fatal cardiac arrhythmias when **ECT** is used in NMS.

7. Nifedipine's efficacy was reported in a few cases. Controlled trials with this agent have not been done to date. The possible mode of action is based on its calcium-channel-blocking activities, with a consequent reduction in intracellular calcium.

Table 20.1 Some of the features (nonspecific) that can aid in differentiating NMS from lethal catatonia

Possible differentiating feature	NMS	Lethal catatonia
Appears while on antipsychotics	Practically always	Not necessarily
Hyperthermia *	Often prior to the stuporus state	Often prior to or during the excitement phase
Muscle rigidity	Evident	Evident
Elevated white blood cell count	Yes	No
Elevated serum CK (creatine phosphokinase)	Yes	Yes
Differentiating symptoms	The catatonic symptoms (listed in the right column) appear very rarely (if at all) in NMS	Often observed: echo phenomena; bizarre postures; ambitendency

* The timing might distinguish up to 75% of cases.

20.2 Tardive dyskinesia (TD) (1)

Treatment strategies (based on published data)

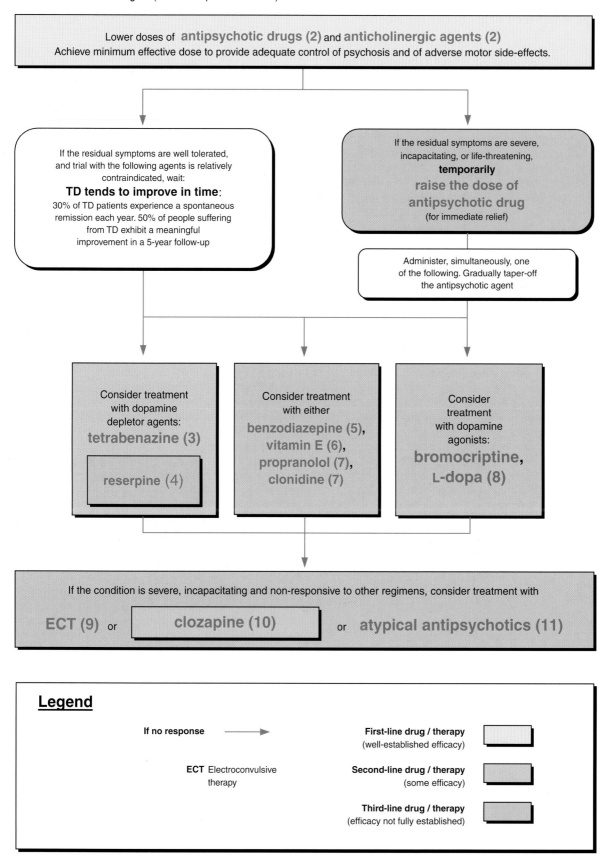

Lower doses of **antipsychotic drugs (2)** and **anticholinergic agents (2)**
Achieve minimum effective dose to provide adequate control of psychosis and of adverse motor side-effects.

If the residual symptoms are well tolerated, and trial with the following agents is relatively contraindicated, wait:
TD tends to improve in time:
30% of TD patients experience a spontaneous remission each year. 50% of people suffering from TD exhibit a meaningful improvement in a 5-year follow-up

If the residual symptoms are severe, incapacitating, or life-threatening,
temporarily
raise the dose of antipsychotic drug
(for immediate relief)

Administer, simultaneously, one of the following. Gradually taper-off the antipsychotic agent

Consider treatment with dopamine depletor agents:
tetrabenazine (3)
reserpine (4)

Consider treatment with either
benzodiazepine (5),
vitamin E (6),
propranolol (7),
clonidine (7)

Consider treatment with dopamine agonists:
bromocriptine,
L-dopa (8)

If the condition is severe, incapacitating and non-responsive to other regimens, consider treatment with
ECT (9) or **clozapine (10)** or **atypical antipsychotics (11)**

Legend

If no response →

ECT Electroconvulsive therapy

First-line drug / therapy
(well-established efficacy)

Second-line drug / therapy
(some efficacy)

Third-line drug / therapy
(efficacy not fully established)

Notes about the numbered items in the scheme

Clinical Aspects

1a. Tardive dyskinesia (TD) is late onset of involuntary, repetitive and purposeless movements that occur, presumably, in predisposed people. The prevalence is about 5–20% of chronic neuroleptics treated. The prevalence is about 70% in the high-risk population:

- Elderly.
- Female (1.7 to 1 over male).
- Comorbidity of mood disorder.
- Diabetes mellitus.
- Concurrent brain injury.
- Increased total duration and dosage of neuroleptic treatment.
- Concomitant anticholinergic treatment.

TD can appear at any time following the administration of neuroleptics – usually within weeks to a few years. The mean time for appearance is 7 years.

b. To date, only **clozapine** (and perhaps other new **atypical antipsychotics** or **sulpiride**) have minimal or diminished capacity to cause TD.

c. It is estimated that chronic antagonism of the dopaminergic receptors in the nigrastriatal pathway causes the receptors to become hypersensitive. Therefore the main treatment rationale, in many cases, is to downregulate the supposed upregulated receptors (via administration of dopamine agonists) or to suppress dopaminergic transmission in presynaptic nerve terminals by depleting the dopaminergic stores.

Treatment

2. Increased antipsychotic dose is beneficial in the short term only, since later worse dyskinesias may appear. Therefore lower the antipsychotic dose to the minimum effective dose that will, on the one hand, control the psychosis, and, on the other hand, will suppress or not aggravate the TD. **Anticholinergic** agents tend to enhance the dyskinesia, and should be avoided if possible.

3,4. **Tetrabenazine** is a biogenic-amine depletor agent (including dopamine) (see Section 1.11). Both **tetrabenazine** and **reserpine** antagonize the vesicular monoamine transporter type 2 (VMAT2) and inhibit the uptake of biogenic amines into intracellular vesicles. A consequent reduction in biogenic amine availability for exocytosis is evident, and the net concentration of biogenic amines in the synaptic cleft is decreased. **Tetrabenazine** is probably the most efficient agent for the treatment of TD (**3**). Beneficial effects are reported in up to 50% of patients. Its mechanism of action is not totally clear, but is probably due to its suppression of dopaminergic transmission in presynaptic nerve terminals in the nigrastriatal pathway. **Reserpine** has a similar mode of action, but its efficacy is not well established (**4**).

5. One of the theories regarding the pathogenesis of TD is of γ-aminobutyric acid (GABA) hypofunction which leads to enhanced dopaminergic transmission in various regions. **Benzodiazepines**, as GABA agonists, have been reported to improve some of the dyskinetic movements in TD.

6. Vitamin E was reported in several reports to have beneficial effects in TD, maybe due to its activity as an antioxidant. To date, these findings have not been replicated in large well-controlled studies.

7. The use of adrenergic agents such as **propranolol** or **clonidine** has been suggested, but only anecdotal reports have shown their beneficial effects and there are no replications of these findings.

8. Upregulated and oversensitive dopaminergic receptors are believed to be among the factors associated with the production of TD. Dopamine agonists such as L-**dopa** and **bromocriptine** downregulate the postsynaptic receptors. Their clinical efficacy is not well established and sometimes contradictory. It seems that L-**dopa** is most efficient if given early in the course of the disorder.

9. Electroconvulsive therapy (**ECT**) has been anecdotally reported to improve dyskinetic movements.

10. Clozapine does not cause TD, and in a few cases changing the antipsychotic drug to **clozapine** significantly reduced dyskinetic movements. However, the use of **clozapine** in TD should be reserved for severe and non-responsive cases due to its possible serious adverse side-effects.

11. The efficacy of the other atypical antipsychotic drugs (**olanzapine, risperidone, sertindole**) has not been studied to date, in this disorder.

20.3 Akathisia (1)

Treatment strategies (based on published data)

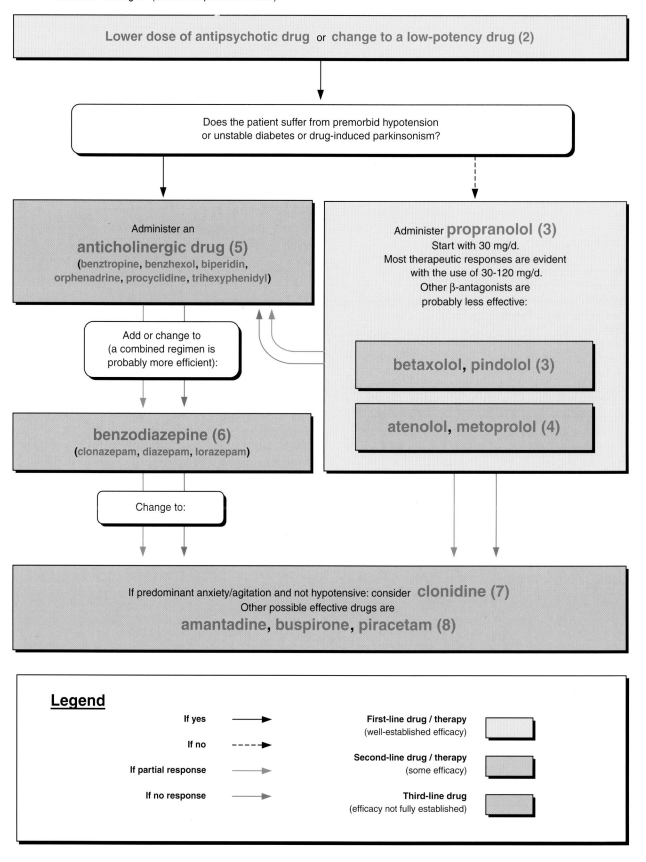

Lower dose of antipsychotic drug or change to a low-potency drug (2)

Does the patient suffer from premorbid hypotension or unstable diabetes or drug-induced parkinsonism?

Administer an
anticholinergic drug (5)
(benztropine, benzhexol, biperidin, orphenadrine, procyclidine, trihexyphenidyl)

Administer **propranolol (3)**
Start with 30 mg/d.
Most therapeutic responses are evident with the use of 30-120 mg/d.
Other β-antagonists are probably less effective:

betaxolol, pindolol (3)

atenolol, metoprolol (4)

Add or change to
(a combined regimen is probably more efficient):

benzodiazepine (6)
(clonazepam, diazepam, lorazepam)

Change to:

If predominant anxiety/agitation and not hypotensive: consider **clonidine (7)**
Other possible effective drugs are
amantadine, buspirone, piracetam (8)

Legend

If yes	⟶	First-line drug / therapy (well-established efficacy)
If no	----▶	
If partial response	⟶	Second-line drug / therapy (some efficacy)
If no response	⟶	Third-line drug (efficacy not fully established)

Notes about the numbered items in the scheme

Clinical Aspects

1. Akathisia is a side-effect caused mostly by the use of **antipsychotic drugs** (**APDs**). While all **APDs** can cause akathisia, the incidence is increased with the use of **high-potency agents**. The exact incidence of akathisia due to the use of **atypical antipsychotics** is not known (**clozapine** has been shown to cause akathisia, but data about the other newly developed **atypical antipsychotics** are lacking). There is no well-accepted definition of akathisia, although most clinicians agree on the fact that there two main components to the disorder:

    a. A subjective feeling of inner restlesness that results in a need to engage in a motor activity, usually of the lower extremities.

    b. An objective component witnessed by the examiner that consists of characteristic movements such as pacing constantly or inability to stand still, sit or lie at the same position for more that few minutes. The pathophysiology of akathisia is not yet fully understood.

The dopaminergic and adrenergic systems are presumed to have a key role in the evolvement of akathisia, particularly due to two observations:

    a. Most drugs capable of inducing akathisia have at least some capacity to antagonize the central D_2 dopaminergic receptors.

    b. The best treatment results for akathisia are achieved with the use of central β-adrenergic antagonists.

Noradrenergic projections from the locus ceruleus to limbic structures and the diencephalo-spinal-cord pathway are presumed to be the most important pathways associated with the pathophysiology of akathisia. The suppressed dopaminergic system along with an overactive noradrenergic system, is believed, at least by some investigators, to be the consequence of inhibited presynaptic D_2 dopaminergic receptors located on noradrenergic nerve terminals (due to the use of antipsychotics). These are heteroreceptors that suppress the release of norpinephrine from presynaptic nerve terminals; hence their blockage by antipsychotic drugs increase the amount of norepinephrine released into the synaptic cleft. Other proposals have been made to explain the evolution of akathisia such as an imbalanced dopaminergic–cholinergic transmission that causes a compensatory increase in either norepinephrine or serotonin release (see Section 6.1 for further details).

The association between low serum iron and akathisia, low serum ferritin concentrations and akathisia, and significant inverse correlation between serum iron levels and akathisia rating have all been implicated. Even so, other studies have not been able to replicate these findings, and contradictory results have often been obtained.

Treatment

2. Since akathisia is associated with the use of **high-potency antipsychotics**, and higher doses might increase the risk of developing the disorder, it is presumed that lowering the dose of the **APDs** or changing to a low-potency drug might suppress the symptoms. However, the efficacy of such practice has not been studied enough.

3,4. β-**adrenergic antagonists** are often helpful and usually well tolerated for the treatment of akathisia. Their efficacy rate is not known, but they are assumed to be the most beneficial drugs for treating akathisia. Most data suggests that the more-lipophilic drugs (**propranolol, pindolol, betaxolol**) (**3**) are the most effective, while the most-hydrophilic (**metoprolol, nadolol**) are practically inefficient (**4**). Since passage through the blood–brain barrier is probably directly correlated with the lipophilicity of a drug, these observations imply that a central mechanism is a predominant factor in inducing akathisia. These drugs should be avoided, as much as possible, in patients with diabetes mellitus or known hypotension (β-**adrenergic antagonists** can impair serum glucose regulation and further lower blood pressure).

5. All of the listed **anticholinergic drugs** have been reported to exert beneficial effects in treating akathisia, and they are most efficient when there is concomitant **APD**-induced parkinsonism. The overall efficacy of these drugs is unsatisfactory.

6. Benzodiazepines (**BDZs**) have been only anecdotally reported to improve akathisia, and in most of these cases they were co-administered with an anticholinergic drug. For that reason it seems that a combined **BDZ–anticholinergic drug** is a more efficient regimen than **BDZs** alone. Even so, the overall efficacy of this combination is unsatisfactory.

7. Clonidine has not been well investigated in this disorder, but there are a few reports that suggest that it has a substantial capacity to improve akathisia. **Clonidine** is a sedative drug and it might also cause hypotension, it should only be used for agitated or anxious patients without known hypotension.

8. Amantadine and **piracetam** were anecdotally reported to be efficient for akathisia. **Buspirone** was shown to either improve or aggrevate akathisia.

20.4 Delirium (1)

Treatment strategies (based on published data)

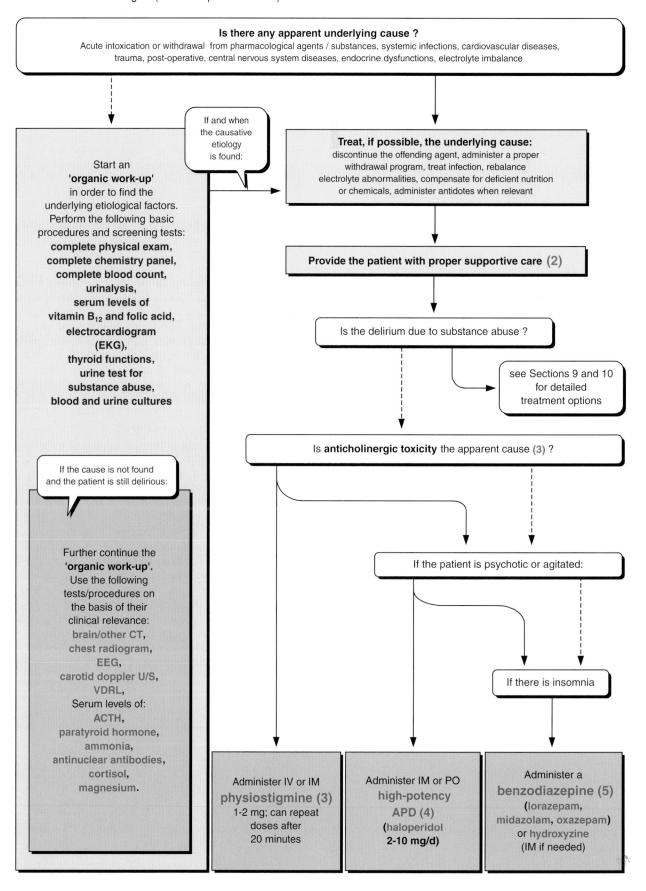

Notes about the numbered items in the scheme

Clinical Aspects

1a. Delirium is a clinical syndrome, known by a variety of different names: 'acute confusional state', 'toxic/metabolic encephalopathy' or 'acute brain syndrome'. Its core features are as follows:

- Impaired consciousness, with reduced ability to focus, sustain or shift attention.
- Multiple cognitive impairments (memory, orientation, language).
- Perceptual disturbance that cannot be accounted for by another mental disorder, including dementia.
- Psychiatric symptoms, including mood disturbances, anxiety and behavioral abnormalities.
- Neurologic symptoms (tremor, nystagmus, impaired coordination, urinary incontinence).
- The above-mentioned symptoms tend to develop over a short period of time.
- Symptoms tend to fluctuate during the course of the day (worse at night).
- There is evidence that the delirium is caused by a direct physiological consequence of a general medical condition.

b. Delirium can be caused by numerous etiologies, about 85% of which are extracranial. The mechanism is unclear, but the final common pathway may be decreased cholinergic activity, especially in the dorsal tegmental area of the brainstem's reticular formation (belived to be one of the major brain sites in charge of regulating attention and arousal). Even so, other neurotransmitter abnormalities have been suggested to be involved in delirium.

c. About 1–20% of general hospital inpatients suffer from delirium during their hospitalization periods. The major risk factors for developing the syndrome are

- advanced age (at ages over 65, the incidence in general hospital inpatients rises to 40%);
- prexisting brain disorder;
- malnutrition;
- previous history of delirium;
- concomitant systemic disorders (mainly diabetes and cancer).

d. The prognosis is usually poor, since the 3-month mortality rate of these patients is estimated at about 25–35% while the 1-year mortality rates of patients who had a delirious episode could rise up to 50%.

Treatment

2. The key aspect of treating delirium is the provision of adequate supportive care while administering specific therapy for the underlying cause. Take safety measures to ensure that no accidental falls or damages to important medical procedures are made by the patient. Restraints might be needed. The delirious patient should not be sensory-deprived or sensory-over-stimulated. Provide the patient with familiar surroundings that includes well-known people, familiar objects, meals and daily activities.

3. The possiblity of an anticholinergic toxicity should be ruled out, especially if the patient has been using pharmacological agents with an anticholinergic capacity (**low-potency antipsychotics**, specific **anticholinergic agents**, **tricyclic antidepressants**, **digoxin**, **theophylline**, **warfarin**, **nifedipine**, **cimetidine**). When an anticholinergic toxicity is evident, the use of the acetylcholineesterase inhibitor **physiostigmine** might be indicated. **Physiostigmine** raises the amount of acetylcholine available for synaptic transmission and thus reduces the anticholinergic symptoms – a core feature of delirium. It can be given either IV (2 mg; effects are evident in about 2 minutes, and can be repeated in 20 minutes) or IM with repeated doses every 30–60 minutes.

4. For psychotic or very agitated patients, use high-potency antipsychotics such as **haloperidol** due to their relative lack of anticholinergic effects along with no prominent effects on the cardiovascular system, and especially their minimal hypotensive capacity. In the elderly, doses of 0.5 mg bid might be sufficient, while younger people might require higher doses.

5. To treat insomnia the use of benzodiazepines such as **lorazepam**, **oxazepam** or **midazolam** is recommended. These agents have short half-lives and no active metabolites and are metabolized by glucuronidation, a relatively well-preserved mechanism in the elderly. **Lorazepam** also has the advantage of being administered, if needed, IM.

1. Basic aspects related to drug action

Amara SG, Kuhar MJ (1993) Neurotransmitter transporters: recent progress, *A Rev Neurosci* **16**:73–93.

Amrein R, Guentert TW, Dingemanse J, et al (1992) Interactions of moclobemide with concomitantly administered medication: evidence from pharmacological and clinical studies, *Psychopharmacol* **106**(suppl):S24–31.

Arranz MJ, Dawson E, Shaikh S, et al (1995) Cytochrome P4502D6 gene type does not determine response to clozapine, *Br J Clin Pharmacol* **39**:417–420.

Barbhaiya RH, Shukla UA, Greene DS, et al (1996) Investigation of pharmacokinetic and pharmacodynamic interactions after coadministration of nefazodone and haloperidol, *J Clin Psychopharmacol* **16**:26–34.

Baron BM, Ogden AM, Siegel BW, et al (1988) Rapid down regulation of beta adrenoreceptors by coadministration of desipramine and flouxetine, *European J Clin Pharmacol* **154**:125–134.

Bauman P, Bertschy G (1993) Pharmacodynamic and pharmacokinetic interactions of selective serotonin re-uptake inhibiting antidepressants (SSRIs) with other psychotropic drugs, *Nordic J of Psychiatry* **47**(suppl 30):13–19.

Beasley CM, Sanger W, Satterlee G, et al (1996) Olanzapine versus placebo: results of a double-blind, fixed-dose olanzapine trial, *Psychopharmacol (Berl)* **124**:159–167.

Beasley CM, Tollefson G, Tran P, et al (1996) Olanzapine versus placebo and haloperidol: acute phase results of the North American double-blind olanzapine trial, *Neuropsychopharmacol* **14**:111–123.

Benedetti MS, Dostert P (1992) Monoamine oxidase: from physiology and pathophysiology to the design and clinical application of reversible inhibitors, *Adv Drug Res* **23**:67–125.

Bennie EH, Mullin JM, Martindale JJ (1995) A double-blind multicenter trial comparing sertraline and fluoxetine in outpatients with major depression, *J Clin Psychiatry* **56**:229–237.

Blackwell B (1963) Hypertensive crisis due to monoamine-oxidase inhibition, *Lancet* **ii**:849–851.

Brodribb TR, Downey M, Gilbar PJ (1994) Efficacy and adverse effects of moclobemide, *Lancet* **343**:475.

Brooks D, Prothero W, Bouras N, et al (1984) Trazodone: a comparison of single night-time and divided daily dosage regimens, *Psychopharmacol* **84**:1–8.

Brosen K, Skjelbo E, Rasmussen BB, et al (1993) Fluvoxamine is a potent inhibitor of cytochrome P450 1A2, *Biochem Pharmacol* **45**:1211–1214.

Casey DE (1997) The relationship of pharmacology to side effects, *J Clin Psychiatry* **58**(suppl 10):55–62.

Cavanaugh SV (1991) Drug-drug interactions of fluoxetine with tricyclics, *Psychosomatics* **31**:273–276.

Cesura AM, Pletscher A (1992) The new generation of monoamine oxidase inhibitors, *Progr Drug Res* **38**:174–297.

Cowen PJ, Power AC (1993) Combination treatment of depression, *Br J Psychiatry* **162**:266–267.

Crewe HK, Lennard MS, Tucker GT, et al (1991) The effect of paroxetine and other specific 5HT re-uptake inhibitors on cytochrome P450IID6 activity in human liver microsomes, *Br J Clin Pharmacol* **32**:658–659P.

Darchen F, Scherman D, Henry JP (1989) Reserpine binding to chromaffin granules suggests the existence of two conformations of the monoamine transporter, *Biochemistry, NY* **28**:1692–1697.

De Jonghe F, Swinkels JA (1992) The safety of antidepressants, *Drugs* **43**(suppl 2):40–47.

de Oliveira IR, Do Prado-Lima PAS, Samuel-Lajeunesse B (1989) Monitoring of tricyclic antidepressant plasma levels and clinical response: a review of the literature. Part 1, *Psychiatry Psychobiol* **4**:43–60.

DeVane CL (1994) Pharmacogenetics and drug metabolism of newer antidepressant agents, *J Clin Psychiatry* **55**(12, suppl):38–45.

Devinsky O, Honigfeld G, Patin J (1991) Clozapine-related seizures, *Neurology* **41**:369–371.

Ereshefsky L, Riesenman C, Lam YWF (1995) Antidepressant drug interactions and the cytochrome P450 system: the role of CYP2D6, *Clin Pharmacokinet* **29**(suppl 1):10–19.

Ereshefsky L, Riesenman C, Lam YWF (1996) Serotonin selective re-uptake inhibitor drug interactions and the cytochrome P450 system, *J Clin Psychiatry* **57**(suppl 8):17–25.

Erickson JD, Eiden LE (1993) Functional identification and molecular cloning of a human brain vesicle monoamine transporter, *J Neurochem* **61**:2314–2317.

Fava M, Rosensbaum JF, McGrath PJ, et al (1994) Lithium and tricyclic augmentation of fluoxetine treatment for resistant major depression: a double-blind, controlled study, *Am J of Psychiatry* **151**:1372–1374.

Fleishaker JC, Hulst LK (1994) A pharmacokinetic and pharmacodynamic evaluation of the combined administration of alprazolam and fluvoxamine, *Eur J Clin Pharmacol* **46**:35–39.

Goff DC, Midha KK, Brotman AW, et al (1991) Elevation of plasma concentrations of haloperidol after addition of fluoxetine, *Am J Psychiatry* **148**:790–792.

Goldstein JA, de Morais SMF (1994) Biochemistry and molecular biology of the human CYP2C subfamily, *Pharmacogenetics* **4**:285–299.

Goodnick PJ (1994) Pharmacokinetic optimisation of therapy with newer antidepressants, *Clin Pharmacokinet* **27**(4):307–330.

Gram LF, Hansen MGJ, Sindrup SH, et al (1993) Citalopram: Interaction studies with levomepromazine, imipramine and lithium, *Therapeutic Drug Monitoring* **15**:18–24.

Greene DS, Salazar DE, Dockens RC, et al (1995) Coadministration of nefazodone and benzodiazepines, III: a pharmacokinetic interaction study with alprazolam, *J Clin Psychopharmacol* **15**:399–408.

Guentert TW, Mayersohn M (1994) Clinical-pharmacokinetic profile of moclobemide and its comparison with other MAO-inhibitors, *Rev Contemp Pharmacother* **5**:19–34.

Harvey AT, Preskorn SH (1996) Cytochrome P450 enzymes: interpretation of their interactions with selective serotonin re-uptake inhibitors: part 1, *J Clin Psychopharmacol* **16**:273–285.

Henry JP, Botton D, Sagne C, et al (1994) Biochemistry and molecular biology of the vesicular monoamine transporter from chromaffin granules, *J exp Biol* **196**:251–262.

Hiemke C, Weigmann H, Hartter S, et al (1994) Elevated levels of clozapine in serum after addition of fluvoxamine, *J Clin Psychopharmacol* **14**:279–281.

Jue SG, Dawson GW, Brogden RN (1982) Amoxapine: a review of its pharmacology and efficacy in depressed states, *Drugs* **24**:1–23.

Kane JM, Honigfeld G, Singer J (1988) Clozapine for the treatment-resistant schizophrenic: a double-blind comparison with chlorpromazine, *Arch Gen Psychiatry* **45**:789–796.

Kasper S, Fuger J, Moller HJ (1992) Comparative efficacy of antidepressants, *Drugs* **43**(suppl 2):11–23.

Kerr BM, Thummel KE, Wurden CJ, et al (1994) Human liver carbamazepine metabolism: role of CYP3A4 and CYP2C8 in 10,11–epoxide formation, *Biochem Pharmacol* **47**:1969–1979.

Krishna DR, Klotz U (1994) Extrahepatic metabolism of drugs in humans, *Clin Pharmacokinet* **26**:144–160.

Kronbach T, Mathys D, Umeno M, et al (1989) Oxidation of midazolam and triazolam by human liver cytochrome P450IIIA4, *Mol Pharmacol* **36**:89–96.

Langer SZ (1997) 25 years since the discovery of presynaptic receptors: present knowledge and future perspectives, *TiPS* **18**:95–99.

Leinonen E, Lillsunde P, Laukkanen V, et al (1991) Effects of carbamazepine on serum antidepressant concentrations in psychiatric patients, *J Clin Psychopharmacol* **11**:313–318.

Lemoine A, Gautier JC, Azoulay D, et al (1993) Major pathway of imipramine metabolism is catalyzed by cytochromes P450 1A2 and P450 3A4 in human liver, *Mol Pharmacol* **43**:827–832.

Levy RH (1995) Cytochrome P450 isoenzymes and anti-epileptic drug interactions, *Epilepsia* **36**(suppl 5): S8–S13.

Lydiard RB, Anton RF, Cunningham T (1993) Interactions between sertraline and tricyclic antidepressants, *Am J Psychiatry* **150**:1125–1126.

Maguire KP, Norman TR, Burrows GD, et al (1982) A pharmacokinetic study of mianserin, *Eur J Clin Pharmacol* **21**:517–520.

Mayersohn M, Guentert TW (1995) Clinical pharmacokinetics of the monoamine oxidase-A inhibitor moclobemide, *Clin Pharmacokinet* **29**(5):292–332.

Nelson DR, Kamataki T, Waxman DJ, et al (1993) The P450 superfamily: update on new sequences, gene mapping, accession numbers, early trivial names of enzymes, and nomenclature, *DNA Cell Biol* **12**:1–51.

Nemeroff CB (1991) Augmentation regimens for depression, *J Clin Psychiatry* **52**(May suppl):21–27.

Nemeroff CB, DeVane CL, Pollock BG (1996) Newer antidepressants and the cytochrome P450 system, *Am J Psychiatry* **153**:311–320.

Neuvonen PJ, Pohjola-Sintonen S, Vuori E (1993) Five fatal cases of serotonin syndrome after moclobemide-citalopram or moclobemide-clomipramine overdoses, *Lancet* **342**:1419.

Otton SV, Ball SE, Cheung SW, et al (1994) Comparative inhibition of the polymorphic enzyme CYP2D6 by venlafaxine and other 5–HT uptake inhibitors [abstract], *Clin Pharmacol Ther* **55**:141.

Otton SV, Wu D, Joffe RT, et al (1993) Inhibition by fluoxetine of cytochrome P450 2D6 activity, *Clin Pharmacol Ther* **53**:401–409.

Perucca E, Gatti G, Spina E (1994) Clinical pharmacokinetics of fluvoxamine, *Clin Pharmacokinet* **27**(3):175–190.

Peter D, Jimenez J, Liu Y, et al (1994) The chromaffin granule and synaptic vesicle amine transporters differ in substrate recognition and sensitivity to inhibitors, *J Biol Chem* **269**:7231–7237.

Peuskens J (1995) Risperidone in the treatment of patients with chronic schizophrenia: a multi-centre, double-blind, parallel-group study versus haloperidol, *Br J Psychiatry* **166**:712–726.

Preskorn SH (1993) Pharmacokinetics of antidepressants: why and how they are relevant to treatment, *J Clin Psychiatry* **54**(Sept suppl):14–34.

Preskorn SH, Magnus RD (1994) Inhibition of hepatic P450 isoenzymes by serotonin selective re-uptake inhibitors: in vitro and in vivo findings and their implications for patient care, *Psychopharmacol Bull* **30**:251–259.

Reddig S, Minnema AM, Tandon R (1993) Neuroleptic malignant syndrome and clozapine, *Ann Clin Psychiatry* **5**:25–27.

Ring BJ, Binkley SN, Vandenbranden M, et al (1996) In vitro interaction of the antipsychotic agent olanzapine with human cytochromes P450 CYP2C9, CYP2C19, CYP2D6, and CYP3A, *Br J Clin Pharmacol* **41**:181–186.

Rudorfer MV, Manji HK, Potter WZ (1994) Comparative tolerability profiles of the new versus older antidepressants, *Drug Saf* **10**:18–46.

Saller CF, Salama AL (1993) Seroquel: biochemical profile of a potential atypical antipsychotic, *Psychopharmacol (Berl)* **112**:285–292.

Scherman D, Gasnier B, Jaudon P, et al (1988) Hydrophobicity of the tetrabenazine-binding site of the chromaffin granule monoamine transporter, *Molec Pharmac* **33**:72–77.

Scherman D, Henry JP (1984) Reserpine binding to bovine chromaffin granule membranes: characterization and comparison with dihydrotetrabenazine binding, *Molec. Pharmac* **25**:113–122.

Shami M, Elliot HL, Kelman AW, et al (1983) The pharmacokinetics of mianserin, *Br J Clin Pharmacol* **15**:313S–322S.

Shen, WW (1995) Cytochrome P450 monooxygenases and interactions of psychotropic drugs: a five-year update, *Int'l J Psychiatry in Medicine* **25**:277–290.

Spar JE (1987) Plasma trazodone concentrations in elderly depressed inpatients: cardiac effects and short-term efficacy, *J Clin Psychopharmacol* **7**:406–409.

Taylor D (1995) Selective serotonin re-uptake inhibitors and tricyclic antidepressants in combination: interactions and therapeutic uses, *Br J Psychiatry* **167**:575–580.

Taylor D, Lader M (1996) Cytochromes and psychotropic drug interactions, *Br J Psychiatry* **168**:529–532.

Tollefson GD, Beasley CM Jr, Tran PV, et al (1997) Olanzapine vs haloperidol in the treatment of schizophrenia, schizoaffective and schizophreniform disorders: results of an international collaborative trial, *Am J Psychiatry* **154**:457–465.

Tran PV, Dellva MA, Tollefson GD, et al (1997) Extrapyramidal symptoms and tolerability of olanzapine vs haloperidol in the acute treatment of schizophrenia, *J Clin Psychiatry* **58**:205–211.

van Harten J (1993) Comparative pharmacokinetics of selective serotonin re-uptake inhibitors, *Clin Pharmacokinet* **24**:203–220.

van Harten J (1995) Overview of the pharmacokinetics of fluvoxamine, *Clin Pharmacokinet* **29**(suppl 1):1–9.

van Kammen DP, McEvoy JP, Targum S, et al (1996) A randomized, controlled, dose-ranging trial of sertindole in patients with schizophrenia, *Psychopharmacol (Berl)* **124**:168–175.

van Tol HHM, Bunzow JR, Guan H, et al (1991) Cloning of the gene for a human dopamine D receptor with high affinity for the antipsychotic clozapine, *Nature* **350**:610–614.

von Moltke LL, Greenblatt DJ, Schmider J, et al (1995) Metabolism of drugs by cytochrome P450 3A isoforms: implications for drug interactions in psychopharmacology, *Clin Pharmacokinet* **29**(suppl 1):33–44.

Webster P, Wijerame C (1994) Risperidone-induced neuroleptic malignant syndrome, *Lancet* **344**:1228–1229.

Wilens TE, Biederman J, Baldessarini RJ, et al (1992) Fluoxetine inhibits desipramine metabolism, *Arch Gen Psychiatry* **49**:752.

Youdim MBH, Finberg JPM (1990) New directions in monoamine oxidase A and B: selective inhibitors and substrates, *Biochem Pharmacol* **41**:155–162.

Zimmer R, Gieschke R, Fischbach R, et al (1990) Interaction studies with moclobemide, *Acta Psychiatr Scand* **82**(suppl 360):84–86.

2. Antidepressants and mood stabilizers

Alexanderson B, Evans DAP, Sj?qvist F (1969) Steady-state plasma levels of nortriptyline in twins: influence of genetic factors and drug therapy, *BMJ* **2**:764–768.

Ascher JA, Cole JO, Colin JN, et al (1995) Bupropion: a review of its mechanism of antidepressant activity, *J Clin Psychiatry* **56**:395–401.

Aston-Jones G, Chiang C, Alexinsky T (1991) Discharge of noradrenergic locus coeruleus neurons in behaving rats and monkeys suggests a role in vigilance, *Prog Brain Res* **88**:501–520.

Balon R, Berchou R (1986) Hematologic side effects of psychotropic drugs, *Psychosomatics* **27**:119–127.

Banerjee SP, Kung LS, Chanda SK, Riggi SJ, et al (1977) Development of beta-adrenergic receptor subsensitivity by antidepressants, *Nature* **268**:455–456.

Bannister SJ, Houser VP, Hulse JD, et al (1989) Evaluation of the potential for interactions of paroxetine with diazepam, cimetidine, warfarin and digoxin, *Acta Psychiatr Scand* **80**(suppl 350):102–106.

Baron BM, Ogden AM, Siegel BW, et al (1988) Rapid down regulation of beta adrenoreceptors by coadministration of desipramine and flouxetine, *Eur J Clin Pharmacol* **154**:125–134.

Baumann P (1992) Clinical pharmacokinetics of citalopram and other selective serotonergic re-uptake inhibitors, *Int Clin Psychopharmacol* **6**(suppl 5):13–20.

Benedetti MS, Dostert P (1992) Monoamine oxidase: from physiology and pathophysiology to the design and clinical application of reversible inhibitors, *Adv Drug Res* **23**:67–125.

Berendsen RRG, Broekamp CLE, van Delft AML (1995) Down regulation of 5-HT2A receptors after chronic treatment with remeron, *Eur Neuropsychopharmacol* **5**:306.

Berridge MJ (1993) Inositol triphosphate and calcium signaling, *Nature* **361**:315–325.

Berry MD, Juorio AV, Paterson IA (1994) The functional role of monoamine oxidases A and B in the mammalian central nervous system, *Prog Neurobiol* **42**:375–391.

Bertilsson L, Dahl M-L, Tybring G (1997) Pharmacogenetics of antidepressants: clinical aspects, *Acta Psychiatr Scand Suppl* **96**(suppl. 391):14–21.

Blackwell B (1963) Hypertensive crisis due to monoamine-oxidase inhibition, *Lancet* **ii**:849–851.

Blier P, de Montigny C (1994) Current advances and trends in the treatment of depression, *Trends Pharmacol Sci* **15**:220–226.

Blier P, de Montigny C, Chaput Y (1987) Modifications of the serotonin system by antidepressant treatments: implications for the therapeutic response in major depression, *J Clin Psychopharmacol* **7**(supp):24S–35S.

Bolden-Watson C, Richelson E (1993) Blockade by newly-developed antidepressants of biogenic amine uptake into rat brain synaptosomes, *Life Sci* **52**:1023–1029.

Boyer WF, Blumhardt CL (1992) The safety profile of paroxetine, *J Clin Psychiatry* **53**(2,suppl):61–66.

Boyer WF, Feighner JP (1991) Side effects of the selective serotonin re-uptake inhibitors. In: Feighner JP, Boyer WF, eds. *Selective Serotonin Re-uptake Inhibitors.* Chichester, England: John Wiley & Sons: 122–152.

Brodribb TR, Downey M, Gilbar PJ (1994) Efficacy and adverse effects of moclobemide, *Lancet* **343**:475.

Brooks D, Prothero W, Bouras N, et al (1984) Trazodone: a comparison of single night-time and divided daily dosage regimens, *Psychopharmacol* **84**:1–8.

Brosen K, Skjelbo E, Rasmussen BB, et al (1993) Fluvoxamine is a potent inhibitor of cytochrome P4501A2, *Biochem Pharmacol* **45**:1211–1214.

Burrows GD, Kremer CME (1997) Mirtazapine: clinical advantages in the treatment of depression, *J Clin Psychopharmacol* **17**(suppl 1):34S–39S.

Butler MO, Morinobu S, Duman RS (1993) Chronic electroconvulsive seizures increase the expression of serotonin2 receptor mRNA in rat frontal corte, *J Neurochem* **61**:1270–1276.

Casebolt TL, Jope RS (1991) Effects of chronic lithium treatment on protein kinase C and cyclic AMP-dependent protein phosphorylation, *Biol Psychiatry* **29**:233–243.

Cesura AM, Pletscher A (1992) The new generation of monoamine oxidase inhibitors, *Progr Drug Res* **38**:174–297.

Charney DS, Menkes DB, Heninger GR (1981) Receptor sensitivity and the mechanism of action of antidepressant treatment: implications for the etiology and therapy of depression, *Arch Gen Psychiatry* **38**:1160–1180.

Cooper BR, Wang CM, Cox RF, et al (1994) Evidence that the acute behavioral and electrophysiological effects of bupropion (Wellbutrin) are mediated by a noradrenergic mechanism, *Neuropsychopharmacol* **11**:133–141.

Cusack B, Nelson A, Richelson E, et al (1994) Binding of antidepressants to human brain receptors: focus on newer generation compounds, *Psychopharmacology (Berlin)* **114**:559–565.

Dahl SG (1986) Plasma level monitoring of antipsychotic drugs, *Clin Pharmacokinet* **11**:36–61.

Davidson JRT (1994/1995) Sexual dysfunction and antidepressants, *Depression* **2**:233–240.

Davis R, Wilde MI (1996) Mirtazapine. A review of its pharmacology and therapeutic potential in the management of major depression, *CNS Drugs* **5**:389–402.

de Oliveira IR, Do Prado-Lima PAS, Samuel-Lajeunesse B (1989) Monitoring of tricyclic antidepressant plasma levels and clinical response: a review of the literature. Part 1 *Psychiatry Psychobiol* **4**:43–60.

deBoer T (1996) The pharmacologic profile of mirtazapine, *J Clin Psychiatry* **57**(suppl 4):19–25.

deBoer T, Ruigt GSF, Berendsen HHG (1995) The alpha-2 selective adrenoceptor antagonist Org 3770 (mirtazapine, remeron) enhances noradrenergic and serotonergic transmission, *Hum Psychopharmacol* **10**:S107–S118.

Dechant KL, Clissold SP (1991) Paroxetine: a review of its pharmacodynamic and pharmacokinetic properties, and therapeutic potential in depressive illness, *Drugs* **41**:225–253.

Delgado PL, Price LH, Miller HL (1991) Rapid serotonin depletion as a provocative challenge test for patients with major depression: relevance to antidepressant action and the neurobiology of depression, *Psychopharmacol Bull* **27**:321–330.

Delgado PL, Price LH, Miller HL, et al (1994) Serotonin and the neurobiology of depression, *Arch Gen Psychiatry* **51**:865–874.

Di Mascio M, Esposito E (1997) The degree of inhibition of dopaminergic neurons in the ventral tegmental area induced by selective serotonin re-uptake inhibitors is a function of the density-power spectrum of the interspike interval, *Neurosci* **79**(4):957–961.

Dubovsky SL (1994) Beyond the serotonin re-uptake inhibitors: rationales for the development of new serotonergic agents, *J Clin Psychiatry* **55**(2,suppl): 34–44.

Duman RS, Heninger GR, Nestler EJ (1997) A molecular and cellular theory of depression, *Arch Gen Psychiatry* **54**:597–606.

Duman RS, Nestler EJ (1995) Signal transduction pathways for catecholamine receptors. In: Meltzer H, ed. *Psychopharmacology: the fourth generation of progress.* New York, NY: Raven Press:303–320.

Duman RS, Vaidya VA, Nibuya M, et al (1995) Stress, antidepressant treatments, and neurotrophic factors: molecular and cellular mechanisms, *Neuroscientist* **1**:351–360.

Edwards JG, Goldie A, Papayanni-Papasthatis S (1989) Effects of paroxetine on the electrocardiogram, *Psychopharmacol* **97**:96–98.

Fisch C (1985) Effect of fluoxetine on the electrocardiogram, *J Clin Psychiatry* **46**(3,sec 2):42–44.

Frank E, Kupfer DJ, Perel JM, et al (1993) Comparison of full-dose versus half-dose pharmacotherapy in the maintenance treatment of recurrent depression, *J Affect Dis* **27**:139–145.

Frazer A (1997) Antidepressants, *J Clin Psychiatry* **58**(suppl 6):9–25.

Frazer A (1997) Pharmacology of antidepressants, *J Clin Psychopharmacol* **17**(suppl 1):2S–18S.

Fulton B, Benfield P (1996) Moclobemide: an update of its pharmacological properties and therapeutic use, *Drugs* **52**(3, Sept):450–474.

Gardner EA, Johnston JA (1985) Bupropion: an antidepressant without sexual pathophysiological action, *J Clin Psychopharmacol* **5**:24–29.

Giardina EGV, Barnard JT, Johnson LL, et al (1986) The anti-arrhythmic effect of nortriptyline in cardiac patients with ventricular premature depolarizations, *J Am Coll Cardiol* **7**:1363–1369.

Giardina EGV, Cooper TB, Suckow RF, et al (1987) Cardiovascular effects of doxepin in cardiac patients with ventricular arrhythmias, *Clin Pharmacol Ther* **42**:20–27.

Glassman AH, Bigger JT Jr (1981) Cardiovascular effects of therapeutic doses of tricyclic antidepressants: a review, *Arch Gen Psychiatry* **38**:815–820.

Golden RN, DeVane CL, Laizure SC, et al (1988) Bupropion in depression, II: the role of metabolites in clinical outcome, *Arch Gen Psychiatry* **45**:145–149.

Grimsley SR, Jann MW (1992) Paroxetine, sertraline, and fluvoxamine: new selective serotonin re-uptake inhibitors, *Clin Pharm* **11**:930–957.

Guentert TW, Mayersohn M (1994) Clinical-pharmacokinetic profile of moclobemide and its comparison with other MAO-inhibitors, *Rev Contemp Pharmacother* **5**:19–34.

Guy S, Silke B (1990) The electrocardiogram as a tool for therapeutic monitoring: a critical analysis, *J Clin Psychiatry* **51**(12, suppl B):37–39.

Haria M, Fitton A, McTavish D (1994) Trazodone: a review of its pharmacology, therapeutic use in depression and therapeutic potential in other disorders, *Drugs & Aging* **4**(4):331–355.

Harris MG, Benfield P (1995) Fluoxetine: a review of its pharmacodynamic and pharmacokinetic properties, and therapeutic use in older patients with depressive illness, *Drugs & Aging* **6**(1):64–84.

Herman JB, Brotman AW, Pollack MH, et al (1990) Fluoxetine-induced sexual dysfunction, *J Clin Psychiatry* **51**:25–27.

Holliday SM, Benfield P (1995) Venlafaxine: a review of its pharmacology and therapeutic potential in depression, *Drugs* **49**(2):280–294.

Hudson CJ, Young LT, Li PP, et al (1993) CNS signal transduction in the pathophysiology and pharmacotherapy of affective disorders and schizophrenia, *Synapse* **13**:278–293.

Jackson WK, Roose SP, Glassman AH (1987) Cardiovascular toxicity and tricyclic antidepressants, *Biomed Pharmacother* **41**:377–382.

Kalus O, Asnis GM, Van Praag HM (1989) The role of serotonin in depression, *Psychiatr Ann* **19**:348–353.

Kang H, Schuman EM (1995) Long-lasting neurotrophin-induced enhancement of synaptic transmission in the adult hippocampus, *Science* **267**:1658–1662.

Kasper S (1995) Clinical efficacy of mirtazapine: a review of meta-analyses of pooled data, *Int Clin Psychopharmacol* **10**(suppl 4):25–35.

Khan MC (1995) A randomised, double-blind, placebo-controlled 5–weeks' study of Org 3770 (mirtazapine) in major depression, *Hum Psychopharmacol* **10**:S119–S124.

Kuhs H, Rudolf GAE (1990) Cardiovascular effects of paroxetine, *Psychopharmacol* **102**:379–382.

Kupfer DJ, Frank E, Perel JM, et al (1992) Five-year outcome for mainte-– nance therapies in recurrent depression, *Arch Gen Psychiatry* **49**:769–773.

Laird, LK, Lydiard RB, Morton WA, et al (1993) Cardiovascular effects of imipramine, fluvoxamine, and placebo in depressed outpatients, *J Clin Psychiatry* **54**:224–228.

Lenox RH, Watson DG, Patel J, et al (1992) Chronic lithium administration alters a prominent PKC substrate in rat hippocampus, *Brain Res* **570**:333–340.

Levine ES, Dreyfus CF, Black IB, et al (1995) Brain-derived neurotrophic factor rapidly enhances transmission in hippocampal neurons via postsynaptic tyrosine kinase receptors, *Proc Natl Acad Sci USA* **92**:8074–8077.

Li PP, Sibony D, Green MA, et al (1993) Lithium modulation of phosphoinositide signaling system in rat cortex: selective effect on phorbol ester binding, *J Neurochem* **61**:1722–1730.

Lo DC (1995) Neurotrophic factors and synaptic plasticity, *Neuron* **15**:979–981.

Lund J, Thayssen P, Mengel H, et al (1982) Paroxetine: pharmacokinetics and cardiovascular effects after oral and intravenous single doses in man, *Acta Pharmacol Toxicol (Copenh)* **51**:351–357.

Maguire KP, Norman TR, Burrows GD, et al (1982) A pharmacokinetic study of mianserin, *Eur J Clin Pharmacol* **21**:517–520.

Magyar K, Szende B, Lengyel J, et al (1996) The pharmacology of B-type selective monoamine oxidase inhibitors; milestones in (()-deprenyl research, *J Neural Transm* **48**(suppl):29–43.

Mamounas LA, Blue ME, Siuciak JA, et al (1995) BDNF promotes the survival and sprouting of serotonergic ain the rat brain, *J Neurosci* **15**:7929–7939.

Manji HK, Etcheberrigaray R, Chen G, et al (1993) Lithium decreases membrane- associated protein kinase C in hippocampus: selectivity for the a isozyme, *J Neurochem* **61**:2303–2310.

Manji HK, Potter WZ, Lenox RH (1995) Signal transduction pathways: molecular targets for lithium's actions, *Arch Gen Psychiatry* **52**:531–543.

Menkes DB, Rasenick MM, Wheeler MA, et al (1983) Guanosine triphosphate activation of brain adenylate cyclase: enhancement by long-term antidepressant treatment, *Science* **129**:65–67.

Meyer TE, Habener JF (1993) Cyclic adenosine 3',5'-monophosphate response element-binding protein (CREB) and related transcription-activating deoxyribonucleic acid-binding proteins, *Endocr Rev* **14**:269–290.

Miller HL, Delgado PL, Salomon RM, et al (1996) Clinical and biochemical effects of catecholamine depletion on antidepressant- induced remission of depression, *Arch Gen Psychiatry* **53**:117–128.

Montgomery SA (1995) Safety of mirtazapine: a review, *Int Clin Psychopharmacol* **10**(suppl 4):37–45.

Montgomery SA, Henry J, McDonald G, et al (1994) Selective serotonin re-uptake inhibitors: meta-analysis of discontinuation rates, *Int Clin Psychopharmacol* **9**:47–53.

Morton WA, Sonne SC, Verga MA (1995) Venlafaxine: a structurally unique and novel antidepressant, *Ann Pharmacother* **29**:387–395.

Nakamura S (1990) Antidepressants induce regeneration of catecholaminergic axon terminals in the rat cerebral cortex, *Neurosci Lett* **111**:64–68.

Nelson JC (1997) Safety and tolerability of the new antidepressants, *J Clin Psychiatry* **58**(suppl 6):26–31.

Nemeroff CB (1994) Evaluation of new drugs: the clinical pharmacology and use of paroxetine, a new selective serotonin re-uptake inhibitor, *Pharmacother* **14**(2):127–138.

Nemeroff CB, De Vane CL, Pollock BG (1996) Newer antidepressants and the cytochrome P450 system, *Am J Psychiatry* **153**:311–320.

Nibuya M, Nestler EJ, Duman RS (1996) Chronic antidepressant administration increases the expression of cAMP response element-binding protein (CREB) in rat hippocampus, *J Neurosci* **16**:2365–2372.

Nierenberg AA, Amsterdam JD (1990) Treatment-resistant depression: definition and treatment approaches, *J Clin Psychiatry* **51**(suppl 6):39–47.

Nolen WA, Haffmans J (1989) Treatment resistant depression. Review of the efficacy of various biological treatments, specifically in major depression resistant to cyclic antidepressants, *Int Clin Psychopharmacol* **4**:217–228.

Nomikos GG, Damsma G, Wenkstern D, et al (1989) Acute effects of bupropion on extracellular dopamine concentrations in rat striatum and nucleus accumbens studied by in vivo microdialysis, *Neuropsychopharmacol* **2**:273–279.

Nutt, DJ, Glue, P. (1989) Monoamine oxidase inhibitors: rehabilitation from recent research? *British Journal of Psychiatry*, **154**:287–291.

Nutt, DJ, Pinder, RM. (1996) α_2-adrenoceptors and depression. Eds: E Szabadi, RM Pinder. *Supplement to J Psychopharmacology* **10**(3):35–42.

Potter WZ (1996) Adrenoceptors and serotonin receptor function: relevance to antidepressant mechanisms of action, *J Clin Psychiatry* **57**(suppl 4):4–8.

Preskorn SH (1993) Pharmacokinetics of antidepressants: why and how they are relevant to treatment, *J Clin Psychiatry* **54**(9, suppl):14–34.

Preskorn SH (1995) Comparison of the tolerability of bupropion, fluoxetine, imipramine, nefazodone, paroxetine, sertraline and venlafaxine, *J Clin Psychiatry* **56**(suppl 6):12–21.

Preskorn SH, Fast GA (1991) Therapeutic drug monitoring for antidepressants: efficacy, safety and cost effectiveness, *J Clin Psychiatry* **52**(6,suppl):23–33.

Preskorn, SH (1997) Clinically relevant pharmacology of selective serotonin re-uptake inhibitors: an overview with emphasis on pharmacokinetics and effects on oxidative drug metabolism, *Clin Pharmacokinet* **32**(suppl 1):1–21.

Richelson E (1994) The pharmacology of antidepressants at the synapse: focus on newer compounds, *J Clin Psychiatry* **55**(9,suppl A):34–39.

Riederer P, Konradi C, Hebenstreit G, et al (1989) Neurochemical perspectives to the function of monoamine oxidase, *Acta Neurol Scand* **126**:41–45.

Robinson DS, Roberts DL, Smith JM, et al (1996) The safety profile of nefazodone, *J Clin Psychiatry* **57**(suppl 2):31–38.

Roose SP, Dalack GW, Glassman AH, et al (1991) Cardiovascular effects of bupropion in depressed patients with heart disease, *Am J Psychiatry* **148**:512–516.

Roose SP, Glassman AH (1989) Cardiovascular effects of tricyclic antidepressants in depressed patients with and without heart disease, *J Clin Psychiatry Monograph* **7**(2):1–18.

Roose SP, Glassman AH (1994) Antidepressant choice in the patient with cardiac disease: lessons from the cardiac arrhythmia suppression trial (CAST) studies, *J Clin Psychiatry* **55**(9, suppl A):83–87.

Roose SP, Glassman AH, Giardina EGV, et al (1987) Tricyclic antidepressants in depressed patients with cardiac conduction disease, *Arch Gen Psychiatry* **44**:273–275.

Rudorfer MV, Manji HK, Potter WZ (1994) Comparative tolerability profiles of the newer versus older antidepressants, *Drug Saf* **10**:18–46.

Sedgwick EM, Cilasun J, Edwards JG (1987) Paroxetine and the electroencephalogram, *J Psychopharmacol* **1**:31–34.

Segraves RT (1992) Overview of sexual dysfunction complicating the treatment of depression, *J Clin Psychiatry Monograph* **19**:4–10.

Segraves RT (1992) Overview of sexual dysfunction complicating the treatment of depression, *J Clin Psychiatry Monograph* **10**(2):4–10.

Shami M, Elliot HL, Kelman AW, et al (1983) The pharmacokinetics of mianserin, *Br J Clin Pharmacol* **15**:313S–322S.

Sher M, Krieger NJ, Juergens S (1983) Trazodone and priapism, *Am J Psychiatry* **140**:1362–1363.

Sitsen JMA, Zivkov M (1995) Mirtazapine: clinical profile, *CNS Drugs* **4**(suppl 1):39–48.

Siuciak JA, Lewis D, Wiegand SJ, et al (1996) Antidepressant-like effect of brain-derived neurotrophic factor, *Pharmacol Biochem Behav* **56**:131–137.

Skerritt U, Evans R, Montgomery SA (1997 Mar.) Selective serotonin re-uptake inhibitors in older patients: a tolerability perspective, *Drugs & Aging* **10**(3):209–218.

Skowron DM, Stimmer GL (1992) Antidepressants and the risk of seizures, *Pharmacotherapy* **12**:18–22.

Spar JE (1987) Plasma trazodone concentrations in elderly depressed inpatients: cardiac effects and short-term efficacy, *J Clin Psychopharmacol* **7**:406–409.

Sternbach H (1991) The serotonin syndrome, *Am J Psychiatry* **148**:705–713.

Stimmel GL, Dopheide JA, Stahl SM (1997) Mirtazapine: an antidepressant with noradrenergic and specific serotonergic effects, *Pharmacotherapy* **17**(1):10–21.

Tanigaki N, Manno K, Sugihara K, et al (1987) Specific inhibitory action of a novel antidepressant paroxetine on 5–HT uptake, *Nippon Yakurigaku Zasshi* **89**:175–180.

Taylor DP, Carter RB, Eison AS, et al (1995) Pharmacology and neurochemistry of nefazodone: a novel antidepressant drug, *J Clin Psychiatry* **56**(suppl 6):3–11.

Tollefson GD (1991) Antidepressant treatment and side effect considerations, *J Clin Psychiatry* **52**:S4–S13.

Vohra J, Burrows GD, Hunt D, et al (1975) The effect of toxic and therapeutic doses of tricyclic antidepressant drugs on intracardiac conduction, *Eur J Cardiol* **3**:219–227.

Wachtel H (1983) Potential antidepressant activity of rolipram and other selective cyclic adenosine 3',5'-monophosphate phosphodiesterase inhibitors, *Neuropharmacol* **22**:267–272.

Warner MD, Peabody CA, Whiteford HA, et al (1987) Trazodone and priapism, *J Clin Psychiatry* **48**:244–245.

Warrington SJ (1991) Clinical implications of the pharmacology of sertraline, *Int Clin Psychopharmacol* **6**(suppl 2): 11–21.

Warrington SJ, Padgham C, Lader M (1989) The cardiovascular effects of antidepressants, *Psychol Med* **19**(suppl 16):1–40.

Youdim MBH, Finberg JPM (1990) New directions in monoamine oxidase A and B: selective inhibitors and substrates, *Biochem Pharmacol* **41**:155–162.

Zajecka J, Fawcett J, Schaff M, et al (1991) The role of serotonin in sexual dysfunction: fluoxetine-associated orgasm dysfunction, *J Clin Psychiatry* **52**:66–68.

3. Antipsychotics

Andersson JL, Marcus M, Svensson TH (1993) (1–Adrenoceptor antagonism modulates the changes in firing pattern and transmitter release induced by a selective dopamine (DA)-D2–antagonist in the mesolimbic but not in the nigrostriatal DA system, *Soc Neurosci Abstr* **19**:1374.

Ashby CR Jr., Wang RY (1990) Effects of antipsychotic drugs on 5–HT2 receptors in the medial prefrontal cortex: microiontophoretic studies, *Brain Res* **506**:346–348.

Bett JHN, Holt GW (1983) Malignant ventricular tachyarrhythmia and haloperidol, *Br Med J* **287**:1264.

Bolden-Watson C, Watson MA, Murray KD, al (1993) Haloperidol but not clozapine increases neurotensin receptor mRNA levels in rat substantia nigra, *J Neurochem* **61**: 1141–1143.

Breier A, Buchanan RW, Waltrip RW, et al (1993) Clozapine's superior efficacy is related to its noradrenergic properties, *Soc Neurosci Abstr* **19**:856.

Buckland PR, O'Donovan MC, McGuffin P (1993) Clozapine and sulpiride up-regulate dopamine-D(3) receptor messenger RNA levels, *Neuropharmacol* **32**:901–907.

Buvat J, Lemaire A, Buvat-Herbaut M, et al (1985) Hyperprolactinemia and sexual function in men, *Horm Res* **22**:196–203.

Byerly MJ, DeVane CL (1996) Pharmacokinetics of clozapine and risperidone: a review of recent literature, *J Clin Psychopharmacol* **16**:177–187.

Bymaster FP, Rasmussen K, Calligaro DO, et al (1997) In vitro and in vivo biochemistry of olanzapine: a novel, atypical antipsychotic drug, *J Clin Psychiatry* **58**(suppl 10):28–36.

Casey DE (1989) Clozapine: neuroleptic-induced EPS and tardive dyskinesia, *Psychopharmacol* (Berl) **99**:S47–S53.

Casey DE (1993) Serotonergic and dopaminergic aspects of neuroleptic-induced extrapyramidal syndromes in non-human primates, *Psychopharmacol* **112**(1,suppl):S55–S59.

Casey DE (1996) Side effect profiles of new antipsychotic agents, *J Clin Psychiatry* **57**(suppl 11):40–45.

Chakos MH, Lieberman JA, Alvir J, et al (1995) Caudate nuclei volumes in schizophrenic patients treated with typical antipsychotics or clozapine, *Lancet* **345**:456–457.

Coffey L (1994) Options for the treatment of negative symptoms of schizophrenia, *CNS Drugs* **1**:107–118.

Cohen BM, Keck PE, Satlin A, et al (1991) Prevalence and severity of akathisia in patients on clozapine, *Biol Psychiatry* **29**:1215–1219.

Cohen BM, Lipinski JF (1986) In vivo potencies of antipsychotic drugs in blocking alpha I noradrenergic and dopamine D2 receptors: implications for drug mechanisms of action, *Life Sci* **39**:2571–2580.

Dahl SG (1986) Plasma level monitoring of antipsychotic drugs, *Clin Pharmacokinet* **11**:36–61.

Davis KL, Kahn RS, Ko G, et al (1991) Dopamine in schizophrenia: a review and reconceptualization, *Am J Psychiatry* **148**:1474–1486.

Devinsky O, Honigfeld G, Patin J (1991) Clozapine-related seizures, *Neurology* **41**:369–371.

Dewey SL, Smith GS, Logan J, et al (1995) Serotonergic modulation of striatal dopamine measured with positron emission tomography (PET) and in vivo microdialysis, *J Neurosci* **15**:821–829.

Dubovsky SL, Thomas M (1995) Serotonergic mechanisms and current and future psychiatric practice, *J Clin Psychiatry* **56**:38–48.

Ellenbroek BA (1993) Treatment of schizophrenia: a clinical and preclinical evaluation of neuroleptic drugs, *Pharmacol Ther* **57**:1–78.

Ellenbroek BA, Prinssen EPM, Cools AR (1994) The role of serotonin receptor subtypes in the behavioural effects of neuroleptic drugs – a paw test study in rats, *Eur J Neurosci* **6**:1–8.

Ereshevsky L, Lacombe S (1993) Pharmacological profile of risperidone, *Can J Psychiatry* **38**(3, suppl):S80–S88.

Eshel G, Ross SB, Kelder D, et al (1990) Alpha-1 (but not alpha-2)-adrenoceptor agonists in combination with the dopamine D2 agonist quinpirole produce locomotor stimulation in dopamine-depleted mice, *Pharmacol Toxicol* **67**:123–131.

Esposito E, Pagannone S, Prisco S (1993) Serotonin-dopamine interaction in the rat ventral tegmental area: an electrophysiological study in vivo, *Soc Neurosci Abstr* **19**:1372.

Farde L, Nordstrom AL, Nyberg S, et al (1994) D1–,D2–, 5–HT2–receptor occupancy in clozapine-treated patients, *J Clin Psychiatry* **55**(suppl B):67–69.

Farde L, Nordstrom AL, Wiesel FA, et al (1992) Positron emission tomographic analysis of central D1 and D2 dopamine receptor occupancy in patients treated with classical neuroleptics and clozapine: relation to extrapyramidal side effects, *Arch Gen Psychiatry* **49**:538–544.

Fayer SA (1986) Torsades de pointes ventricular tachyarrhythmia associated with haloperidol, *J Clin Psychopharmacol* **6**:375–376.

Fitzgerald LW, Deutch AY, Gasic G, et al (1995) Regulation of cortical and subcortical glutamate receptor subunit expression by antipsychotic drugs, *J Neurosci* **15**(3 Pt 2):2453–2461.

Fowler NO, McCall D, Chou TC, et al (1976) Electrocardiographic changes and cardiac arrhythmias in patients receiving psychotropic drugs, *Am J Cardiol* **37**:223–230.

Gardos G, Cole JO (1977) Weight reduction in schizophrenics by molindone, *Am J Psychiatry* **134**:302–304.

Gerlach J (1991) New antipsychotics: classification, efficacy, and adverse effects, *Schizophr Bull* **17**:289–309.

Gerlach J, Peacock L (1995) New antipsychotics: the present status, *Int Clin Psychopharmacol* **10**:39–48.

Goff DC, Midha KK, Saridsegal O, et al (1995) A placebo-controlled trial of fluoxetine added to neuroleptic in patients with schizophrenia, *Psychopharmacol (Berl)* **117**:417–423.

Goldberg TE, Weinberger DR (1994) The effects of clozapine on neurocognition: an overview, *J Clin Psychiatry* **55**(suppl B): 88–90.

Goldstein JM (1995) Pre-clinical pharmacology of new atypical antipsychotics in late stage development, *Exp Opinion Invest Drugs* **4**:291–298.

Grace AA (1992) The depolarization block hypothesis of neuroleptic action: implications for the etiology and treatment of schizophrenia, *J Neural Transm Suppl* **36**:91–131.

Graham SR, Kokkinidis L (1993) Clozapine inhibits limbic system kindling: implications for antipsychotic action, *Brain Res Bull* **30**:597–605.

Gunne LM, Andren PE (1993) An animal model for coexisting tardive dyskinesia and tardive Parkinsonism -a glutamate hypothesis for tardive dyskinesia, *Clin Neuropharmacol* **16**:90–95.

Gupta SK, Mishra RK (1992) Effects of chronic treatment of haloperidol and clozapine on levels of G-protein subunits in rat striatum, *J Mol Neurosci* **3**:197–201.

Gygi SP, Gibb JW, Hanson GR (1994) Differential effects of antipsychotic and psychotomimetic drugs on neurotensin systems of discrete extrapyramidal and limbic regions, *J Pharmacol Exp Ther* **270**:192–197.

Hashimoto T, Kitamura N, Kajimoto Y, et al (1993) Differential changes in serotonin 5–HT(1A) and 5–HT(2) receptor binding in patients with chronic schizophrenia, *Psychopharmacol* **112**(1, suppl):S35–S39.

Hiroi N, Graybiel AM (1993) Typical and atypical neuroleptics stimulate contrasting patterns of neuropeptide and Fos/FRA expression in the striatum, *Soc Neurosci Abstr* **19**:129.

Hollister LE (1994) New psychotherapeutic drugs, *J Clin Psychopharmacol* **14**:50–63.

Hoyberg OJ, Fensbo C, Remvig J, et al (1993) Risperidone versus perphenazine in the treatment of chronic schizophrenic patients with acute exacerbations, *Acta Psychiatr Scand* **88**:395–402.

Hyttel J, Arnt J, Costall B, et al (1992) Pharmacological profile of the atypical neuroleptic sertindole, *Clin Neuropharmacol* **15**:267a-268a.

Hyttel J, Larsen JJ, Christensen AV, et al (1991) Receptor-binding profiles of neuroleptics, *Psychopharmacol Suppl* **2**:8509.

Ikeguchi K, Kuroda A (1995) Mianserin treatment of patients with psychosis induced by antiparkinsonian drugs, *Eur Arch Psychiatr Clin Neurosci* **244**:320–324.

Javitt DC, Zukin SR (1990) The role of excitatory amino acids in neuropsychiatric illness, *J Neuropsychiatr Clin Neurosci* **2**:44–52.

Jolicoeur FB, Gagne MA, Rivest R, et al (1993) Atypical neuroleptic-like behavioral effects of neurotensin, *Brain Res Bull* **32**:487–491.

Kapur S, Remington G (1996) Serotonin-dopamine interaction and its relevance to schizophrenia, *Am J Psychiatry* **153**:466–476.

Karler R, Calder LD, Thai LH, et al (1995) The dopaminergic, glutamatergic, GABAergic bases for the action of amphetamine and cocaine, *Brain Res* **671**:100–104.

Kemper AJ, Dunlap R, Pietro DA (1983) Thioridazine-induced torsades de pointes. Successful therapy with isoproterenol, *JAMA* **249**:2931–2934.

Kinkead B, Owens MJ, Nemeroff CB (1993) The effects of sertindole on regional CNS neurotensin concentrations in the rat brain, *Soc Neurosci Abstr* **19**:856.

Kinon BJ, Lieberman JA (1996) Mechanisms of action of atypical antipsychotic drugs: a critical analysis, *Psychopharmacol* **124**:2–34.

Kriwisky M, Perry GY, Tarchitsky D, et al (1990) Haloperidol-induced torsades de pointes, *Chest* **98**:482–484.

Kronig MH, Munne RA, Szymanski S, et al (1995) Plasma clozapine levels and clinical response for treatment-refractory schizophrenic patients, *Am J Psychiatry* **152**:179–182.

Krupp P, Barnes P (1992) Clozapine-associated agranulocyt: risk and aetiology, *Br J Psychiatry* **160**(suppl 17):38–40.

Lader M (1988) Beta-adrenoceptor antagonists in neuropsychiatry: an update, *J Clin Psychiatry* **49**:213–223.

Lang A, Vasar E, Soosaar A, et al (1992) The involvement of sigma and phencyclidine receptors in the action of antipsychotic drugs, *Pharmacol Toxicol* **71**:132–138.

Lappalainen J, Hietala J, Koulu M, et al (1990) Neurochemical effects of chronic co-administration of ritanserin and haloperidol: comparison with clozapine effects, *Eur J Pharmacol* **190**:403–407.

Lawrence KR, Nasraway SA (1997) Conduction disturbances associated with administration of butyrophenone antipsychotics in the critically ill: a review of the literature, *Pharmacotherapy* **17**(3):531–537.

Leysen JE, Janssen PMF, Schotte A, et al (1993) Interaction of antipsychotic drugs with neurotransmitter receptor sites in vitro and in vivo in relation to pharmacological and clinical effects: role of 5HT2 receptors, *Psychopharmacol (Berl)* **112**:S40–S54.

Leysen JE, Megens AAHH, Janssen PMF, et al (1994) Finely balanced 5HT2/D2–antagonism: a crucial factor for the treatment of schizophrenia (abstract), *Neuropsychopharmacol* **10**(3S, part 1):467S.

Litwin LC, Goldstein JM (1994) Effects of neurotensin on mid-brain dopamine neuronal activity, *Drug Dev Res* **32**:6–12.

Marder SR, Meibach RC (1994) Risperidone in the treatment of schizophrenia, *Am J Psychiatry* **151**:825–835.

Meltzer H (1991) The mechanism of action of novel atypical antipsychotic drugs, *Schizophr Bull* **17**:262–287.

Meltzer HY, Matsubara S, Lee JC (1989) Classification of typical and atypical antipsychotic drugs on the basis of dopamine D-1, D-2 and serotonin2 pKi values, *J Pharmacol Exp Ther* **251**:238–246.

Meltzer HY, Matsubara S, Lee J-C (1989a) The ratios of serotonin2 and dopamine2 affinities differentiate atypical and typical antipsychotic drugs, *Psychopharmacol Bull* **25**:390–392.

Merchant KM, Dorsa DM (1993) Differential induction of neurotensin and c-fos gene expression by typical versus atypical antipsychotics, *Proc Natl Acad Sci USA* **90**:3447–3451.

Metzger E, Friedman R (1993) Prolongation of the corrected QT interval and torsades de pointes cardiac arrhythmia associated with intravenous haloperidol in the medically ill, *J Clin Psychopharmacol* **13**:128–132.

Migler BA, Warawa EJ, Malick JB (1993) Seroquel: behavioral effects in conventional and novel tests for atypical antipsychotic drugs, *Psychopharmacol* **112**:299–307.

Moghaddam B, Bunney BS (1990) Acute effects of typical and atypical antipsychotic drugs on the release of dopamine from prefrontal cortex, nucleus accumbens, and striatum of the rat: an in vivo micro-dialysis study, *J Neurochem* **54**:1755–1760.

Moore NA, Leander JD, Benvenga MJ, et al (1997) Behavioral pharmacology of olanzapine: a novel antipsychotic drug, *J Clin Psychiatry* **58**(suppl 10):37–44.

Muller-Spahn F (1992) Risperidone in the treatment of chronic schizophrenic patients: an international double-blind parallel-group study versus haloperidol (International Risperidone Research Group), *Clin Neuropharmacol* **15**(suppl 1, part A): 90A-91A.

Nutt, DJ. (1994) Putting the 'A' in atypical: does α₂ adrenoceptor antagonism account for the therapeutic advantage of new antipsychotics. *J Psychopharmacology* **8**(4):193–195.

Ogren SO, Archer T (1994) Effects of typical and atypical antipsychotic drugs on two-way active avoidance – relationship to dopamine receptor blocking profile, *Psychopharmacol* **114**:383–391.

Ohuoha DC, Hyde TM, Kleinman JE (1993) The role of serotonin in schizophrenia: an overview of the nomenclature, distribution and alterations of serotonin receptors in the central nervous system, *Psychopharmacol (Berl)* **112**(suppl 1): S5–S15.

Peuskens J (1995) Risperidone in the treatment of patients with chronic schizophrenia: a multi-national, multi-centre, double-blind, parallel-group study versus haloperidol, *Br J Psychiatry* **166**:712–726.

Pilowsky LS, Costa DC, Ell PJ, et al (1992) Clozapine, single photon emission tomography, and the D2 dopamine receptor blockade hypothesis of schizophrenia, *Lancet* **340**:199–202.

Ramirez OA, Wang RY (1986) Locus coeruleus norepinephrine-containing neurons: effects produced by acute and subchronic treatment with antipsychotic drugs and amphetamine, *Brain Res* **362**:165–170.

Rao ML, Moller HJ (1994) Biochemical findings of negative symptoms in schizophrenia and their putative relevance to pharmacologic treatment: a review, *Neuropsychobiology* **30**:160–172.

Reddig S, Minnema AM, Tandon R (1993) Neuroleptic malignant syndrome and clozapine, *Ann Clin Psychiatry* **5**:25–27.

Richelson E (1984) Neuroleptic affinities for human brain receptors and their use in predicting adverse effects, *J Clin Psychiatry* **45**:331–336.

Richelson E (1996) Pre-clinical pharmacology of neuroleptics: focus on new generation compounds, *J Clin Psychiatry* **57**(suppl 11):4–11.

Robertson GS, Fibiger HC (1992) Neuroleptics increase c-fos expression in the forebrain: contrasting effects of haloperidol and clozapine, *Neurosci* **46**:315–328.

Roth BL, Craigo SC, Choudhary MS, et al (1994) Binding of typical and atypical antipsychotic agents to (5–hydroxytryptamine)6 and (5–hydroxytryptamine)7 receptors, *J Pharmacol Exp Ther* **268**:1403–1410.

Saller CF, Czupryna MJ, Salama AI (1990) 5–HT2 receptor blockade by ICI 169,369 and other 5–HT2 antagonists modulates the effects of D-2 dopamine receptor blockade, *J Pharmacol Exp Ther* **253**:1162–1170.

Saller CF, Salama AL (1993) Seroquel: biochemical profile of a potential atypical antipsychotic, *Psychopharmacol (Berl)* **112**:285–292.

Sanchez C, Arnt J, Dragsted N, et al (1991) Neurochemical and in vivo pharmacological profile of sertindole, a limbic-selective neuroleptic compound, *Drug Development and Research* **22**:239–250.

Seeger TF, Seymour PA, Schmidt AW, et al (1995) Ziprasidone (CP-88059): a new antipsychotic with combined dopamine and serotonin receptor antagonist activity, *Pharmacol Exp Ther* **275**:101–113.

Stanton JM (1995) Weight gain associated with neuroleptic medication: a review, *Schizophr Bull* **21**:463–472.

Stockmeier CA, DiCarlo JJ, Zhang Y, et al (1993) Characterization of typical and atypical antipsychotic drugs based on in vivo occupancy of serotonin2 and dopamine2 receptors, *J Pharmacol Exp Ther* **266**:1374–1384.

Stockton ME, Rasmussen K (1996) Electrophysiological effects of olanzapine, a novel atypical antipsychotic on A9 and A10 dopamine neurons, *Neuropsychopharmacol* **14**:97–104.

Tran PV, Dellva MA, Tollefson GD, et al (1997) Extrapyramidal symptoms and tolerability of olanzapine vs haloperidol in the acute treatment of schizophrenia, *J Clin Psychiatry* **58**:205–211.

VanTol HHM, Bunzow JR, Guan H, et al (1991) Cloning of the gene for a human dopamine D receptor with high affinity for the antipsychotic clozapine, *Nature* **350**:610–614.

Webster P, Wijerame C (1994) Risperidone-induced neuroleptic malignant syndrome, *Lancet* **344**:1228–1229.

Webster P, Wijeratne C (1994) Risperidone-induced neuroleptic malignant syndrome, *Lancet* **344**:1228–1229.

White FJ, Wang RY (1983) Differential effects of classical and atypical antipsychotic drugs on A9 and A10 dopamine neurons, *Science* **221**:1054–1057.

Zorn SH, Jones SB, Ward KM, et al (1994) Clozapine is a potent and selective muscarinic M(4) receptor agonist, *Eur J Pharmacol* **269**:R1–R2.

4. Anxiolytics

Adam K, Oswald I (1989) Can a rapidly-eliminated hypnotic cause daytime anxiety? *Pharmacopsychiatry* **22**:115–119.

Arendt RM, Greenblatt DJ, Liebisch DC, et al (1987) Determinants of benzodiazepine uptake: lipophilicity versus binding affinity, *Psychopharmacol* **93**:72–76.

Bell J, Bickford-Wimer PD, de la Garza R, et al (1988) Increased central noradrenergic activity during benzodiazepine withdrawal: an electro-physiological study, *Neuropharmacol* **27**:1187–1190.

Bernstein JG (ed) (1988) Anti-anxiety agents and hypnotics. In: *Drug Therapy in Psychiatry*, ed 2, Littleton, Massachusetts, PSG Publishing Company Inc: 51–77.

Gallager DW, Heninger K, Heninger G (1986) Periodic benzodiazepine antagonist administration prevents benzodiazepine withdrawal symptoms in primates, *Eur J Pharmacol* **132**:31–38.

Golden RN, Brown TM, Tancer ME, et al (1989) Effects of beta-adrenergic blockade on effortful and effortless cognition, *Biol Psychiatry* **25**:130–134.

Gorman JM, Liebowitz MR, Fyer AJ, et al (1989) A neuroanatomical hypothesis for panic disorder, *Am J Psychiatry* **146**:148–161.

Grantham P (1987) Benzodiazepine abuse, *Br J HospitMedicine* **9**:292–300.

Greenblatt DJ (1992) Pharmacology of benzodiazepine hypnotics, *J Clin Psychiatry* **53**:7–13.

Greenblatt DJ, Harmatz JS, Engelhardt N, et al (1989) Pharmacokinetic determinants of dynamic differences among three benzodiazepine hypnotics: flurazepam, temazepam, and triazolam, *Arch Gen Psychiatry* **46**:326–332.

Greenblatt DJ, Shader RI, Abernethy DR (1983) Current status of benzodiazepines, *N Engl J Med* **309**:354–358, 410–416.

Lister RG, Weingartner H, Eckhardt MJ, et al (1988) Clinical relevance of effects of benzodiazepines on learning and memory, *Psychopharmacol* **6**:117–127.

Malizia, Al, Cunningham, VJ, Bell, Cm, Liddle, Pf, Jones, T, Nutt, DJ (1998) Decreased brain GABAₐ-benzodiazepine receptor binding in panic disorder: preliminary results from a quantitative PET study. *Archives Gen Psychiatry* **55**:715–720.

Malizia, AL, Nutt, DJ (1995) Psychopharmacology of benzodiazepines – an update. *Human Psychopharmacology* **10**:S1–S14.

Malazia, AL, Nutt, DJ (1995) The effects of flumazenil in neuropsychiatric disorders. *Clinical Neuropharmacology* **18**(3):215–232.

Miller LG, Greenblatt DJ, Barnhill JG, et al (1988) Chronic benzodiazepine administration. I. Tolerance is associated with benzodiazepine receptor downregulation and decreased (-aminobutyric acidA receptor function, *J Pharmacol Exp Ther* **246**:170–176.

Miller LG, Greenblatt DJ, Paul SM, et al (1987) Benzodiazepine receptor occupancy in vivo: correlation with brain concentrations and pharmacodynamic actions, *J Pharmacol Exp Ther* **240**:516–522.

Monti JM (1989) Effect of zolpidem on sleep in insomnia patients, *Eur J Clin Pharmacol* **36**:461–466.

Munjack DJ, Crocker B, Cabe D, et al (1989) Alprazolam, propranolol, and placebo in the treatment of panic disorder and agoraphobia with panic attacks, *J Clin Psychopharmacol* **9**:22–27.

Murphy SM, Owen R, Tyrer P (1989) Comparative assessment of efficacy and withdrawal symptoms after 6 and 12 weeks' treatment with diazepam or buspirone, *Br J Psychiatry* **154**:529–534.

Noyes R, Gravey MJ, Cook BL, et al (1988) Benzodiazepine withdrawal: a review of the evidence, *J Clin Psychiatry* **49**:382.

Nutt DJ, Glue P (1989) Clinical pharmacology of anxiolytics and antidepressants: a psychopharmacological perspective. *Pharmacology and Therapeutics* **44**:309–334.

Nutt DJ (1990) The pharmacology of human anxiety. *Pharmacology and Therapeutics* **47**:233–266.

Nutt DJ, Lawson CW (1992) Panic attacks: a neurochemical overview of models and mechanisms. *British Journal of Psychiatry* **160**:165–178.

Nutt DJ (1996) The psychopharmacology of anxiety. *Br J Hospital Medicine* **55**(4): 187–191.

Nutt DJ, Wilson SJ (1997) Treating insomnia with hypnotic drugs. *Prescriber* 37–44.

Nutt DJ, Bell C (1998) Serotonin and panic disorder. *Br J Psychiatry* **172**:465–471.

Owen RT, Tyrer P (1983) Benzodiazepine dependence: a review of the evidence, *Drugs* **25**:385–398.

Pecknold JC, Swinson RP, Kuch K, et al (1988) Alprazolam in panic disorder and agoraphobia: results from a multi-center trial. III. Discontinuation effects, *Arch Gen Psychiatry* **45**:429–436.

Rickels K, Schweizer E, Cse WG, et al (1990) Long-term therapeutic use of benzodiazepines. I. Effects of abrupt discontinuation, *Arch Gen Psychiatry* **47**:899–907.

Rickels K. Schweizer E, Weiss S, et al (1993) Maintenance drug treatment for panic disorder. II. Short- and long-term outcome after drug taper, *Arch Gen Psychiatry* **50**:61–68.

Scharf MB, Fletcher K, Graham JP (1988) Comparative amnesic effects of benzodiazepine hypnotic agents, *J Clin Psychiatry* **49**:134–137.

Shader, RI, Greenblatt DJ (1993) Use of benzodiazepines in anxiety disorders, *N Engl J Med* **328**(19):1398–1405.

Vgontzas AN, Kales A, Bixler EO (1995) Benzodiazepine side effects: role of pharmacokinetics and pharmacodynamics, *Pharmacol* **51**:205–223.

Wilkinson G, Balestrieri M, Ruggeri M, et al (1991) Meta-analysis of double-blind placebo-controlled trials of antidepressants and benzodiazepines for patients with panic disorders, *Psychol Med* **21**:991–998.

Woods JH, Katz JL, Winger G (1987) Abuse liability of benzodiazepines, *Pharmacol Rev.* **39**:251–419.

Woods JH, Katz JL, Winger G (1988) Use and abuse of benzodiazepines, *JAMA* **260**:3476.

Woods JH, Katz JL, Winger G (1992) Benzodiazepines: use, abuse, and consequences, *Pharmacol Rev* **44**:151–347.

Woods JH, Winger G (1995) Current benzodiazepine issues, *Psychopharmacol* **118**:107–115.

5. Selected adrenergic drugs

Golden RN, Brown TM, Tancer ME, et al (1989) Effects of beta-adrenergic blockade on effortful and effortless cognition, *Biol Psychiatry* **25**:130–134.

Hollander E, McCarley A (1992) Yohimbine treatment of sexual side effects induced by serotonin re-uptake blockers, *J Clin Psychiatry* **53**:207–209.

Morales A, Condra M, Owen JA, et al (1989) Is yohimbine effective in the treatment of organic impotence? Results from a controlled trial, *J Urology* **137**:1168–1172.

Reid K, Morales A, Harris C, et al (1987) Double-blind trial of yohimbine in treatment of psychogenic impotence, *Lancet* **2**:421–422.

6. Miscellaneous drugs

Alford C, Rombaut N, Jones J, et al (1992) Acute effects of hydroxyzine on nocturnal sleep and sleep tendency the following day: a C-EEG study, *Hum Psychopharmacol* **7**:25–35.

Blessed G, Tomlinson BE, Roth M (1968) The association between quantitative measures of dementia and of senile change in the cerebral gray matter of elderly subjects, *Br J Psychiatry* **114**:797.

Gauthier S, Bouchard R, Lamontagne A, et al (1990) Tetrahydroaminoacridine-lecithin combination treatment in patients with intermediate-stage Alzheimer's disease: results of a Canadian double-blind crossover, multicenter study, *N Engl J Med* **322**:1272.

Gengo FM, Dabronzo J, Yurchak A, et al (1987) The relative antihistaminic and psychomotor effects of hydroxyzine and cetirizine, *Clin Pharmacol Ther* **42**:265–272.

Hill SJ (1990) Distribution, properties, and functional characteristics of three classes of histamine receptor, *Pharmacol Rev* **42**:45–83.

Hollister LE (1975) Hydroxyzine hydrochloride: possible adverse cardiac interactions, *Psychopharmacol Commun* **1**:61–65.

Kay DWK (1989) Genetics, Alzheimer's disease and senile dementia, *Br J Psychiatry* **154**:311.

Levander S, Stahle-B?ckdahl M, H?germark O (1991) Peripheral antihistamine and central sedative effects of single and continuous oral doses of cetirizine and hydroxyzine, *Eur J Clin Pharmacol* **41**:435–439.

Pearce FL (1991) Biological effects of histamine: an overview, *Agents Actions* **33**:4–7.

Simons FER (1994) H1–receptor antagonists: comparative tolerability and safety, *Drug Safety* **10**:350–380.

Simons FER, Simons KJ (1994) The pharmacology and use of H1–receptor-antagonist drugs, *Drug Ther* **330**(23):1663–1669.

Simons KJ, Watson WTA, Martin TJ, et al (1990) Diphenhydramine: pharmacokinetics and pharmacodynamics in elderly adults, young adults, and children, *J Clin Pharmacol* **30**:665–671.

Simons KJ, Watson WTA, Chen XY, et al (1989) Pharmacokinetic and pharmacodynamic studies of the H1–receptor antagonist hydroxyzine in the elderly, *Clin Pharmacol Ther* **45**:9–14.

Singh KP, Pendse VK, Bhandari DS (1975) Cyproheptadine in ventricular arrhythmias, *Indian Heart J* **27**:120–126.

Whalley LJ (1989) Drug treatments of dementia, *Br J Psychiatry* **155**:595.

Woosley RL (1996) Cardiac actions of antihistamines, *Annu Rev Pharmacol Toxicol* **36**:233–252.

7. Drugs affecting sexual functioning

Agmo A, Gomez M (1993) Sexual reinforcement is blocked by infusion of naloxone into the medial preoptic area, *Behav Neurosci* **107**:812–818.

Agmo A, Picker Z (1990) Catecholamines and the initiation of sexual behavior in male rats without sexual experience, *Pharmacol Biochem Behav* **35**:327–334.

Ahlenius S, Hillegaart V, Hjorth S, et al (1991) Effects of sexual interactions on the in vivo rate of monoamine synthesis in forebrain regions of the male rat, *Behav Brain Res* **46**:117–122.

Aizenberg D, Shiloh R, Zemishlany Z, Weizman A (1996) Low-dose imipramine for thioridazine-induced male orgasmic disorder. *Sex Marital Ther* **22**:225–229

Aldridge SH (1982) Drug-induced sexual dysfunction, *Clin Pharmacol* **1**:141–147.

Ananth J (1982) Impotence associated with pimozide, *Amer J Psychiatry* **139**:1374.

Arendash GW, Gorski RA (1983) Effects of discrete lesions of the sexually dimorphic nucleus of the preoptic area or other medial preoptic regions on the sexual behavior of male rats, *Brain Res Bull* **10**:147–154.

Arnott S, Nutt D (1994) Successful treatment of fluvoxamine-induced anorgasmia by cyproheptadine, *Br J Psychiatry* **164**:838–839.

Assalian P (1988) Clomipramine in the treatment of premature ejaculation, *J Sex Res* **24**:213–215.

Balogh S, Hendricks SE, Kang J (1992) Treatment of fluoxetine-induced anorgasmia with amantadine (letter), *J Clin Psychiatry* **53**:212–213.

Balon R, Yeragani VK, Pohl R, et al (1993) Sexual dysfunction during antidepressant treatment, *J Clin Psychiatry* **54**:209–212.

Barfield RJ, Wilson C, McDonald PG (1975) Sexual behavior: extreme reduction of postejaculatory refractory period by midbrain lesions in male rats, *Science* **189**:147–149.

Benelli A, Arletti R, Basaglia R, et al (1993) Male sexual behavior: further studies on the role of alpha-2 antagonists, *Pharmacol Res* **28**:35–45.

Bitran D, Holmes G, Hull E, et al (1986) Dopaminergic regulation of male rat copulatory behavior: relative roles of pre- vs. post-synaptic dopamine receptors in the medial preoptic area, *Soc Neurosci Abstr* **12**:835.

Bloch GJ, Gorski RA (1988) Estrogen/progeterone treatment in adulthood affects the size of several components of the medial preoptic area in the male rat, *J Comp Neurol* **275**:613–622.

Bra, NL, Edwards DA (1984) Medial preoptic connections with midbrain tegmentum are essential for male sexual behavior, *Physiol Behav* **32**:79–84.

Buffum J (1982) Pharmacosexology: the effects of drugs on sexual function; a review, *J Psychoactive Drugs* **14**:5–44.

Buvat J, Lemaire A, Buvat-Herbaut M, et al (1985) Hyperprolactinemia and sexual function in men, *Horm Res* **22**:196–203.

Cohen AJ (1992) Fluoxetine-induced yawning and anorgasmia reversed by cyproheptadine treatment (letter), *J Clin Psychiatry* **53**:174.

Davidson JRT (1994/1995) Sexual dysfunction and antidepressants, *Depression* **2**:233–240.

DeGroat WC, Booth AM (1980) Physiology of male sexual function, *Annals of Internal Medicine* **92**:329–331.

DeLeo D, Magni G (1983) Sexual side effects of antidepressant drugs, *Psychosomatics* **24**:1076–1982.

Edwards DA, Einhorn LC (1986) Preoptic and midbrain control of sexual motivation, *Physiol Behav* **37**:329–335.

Feder R (1991) Reversal of antidepressant activity of fluoxetine by cyproheptadine in three patients, *J Clin Psychiatry* **52**:163–164.

Fernandez-Guasti A, Hansen S, Archer T, et al (1986) Noradrenaline-serotonin interactions in the control of sexual behavior in the male rat: DSP4–induced noradrenaline depletion antagonizes the facilitatory effect of serotonin receptor agonists, 5–MeODMT and lisuride, *Brain Res* **377**:112–118.

Fibiger HC, Phillips AG (1988) Mesocorticolimbic dopamine systems and reward, *Ann NY Acad Sci* **537**:206–215.

Gardner EA, Johnston JA (1985) Bupropion: an antidepressant without sexual pathophysiological action, *J Clin Psychopharmacol* **5**(1):24–29.

Genazzani AR, Trentini GP, Petraglia F, et al (1990) Estrogens modulate the circadian rhythm of hypothalamic beta-endorphin contents in female rats, *Neuroendocrinology* **52**:221–224.

Gitlin MJ (1994) Psychotropic medications and their effects on sexual function: diagnosis, biology, and treatment approaches, *J Clin Psychiatry* **55**:406–413.

Gitlin MJ (1995) Treatment of sexual side-effects with dopaminergic agents, *J Clin Psychiatry* **56**:124.

Gross MD (1982) Reversal by bethanechol of sexual dysfunction caused by anticholinergic antidepressants, *Am J Psychiatry* **139**:1193–1194.

Harrison WM, Rabkin JG, Ehrhardt AA, et al (1986) Effect of antidepressant medication on sexual function: a controlled study, *J Clin Psychopharmacol* **6**(3):144–149.

Harrison WM, Stewart J, Ehrhardt AA, et al (1985) A controlled study of the effects of antidepressants on sexual function, *Psychopharmacol Bull* **21**:85–88.

Hawkins CA, Everitt BJ, Herbert J (1988) The influence of steroid hormones on competing sexual and ingestive behavior in the male rat, *Physiol Behav* **44**:291–300.

Herman JB, Brotman AW, Pollack MH, et al (1990) Fluoxetine-induced sexual dysfunction, *J Clin Psychiatry* **51**:25–27.

Herman JB, Brotman HW, Pollack MH (1990) Fluoxetine-induced sexual dysfunction, *J Clin Psychiatry* **51**:25–27.

Hollander E, McCarley A (1992) Yohimbine treatment of sexual side effects induced by serotonin re-uptake blockers, *J Clin Psychiatry* **53**:207–209.

Hull EM, Eaton RC, Markowski VP, et al (1992) Opposite influence of medial preoptic D1 and D2 receptors on genital reflexes: implications for copulation, *Life Sci* **51**:1705–1713.

Hull EM, Warner RK, Bazzett TJ, et al (1989) D2/D1 ratio in the medial preoptic area affects copulation of male rats, *J Pharmacol Exp Ther* **251**:422–427.

Jani NN, Wise TN (1988) Antidepressants and inhibited female orgasm: a literature review, *J Sex Marital Ther* **14**(4):279.

Kogeorgos J, Alwis C (1986) Priapism and psychotropic medication, *Br J Psychiatry* **149**:241–243.

Kotin J, Wilbert DE, Verburg D, et al (1976) Thioridazine and sexual dysfunction, *Amer J Psychiatry* **133**:82–85.

Kowalski A, Stanley R, Dennerstein L, et al (1985) The sexual side effects of antidepressant medication: a double-blind comparison of two antidepressants in a nonpsychiatric population, *Br J Psychiatry* **147**:413–418.

Langub MCh, Watson RE (1992) Estrogen receptive neurons in the preoptic area of the rat are postsynaptic targets of a sexually dimorphic enkephalinergic fiber plexus, *Brain Res* **573**:61–69.

Marson L, McKenna KE (1992) A role for 5–hydroxytryptamine in descending inhibition of spinal sexual reflexes, *Exp Brain Res* **88**:313–320.

Mas M, Gonzalez-Mora JL, Louilot A, et al (1990) Increased dopamine release in the nucleus accumbens of copulating male rats as evidenced by in vivo voltametry, *Neurosci Lett* **110**:303–308.

McCormick S, Olin J, Brotman AW (1990) Reversal of fluoxetine-induced anorgasmia by cyproheptadine in two patients, *J Clin Psychiatry* **51**:383–384.

Melman A, Henry DP, Felten DL, et al (1980) Alteration of the penile corpora in patients with erectile impotence, *Investigative Urology* **17**:474–477.

Meston CM, Gorzalka BB (1992) Psychoactive drugs and human sexual behavior: the role serotonergic activity, *J Psychoactive Drugs* **24**:1–40.

Mitchell JB, Gratton A (1991) Opioid modulation and sensitization of dopamine release elicited by sexually relevant stimuli: a high-speed chronoamperometric study in freely behaving rats, *Brain Res* **551**:20–27.

Mitchell JE, Popkin MK (1982) Antipsychotic drug therapy and sexual dysfuntion in men, *Amer J Psychiatry* **139**:633–637.

Mitchell JE, Popkin MK (1983) Antidepressant drug therapy and sexual dysfuntion in men: a review, *J Clin Psychopharmacol* **3**:76–79.

Monteiro WO, Noshirvan HF, Marks IM, et al (1987) Anorgasmia from clomipramine in obsessive-compulsive disorder: a controlled trial, *Br J Psychiatry* **151**:107.

Morales A, Condra M, Owen JA, et al (1989) Is yohimbine effective in the treatment of organic impotence? Results from a controlled trial, *J Urology* **137**:1168–1172.

Neuman HF, Reiss H, Northrup JD (1982) Physical basis of emission, ejaculation and orgasm in the male, *Urology* **19**:341–350.

Norden MJ (1994) Buspirone treatment of sexual dysfunction associated with selective serotonin re-uptake inhibitors, *Depression* **2**:109–112.

Othmer E, Othmer SC (1987) Effect of buspirone on sexual dysfunction in patients with generalized anxiety disorder, *J Clin Psychiatry* **48**(5):201.

Pehek EA, Thompson JT, Hull EM (1989) The effects of intracranial administration of the dopamine agonist apomorphine on penile reflexes and seminal emission in the rat, *Brain Res* **500**:325–332.

Pollack MH, Reiter S, Hammerness P (1992) Genitourinary and sexual adverse effects of psychotropic medication, *Int'l J Psychiatry in Medicine* **22**(4):305–327.

Reid K, Morales A, Harris C, et al (1987) Double-blind trial of yohimbine in treatment of psychogenic impotence, *Lancet* **2**:421–422.

Reubens JR (1982) The physiology of normal sexual response in females, *J Psychoactive Drugs* **14**:45–46.

Rosenbaum JF, Pollack MH (1988) Anhedonic ejaculation with desipramine, *Int'l J Psychiatry and Med* **18**(1):85–88.

Schiavi RC, Segraves RT (1985) The biology of sexual function, *Psychiatr Clin North Am* **18**:7–24.

Schwartz MF, Bauman JE, Masters WH (1982) Hyperprolactinemia and sexual disorders in men, *Biol Psychiatry* **17**:861–876.

Segraves RT (1988) Psychiatric drugs and inhibited female orgasm, *J Sex Marital Ther* **14**(3):202.

Segraves RT (1988) Sexual side-effects of psychiatric drugs, *Int J Psychiatry Med* **18**(3):243.

Segraves RT (1992) Overview of sexual dysfunction complicating the treatment of depression, *J Clin Psychiatry Monograph* **10**(2):4–10.

Segraves RT (1993) Treatment-emergent sexual dysfunction in affective disorder: a review, *J Clin Psychiatry* (Monograph series) **11**:57–63.

Segraves, RT (1989) Effects of psychotropic drugs on human erection and ejaculation, *Arch Gen Psychiatry* **46**:275–284.

Shen WW, Sata LS (1990) Inhibited female orgasm resulting from psychotropic drugs: a five-year, updated, clinical review, *J Reprod Med* **35**(1):11.

Sher M, Krieger NJ, Juergens S (1983) Trazodone and priapism, *Am J Psychiatry* **140**:1362–1363.

Sorscher SM, Dilsaver SC (1986) Antidepressant-induced sexual dysfunction in men: due to cholinergic blockade? *J Clin Psychopharmacol* **6**:53–55.

Sovner R (1984) Treatment of tricyclic antidepressant-induced orgasmic inhibition with cyproheptadine, *J Clin Psychopharmacol* **4**:169.

Sullivan G (1988) Increased libido in three men treated with trazodone, *J Clin Psychiatry* **49**:202–203.

▪ Bibliography

Sullivan G, Lukoff D (1990) Sexual side effects of antipsychotic medication: evaluation and interv, *Hosp Community Psychiatry* **41**:1238–1241.

Thompson JW Jr, Ware MR, Blashfield RK (1990) Psychotropic medication and priapism: a comprehensive review, *J Clin Psychiatry* **51**:430–433.

van Furth WR, Wolterink G, van Ree JM (1995) Regulation of masculine sexual behavior: involvement of brain opioids and dopamine, *Brain Research Rev* **21**:162–184.

Warner MD, Peabody CA, Hollister HA, Whiteford HA, et al (1987) Trazodone and priapism, *J Clin Psychiatry* **48**(6):244–245.

Weiss HD (1972) The physiology of human penile erection, *Annals of Internal Medicine* **76**:793–799.

Wenkstern D, Pfaus JG, Fibiger HC (1993) Dopamine transmission increases in the nucleus accumbens of male rats during their first exposure to sexually receptive female rats, *Brain Res* **618**:41–46.

Wieland NG, Wise PM (1990) Estrogen and progesterone regulate opiate receptor densities in multiple brain regions, *Endocrinology* **126**:804–808.

Wise RA, Hoffman DC (1992) Localization of drug reward mechanisms by intracranial injections, *Synapse* **10**:247–263.

Zajecka J, Fawcett J, Schaff M, et al (1991) The role of serotonin in sexual dysfunction: fluoxetine-associated orgasm dysfunction, *J Clin Psychiatry* **52**(2):66–68.

Zarrindast MR, Mamanpush SH, Rashidy-pou A (1994) Morphine inhibits dopaminergic and cholinergic-induced ejaculation in rats, *Gen Pharmacol* **25**:803–808.

8. Other biological treatments

Butler MO, Morinobu S, Duman RS (1993) Chronic electroconvulsive seizures increase the expression of serotonin2 receptor mRNA in rat frontal cortex, *J Neurochem* **61**:1270–1276.

Nutt DJ, Gleiter CH, Glue P (1989) Neuropharmacological aspects of ECT: in serach of the primary mechanism of action. *Convulsive Therapy* **5**:250–260.

Ozawa H, Rasenick MM (1991) Chronic electroconvulsive treatment augments coupling of the GTP-binding protein GS to the catalytic moiety of adenylyl cyclase in a manner similar to that seen with chronic antidepressant drugs, *J Neurochem* **56**:330–338.

Terman M, Terman JS, Quitkin FM, et al (1989) Light therapy for seasonal affective disorder: a review of efficacy, *Neuropsychopharmacol* **2**:1–22.

Wirz-Justice A, Graw P, Kräuchi K, et al (1993) Light therapy in seasonal affective disorder is independent of time of day or circadian phase, *Arch Gen Psychiatry* **50**(12):929–937.

9–10   Abused substances

Albeck JH (1987) Withdrawal and detoxification from benzodiazepine dependence: a potential role for clonozepam, *J Clin Psychiatry* **48**:43.

Altman SJ, Everitt BJ, Glautier S, Markou A, Nutt DJ, Oretti R, Phillips GD, Robbins TW (1996) The biological, social and clinical bases of drug addiction: commentary and debate. *Psychopharmacology* **125**:285–345.

Aniline O, Pitts FN Jr (1981) Phencyclidine (PCP): a review and perspectives, *CRC Crit Rev Toxicol* **10**:145–177.

Benowitz NL (1988) Pharmacologic aspects of cigarette smoking and nicotine addiction, *N Engl J Med* **319**:1318–1330.

Benowitz NL (1991) Pharmacodynamics of nicotine: implications for rational treatment of nicotine addition, *Br J Addict* **86**:495–499.

Covey LS, Glassman AH (1991) A meta-analysis of double-blind placebo-controlled trials of clonidine for smoking cessation, *Br J Addict* **86**:991–998.

Fawcett J, Clark DC, Aagesen CA, et al (1987) A double-blind, placebo-controlled trial of lithium carbonate therapy for alcoholism, *Arch Gen Psychiatry* **44**:248–256.

Fibiger HC, Phillips AG (1988) Mesocorticolimbic dopamine systems and reward, *Ann NY Acad Sci* **537**:206–215.

Gawin FH, Ellinwood EH (1988) Cocaine and other stimulants, *N Engl J Med* **318**:1173.

Gawin FH, Kleber HD, Byck R, et al (1989) Desipramine facilitation of initial cocaine abstinence, *Arch Gen Psychiatry* **46**:117.

Giannini AJ, Folts DJ, Feather JN, et al (1989) Bromocriptine and amantadine in cocaine detoxification, *Psychiatry Res* **29**:11.

Glassman AH, Stetner F, Walsh BT, et al (1988) Heavy smokers, smoking cessation, and clonidine: results of a double-blind randomized trial, *JAMA* **259**:2862–2866.

Glue PW, Nutt DJ (1990) Overexcitement and disinhibition: dynamic neurotransmitter interactions in alcohol withdrawal. *British Journal of Psychiatry* **157**: 491–499.

Karler R, Calder LD, Thai LH, et al (1995) The dopaminergic, glutamatergic, GABAergic bases for the action of amphetamine and cocaine, *Brain Res* **671**:100–104.

Kosten TR (1989) Pharmacotherapeutic interventions for cocaine abuse: matching patients to treatments, *J Nerv Ment Dis* **177**:379.

Kosten TR, Morgan CJ, Kleber HD (1989) Buprenorphine treatment of cocaine abuse, *NIDA Res Monogr Ser* **95**:46.

Kraus ML, Gottleib LD, Horowitz RI, et al (1985) Randomized clinical trial of atenolol in patients with alcohol withdrawal, *N Engl J Med* **313**:905–909.

Lam WC, Sacks HS, Sze PC, et al (1987) Meta-analysis of randomised controlled trials of nicotine chewing-gum, *Lancet* **2**:27–30.

Ling W, Wesson DR (1990) Drugs of abuse – opiates, *West J Med* (special issue on addiction medicine) **152**:565–572.

Liskow BI, Goodwin DW (1987) Pharmacological treatment of alcohol intoxication, withdrawal and dependence: a critical review, *J Stud Alcohol* **48**:356–370.

Malcolm R, Ballenger JC, Sturgis ET, et al (1989) Double-blind controlled trial comparing carbamazepine to oxazepam treatment of alcohol withdrawal, *Am J Psychiatry* **146**:617–621.

Marlatt GA, Gordon JR (1985) *Relapse Prevention: Maintenance Strategies in the Treatment of Addictive Behaviors*, New York: Guildford Press.

Nemeroff CB, DeVane CL, Pollock BG (1996) Newer antidepressants and the cytochrome P450 system, *Am J Psychiatry* **153**:311–320.Covey LS, Glassman AH (1991) A meta-analysis of double-blind placebo-controlled trials of clonidine for smoking cessation, *Br J Addict* **86**:991–998.

Nutt D, Adinoff B, Linnoila M (1988) Benzodiazepines in the treatment of alcoholism, *In* Galanter M, ed. *Recent Developments in Alcoholism*. Vol. 7. Treatment Research. Washington, DC: American Medical Society on Alcoholism:283.

Regier DA, Farmer ME, Rae DS, et al: (1990) Comorbidity of mental disorders with alcohol and drug abuse: results from the epidemiological catchment area (ECA) study, *JAMA* **264**(19):2511–2518.

Rickels K, Schweizer E, Case WG, et al (1990) Long-term therapeutic use of benzodiazepines: effects of abrupt discontinuation, *Arch Gen Psychiatry* **47**:899.

Schweizer E, Rickels K, Case WG, et al (1990) Long-term use of benzodiazepines: effects of gradual tapering, *Arch Gen Psychiatry* **47**:908.

West R, Hajek P, McNeill A (1991) Effect of buspirone on cigarette withdrawal symptoms and short-term abstinence rates in a smokers clinic, *Psychopharmacol* **104**:91–96.

Wise RA, Hoffman DC (1992) Localization of drug reward mechanisms by intracranial injections, *Synapse* **10**:247–263.

11–13   Drug interactions

Arranz MJ, Dawson E, Shaikh S, et al (1995) Cytochrome P4502D6 gene type does not determine response to clozapine, *Br J Clin Pharmacol* **39**:417–420.

Byerly MJ, DeVane CL (1996) Pharmacokinetics of clozapine and risperidone: a review of recent literature, *J Clin Psychopharmacol* **16**:177–187.

Dumortier G, Lochu A, Colen de Melo P, et al (1996) Elevated clozapine plasma concentrations after fluvoxamine initiation, *Am J Psychiatry* **153**:738–739.

Ereshefsky L (1996) Drug-drug interactions involving antidepressants: focus on venlafaxine, *J Clin Psychopharmacol* **16**(suppl):37–53.

Ereshefsky L (1996) Pharmacokinetics and drug interactions: update for new antipsychotics, *J Clin Psychiatry* **57**(suppl 11):12–25.

Ereshefsky L, LeRoy A, Tran-Johnson T, et al (1988) Pharmacokinetic factors affecting antidepressant drug clearance and clinical effect: evaluation of doxepin and imipramine: new data and review, *Clin Chem* **34**:863–880.

Ereshefsky L, Saklad SR, Davis CM, et al (1984) Clinical implications of fluphenazine kinetics. Presented at the American Psychiatric Association, New York NY.

Ereshevsky L, Jann MW, Saklad SR, et al (1985) Effects of smoking on fluphenazine clearance in psychiatric inpatients, *Biol Psychiatry* **20**:329–352.

Funderburg LG, Vertrees JE, True JE, et al (1994) Seizure after the addition of erythromycin to clozapine treatment, *Am J Psychiatry* **151**:1840–1841.

Graves NM (1995) Neuropharmacology and drug interactions in clinical practice, *Epilepsia* **36**(suppl 2):S27–S33.

Harvey AT, Preskorn SH (1996) Cytochrome P450 enzymes: interpretation of their interactions with selective serotonin re-uptake inhibitors: part 1, *J Clin Psychopharmacol* **16**:273–285.

Jann MW, Saklad SR, Ereshefsky L, et al (1986) Effects of smoking on haloperidol and reduced haloperidol plasma concentrations and haloperidol clearance, *Psychopharmacol (Berl)* **90**:468–470.

Levy RH (1995) Cytochrome P450 isoenzymes and anti-epileptic drug interactions, *Epilepsia* **36**(suppl 5): S8–S13.

Miller D (1991) Effects of phenytoin on plasma clozapine concentrations in two patients, *J Clin Psychiatry* **52**:23–25.

Nemeroff CB, DeVane CL, Pollock BG (1996) Newer antidepressants and the cytochrome P450 system, *Amer J Psychiatry* **153**:311–320.

Taylor D (1997) Pharmacokinetic interactions involving clozapine, *Br J Psychiatry* **171**:109–112.

Taylor D, Lader M (1996) Cytochromes and psychotropic drug interactions, *Br J Psychiatry* **168**:529–532.

14. Treatment strategies- mood disorders

Avery DH, Khan A, Dager SR, et al (1991) Morning or evening bright light treatment of winter depression? The significance of hypersomnia, *Biol Psychiatry* **29**:117–126.

Bauer MS, Whybrow PC (1990) Rapid cycling bipolar affective disorder: treatment of refractory rapid cycling with high-dose levothyroxine: a preliminary study, *Arch Gen Psychiatry* **47**:435–440.

Bauer MS, Whybrow PC (1990) Rapid cycling bipolar affective high-dose levothyroxine: a preliminary study, *Arch Gen Psychiatry* **47**:435–440.

Beck AT, Rush AJ, Shaw BF, et al (1979) *Cognitive Therapy of Depression: A Treatment Manual*, New York: Guilford.

Bennie EH, Mullin JM, Martindale JJ (1995) A double-blind multicenter trial comparing sertraline and fluoxetine in outpatients with major depression, *J Clin Psychiatry* **56**:229–237.

Black DW, Winokur G, Nasrallah A (1987) Treatment of mania: a naturalistic study of electroconvulsive therapy versus lithium in 438 patients, *J Clin Psychiatry* **48**:132–139.

Bouchard RH, Pourcher E, Vincent P (1989) Fluoxetine and extrapyramidal side effects, *Am J Psychiatry* **146**:1352.

Bowden CL (1995) Predictors of response to divalproex and lithium, *J Clin Psychiatry* **56**(suppl 3):25–30.

Bowden CL, Brugger AM, Swann AC, et al (Depakote mania study group) (1994) Efficacy of divalproex vs. lithium and placebo in the treatment of mania, *J Amer Med Assoc* **271**:918–924.

Bowden CL, Janicak PG, Orsulak P, et al (1996) Relation of serum valproate concentration to response in mania, *Amer J Psychiatry* **153**(6):765–770.

Calabrese JR, Woyshville MJ (1995) A medication algorithm for treatment of bipolar rapid cycling? *J Clin Psychiatry* **56**(suppl 3):11–18.

Calabrese, JR, Kimmel SE, Woyshville MJ, et al (1996) Clozapine for treatment-refractory mania, *Amer J Psychiatry* **153**(6):759–764.

Chiarello RJ, Cole JO (1987) The use of psychostimulants in general psychiatry, *Arch Gen Psychiatry* **44**:286.

Chou JCY (1991) Recent advances in treatment of acute mania, *J Clin Psychopharmacol* **11**:3–21.

Coryell W, Keller M, Lavori P, et al (1989) Affective syndromes, psychotic features, and prognosis: I. Depression, *Arch Gen Psychiatry* **47**:651–657.

Coryell W, Keller M, Lavori P, et al (1989) Affective syndromes, psychotic features, and prognosis: II. Mania, *Arch Gen Psychiatry* **47**:658–662.

Cowen PJ, Power AC (1993) Combination treatment of depression, *Br J of Psychiatry* **162**:266–267.

Davidson JRT, Giller EL, Zisook S, et al (1988) An efficacy study of isocarboxazid and placebo in depression, and its relationship to depressive nosology, *Arch Gen Psychiatry* **45**:120–127.

Delini-Stula A, Mikkelsen H, Angst J (1995) Therapeutic efficacy of antidepressants in agitated anxious depression: a meta-analysis of moclobemide studies, *J Affective Disorders* **9;35**(1–2):21–30.

Dubovsky SL, Thomas M (1992) Psychotic depression: advances in conceptualization and treatment, *Hospital and Community Psychiatry* **43**(12):733–745.

Frank E, Kupfer DJ, Perel JM, et al (1990) Three-year outcomes for maintenance therapies in recurrent depression, *Arch Gen Psychiatry* **48**:1093–1099.

Frank E, Kupfer DJ, Perel JM, et al (1990) Three-year outcomes from maintenance therapies in recurrent depression, *Arch Gen Psychiatry* **47**:1093–1099.

Frank E, Kupfer DJ, Perel JM, et al (1993) Comparison of full-dose versus half-dose pharmacotherapy in the maintenance treatment of recurrent depression, *J Affect Dis* **27**:139–145.

Friedman RA, Mitchell J, Kocsis JH (1995) Retreatment for relapse following desipramine discontinuation in dysthymia, *Amer J Psychiatry* **152**(6):926–928.

Gelenberg AJ, Kane JM, Keller MB, et al (1989) Comparison of standard and low serum levels of lithium for maintenance treatment of bipolar disorder, *N Engl J Med* **321**:1489–1493.

Georgotis A, McCue RE (1989) Relapse of depressed patients after effective continuation therapy, *J Affective Disord* **17**:159–164.

Gitlin MJ, Swendsen J, Heller TL, et al (1995) Relapse and impairment in bipolar disorder, *Amer J Psychiatry* **152**(11):1635–1640.

Glassman AH, Bigger T Jr (1981) Cardiovascular effects of therapeutic doses of tricyclic antidepressants, *Arch Gen Psychiatry* **38**:815.

Goodwin FK, Prange AJ, Post RM, el at (1982) Potentiation of antidepressant effect by triiodothyronine in tricyclic non-responders, *Am J Psychiatry* **139**:34–38.

Hellerstein DJ, Yanowitch P, Rosenthal J, et al (1993) Randomized double-blind study of fluoxetine versus placebo in the treatment of dysthymia, *Amer J Psychiatry* **150**(8):1169–1175.

Hollon SD, DeRubeis RJ, Evans MD, et al (1992) Cognitive therapy and pharmacotherapy for depression: singly and in combination, *Arch Gen Psychiatry* **49**:774–781.

Hopkins HS, Gelenberg AJ (1994) Treatment of bipolar disorder: how far have we come? *Psychopharmacol Bull* **30**(1):27–38.

Janicak PG, Sharma RP, Easton M, et al (1989) A double-blind, placebo-controlled trial of clonidine in the treatment of acute mania, *Psychopharmacol Bull* **25**:243–245.

Jue SG, Dawson GW, Brogden RN (1982) Amoxapine: a review of its pharmacology and efficacy in depressed states, *Drugs* **24**:1–23.

Kane J (1990) Treatment programme and long-term outcome in chronic schizophrenia, *Acta Psychiatr Scand* **82**(suppl 358):151–157.

Kemali D (1989) A multicenter Italian study of amineptine (survector 100), *Clin Neuropharmacol* **12**(2):S41–S50.

Kline MD (1989) Fluoxetine and anorgasmia, *Am J Psychiatry* **146**:804.

Kocsis JH, Frances AJ, Voss C, et al (1988) Imipramine treatment for chronic depression, *Arch Gen Psychiatry* **45**:253–257.

Kramlinger KG, Post RM (1989) Adding lithium carbonate to carbamazepine: antimanic efficacy in treatment-resistant mania, *Acta Psychiatr Scand* **79**:378–385.

Kramlinger KG, Post RM (1989) The addition of lithium to carbamazepine: antidepressant efficacy in treatment-resistant depression, *Arch Gen Psychiatry* **46**:794–800.

Kupfer DJ, Frank E, Perel JM, et al (1992) Five-year outcome for maintenance therapies in recurrent depression, *Arch Gen Psychiatry* **49**:769–773.

Lam RW, Gorman CP, Michalon M, et al (1995) Multi-center, placebo-controlled study of fluoxetine in seasonal affective disorder, *Amer J Psychiatry* **152**:1765–1770.

Lenzi A, Marazziti D, Raffaelli S, et al (1995) Effectiveness of the combination verapamil and chlorpromazine in the treatment of severe manic or mixed patients, *Progress in Neuropsychopharmacol and Biological Psychiatry* **19**(3):519–528.

Lerner Y, Mintzer Y, Schestatzky M (1988) Lithium combined with haloperidol in schizophrenic patients, *Br J Psychiatry* **153**:359–362.

Levitt JJ, Tsuang MT (1988) The heterogeneity of schizoaffective disorder: implications for treatment, *Am J Psychiatry* **145**:926–936.

Levy AB, Drake ME, Shy KE (1988) EEG evidence of epileptiform paroxysms in rapid cycling bipolar patients, *J Clin Psychiatry* **49**:232–234.

Lewy AJ (1987) Treating chronobiologic sleep and mood disorders with bright light, *Psychiatr Ann* **17**:664–669.

Liebowitz MR, Quitkin FM, Stewart JW, et al (1988) Antidepressant specificity in atypical depression, *Arch Gen Psychiatry* **45**:129–137.

Maj M (1988) Lithium prophylaxis of schizoaffective disorders: a prospective study, *J Affective Disord* **14**:129–135.

Marin DB, Kocsis JH, Frances AJ, et al (1994) Desipramine for the treatment of pure dysthymia versus double depression, *Amer J Psychiatry* **151**(7):1079–1080.

McElroy SL, Keck PE Jr, Pope HG Jr, et al (1991) Correlates of antimanic response to valproate, *Psychopharmacol Bull* **27**:127–133.

McElroy SL, Keck PE, Pope HG, et al (1989) Valproate in psychiatric disorders: literature review and clinical guidelines, *J Clin Psychiatry* **50**(suppl 3):23–29.

Meco G, Marini S, Mariana L, et al (1988) Ritanserin in dysthymic disorders (DSM-III): a double-blind study vesus amitryptyline (abstr), *Psychopharmacology* :282.

Mukherjee S, Sackheim HA, Schnur DB (1994) Electroconvulsive therapy of acute manic episodes: a review of 50 years' experience, *Amer J Psychiatry* **151**:169–176.

Nelson JC, Mazure CM (1986) Lithium augmentation in psychotic depression refractory to combined drug treatment, *Am J Psychiatry* **143**:363–366.

Nemeroff CB (1991) Augmentation regimens for depression, *J Clin Psychiatry* **52**(May suppl):21–27.

Nierenberg AA, Amsterdam JD (1990) Treatment-resistant depression: definition and treatment approaches, *J Clin Psychiatry* **51**(suppl 6):39–47.

NoWA, Haffmans J (1989) Treatment resistant depression. Review of the efficacy of various biological treatments, specifically in major depression resistant to cyclic antidepressants, *Int Clin Psychopharmacol* **4**:217–228.

Petrides G, Dhossche D, Fink M, et al (1994) Continuation ECT: relapse prevention in affective disorders, *Convulsive Therapy* **10**(3):189–194.

Pope HG, McElroy SL, Keck PE, et al (1991) Valproate in the treatment of acute mania: a placebo-controlled study, *Arch Gen Psychiatry* **48**:62–68.

Post RM (1990) Non-lithium treatment for bipolar disorder, *J Clin Psychiatry* **51**:8.

Post RM, Kramlinger KG, Altshuler LL, et al (1990) Treatment of rapid cycling bipolar illness, *Psychopharmacol Bull* **26**:37–47.

Post RM, Rubinow DR, Uhde TW, et al (1989) Dysphoric mania: clinical and biological correlates, *Arch Gen Psychiatry* **46**:353–358.

Post RM, Uhde TW, Roy-Byrne PP, et al (1987) Correlates of antimanic response to carbamazepine, *Psychiatry Res* **21**:71–83.

Prell GD, Green JP (1986) Histamine as a neuroregulator, *Ann Rev Neurosci* **9**:209.

Preskorn SH (1989) Tricyclic antidepressants: the whys and hows of therapeutic drug monitoring, *J Clin Psychiatry* **50**:34.

Prien RF, Gelenberg AJ (1989) Alternatives to lithium for preventive treatment of bipolar disorder, *Am J Psychiatry* **146**:840–848.

Prien RF, Kupfer DJ (1986) Continuation drug therapy for major depressive episodes: How long should it be maintained? *Am J Psychiatry* **143**:18–23.

Prien RF, Kupfer DJ, Mansky PA, et al (1984) Drug therapy in the prevention of recurrences in unipolar and bipolar affective disorders, *Arch Gen Psychiatry* **41**:1096.

Quitkin FM, McGrath PJ, Stewart JW, et al (1989) Phenelzine and imipramine in mood reactive depressives: further delineation of the syndrome of atypical depression, *Arch Gen Psychiatry* **46**:787–793.

Quitkin FM, McGrath PJ, Stewart JW, et al (1990) Atypical depression, panic attacks, and response to imipramine and phenelzine, *Arch Gen Psychiatry* **47**:935–941.

Richelson E, Nelson A (1984) Antagonism by antidepressants of neurotransmitter receptors of normal human brain in vitro, *J Pharmacol Exp Ther* **230**:94.

Ries RK, Wilson L, Bokan JA, et al (1981) ECT in medication-resistant schizoaffective disorder, *Compr Psychiatry* **22**:167–173.

Robinson D, Lerfald SC, Binnett B, et al (1991) Continuation and maintenance treatment of major depression with the monoamine oxidase inhibitor phenelzine: a double-blind placebo-controlled study, *Psychopharmacol Bull* **27**:31–40.

Sack RL, Lewy AJ, White DM, et al (1990) Morning versus evening light treatment for winter depression. Evidence that the therapeutic effects of light are mediated by circadian phase shifts, *Arch Gen Psychiatry* **473**:343–351.

Sackeim H, Prudic J, Devanand DP, et al (1990) The impact of medication resistance and continuation pharmacotherapy on relapse following responses to electroconvulsive therapy in major depression, *J Clin Psychopharmacol* **10**:96–104.

Siris SG, Adan F, Cohen M, et al (1988) Post-psychotic depression and negative symptoms: an investigation of syndromal overlap, *Am J Psychiatry* **145**:1532–1537.

Siris SG, Cutler J, Owen K, et al (1989) Adjunctive imipramine maintenance in schizophrenic patients with remitted post-psychotic depressions, *Am J Psychiatry* **146**:1495–1497.

Siris SG, Morgan V, Fagerstrom R, et al (1987) Adjunctive imipramine in the treatment of post-psychotic depression: a controlled trial, *Arch Gen Psychiatry* **44**:533–539.

Small JG (1990) Anticonvulsants in affective disorders, *Psychopharmacol Bull* **26**:25–36.

Taylor D (1995) Selective serotonin reuptake inhibitors and tricyclic antidepressants in combination: interactions and therapeutic uses, *Br J Psychiatry* **167**:575–580.

Terman M, Terman JS, Quitkin FM, et al (1989) Light therapy for seasonal affective disorder: a review of efficacy, *Neuropsychopharmacol* **2**:1–22.

Thase ME, Mallinger AG, McKnight D, et al (1992) Treatment of imipramine-resistant recurrent depression: a double-blind cross-over study of tranylcypromine for anergic bipolar depression, *Amer J Psychiatry* **149**(2):195–198.

Vanelle JM, Loo H, Galinowski A, et al (1994) Maintenance ECT in intractable manic-depressive disorders, *Convulsive therapy* **10**(3):195–205.

Wehr TA, Sack DA, Rosenthal NE, et al (1988) Rapid cycling affective disorder: contributing factors and treatment responses in 51 patients, *Am J Psychiatry* **145**:179–184.

White K, Simpson GM (1981) Combined MAOI-tricyclic antidepressant treatment: a re-evaluation, *J Clin Psychopharmacol* **1**:264–282.

Wirz-Justice A, Graw P, Kr?uchi K, et al (1993) Light therapy in seasonal affective disorder is independent of time of day or circadian phase, *Arch Gen Psychiatry* **50**(12):929–937.

Zarate CA Jr., Tohen M, Baldessarini RJ (1995a) Clozapine in severe mood disorders, *J Clin Psychiatry* **56**(9):411–417.

Zarate CA Jr., Tohen M, Banov MD, et al (1995b) Is clozapine a mood stabilizer? *J Clin Psychiatry* **56**(3):108–112.

15. Treatment strategies – psychotic disorders

Altamura AC, Mauri MC, Mantero M, et al (1987) Clonazepam/haloperidol combination therapy in schizophrenia: a double-blind study, *Acta Psychiatr Scand* **76**:702–706.

Beasley CM, Sanger W, Satterlee G, et al (1996) Olanzapine versus placebo: results of a double-blind, fixed-dose olanzapine trial, *Psychopharmacol (Berl)* **124**:159–167.

Beasley CM, Tollefson G, Tran P, et al (1996) Olanzapine versus placebo and haloperidol: acute phase results of the North American double-blind olanzapine trial, *Neuropsychopharmacol* **14**:111–123.

Carpenter WT Jr, Conley RR, Buchanan RW, et al (1995) Patient response and resource management: another view of clozapine treatment of schizophrenia, *Amer J Psychiatry* **152**(6):827–832.

Christison GW, Kirch DG, Wyatt RJ (1991) When symptoms persist: choosing among alternative somatic treatments for schizophrenia, *Schizophrenia Bull* **17**:217–245.

Coffey L (1994) Options for the treatment of negative symptoms of schizophrenia, *CNS Drugs* **1**:107–118.

Ereshevsky L (1995) Treatment strategies for schizophrenia, *Psychiatric Annals* **25**:285–296.

Goff DC, Midha KK, Saridsegal O, et al (1995) A placebo-controlled trial of fluoxetine added to neuroleptic inpatients with schizophrenia, *Psychopharmacol (Berl)* **117**:417–423.

Herz MI, Glazer WM, Mostert MA, et al (1991) Intermittent vs maintenance medication in schizophrenia, *Arch Gen Psychiatry* **48**:333–339.

Kane J, Honigfeld G, Singer J, et al (1988) Clozapine for the treatment-resistant schizophrenic: a double-blind comparison with chlorpromazine, *Arch Gen Psychiatry* **45**:789–796.

Kane JM, Honigfeld G, Singer J (1988) Clozapine for the treatment-resistant schizophrenic: a double-blind comparison with chlorpromazine, *Arch Gen Psychiatry* **45**:789–796.

Kendler KS, Hays P (1981) Paranoid psychosis (delusional disorder) and schizophrenia, *Arch Gen Psychiatry* **38**:547–551.

Levinson DF, Simpson GM, Singh H, et al (1990) Fluphenazine dose, clinical response, and extrapyramidal symptoms during acute treatment, *Arch Gen Psychiatry* **47**:761–768.

Lieberman JA, Safferman AZ, Pollack S, et al (1994) Clinical effects of clozapine in chronic schizophrenia: response to treatment and predictors of outcome, *Amer J Psychiatry* **151**(12):1744–1752.

Lindskov R, Baadsgaard O (1985) Delusions of infestation treated with pimozide: a follow-up study, *Acta Derm Venereol* (Stockholm) **65**(3):267–270.

Meltzer HY, Cola P, Way L, et al (1993) Cost effectiveness of clozapine in neuroleptic-resistant schizophrenia, *Amer J Psychiatry* **150**(11):1630–1638.

Meltzer HY, Okayli G (1995) Reduction of suicidality during clozapine treatment of neuroleptic-resistant schizophrenia: impact on risk-benefit assessment, *Amer J Psychiatry* **152**(2):183–190.

Mok H, Yatham LN (1994) Treatment of delusional disorders with clozapine, *Amer J Psychiatry* **151**(9).

Munro A, O'Brien JV, Ross D (1985) Two cases of pure or primary erotomania successfully treated with pimozide, *Canadian J Psychiatry* **30**(8):619–622.

Opjordsmoen S (1989) Delusional disorders. I. Comparative long-term outcome, *Acta Psychiatr Scand* **80**:603–612.

Peuskens J (1995) Risperidone in the treatment of patients with chronic schizophrenia: a multi-centre, double-blind, parallel-group study versus haloperidol, *Br J Psychiatry* **166**:712–726.

Richelson E (1988) Neuroleptic binding to human brain receptors: relation to clinical effects, *Ann NY Acad Sci* **537**:435–442.

Rifkin A, Doddi S, Karajgi B, et al (1991) Dosage of haloperidol for schizophrenia, *Arch Gen Psychiatry* **48**:166–170.

Seeman P (1987) Dopamine receptors and the dopamine hypothesis of schizophrenia, *Synapse*:133–152.

Shiloh R, Zemishlany Z, Aizenberg D, Weizman A (1997) Sulpiride adjunction to clozapine in treatment-resistant schizophrenic patients:liminary case-serious study. *Eur Psychiatry* **12**:152–155.

Shiloh R, Zemishlany Z, Aizenberg D, et al (1997) Sulpiride augmentation in schizophrenic patients partially responsive to clozapine. A double-blind, placebo controlled study. *Br J Psychiatry* **171**:569–73.

Tollefson GD, Beasley CM Jr, Tran PV, et al (1997) Olanzapine vs haloperidol in the treatment of schizophrenia, schizoaffective and schizophreniform disorders: results of an international collaborative trial, *Am J Psychiatry* **154**:457–465.

Ungvari G, Vladar K (1986) Pimozide treatment for delusion of infestation, *Act Nerv Super* (Prague) **28**(2):103–107.

van Kammen DP, McEvoy JP, Targum S, et al (1996) A randomized, controlled, dose-ranging trial of sertindole in patients with schizophrenia, *Psychopharmacol (Berl)* **124**:168–175.

16. Treatment strategies – anxiety disorders

Agras WS (1990) Treatment of social phobias, *J Clin Psychiatry* **51**:(suppl):52–58.

Baer L, Rauch SL, Ballantine HT Jr., et al (1995) Cingulotomy for intractable obsessive-compulsive disorder: prospective long-term follow-up of 18 patients, *Arch Gen Psychiatry* **52**(5):384–392.

Baldwin D, Rudge S (1995) The role of serotonin in depression and anxiety, *Int'l Clin Psychopharmacol* **9**(suppl 4):41–45.

Ballenger JC, Burrows GD, DuPont RL, et al (1988) Alprazolam in panic disorder and agoraphobia: results from a multicenter trial: I. Efficacy in short-term treatment, *Arch Gen Psychiatry* **45**:413–422.

Benjamin J, Levine J, Fux M, et al (1995) A double-blind, placebo-controlled, cross-over trial of inositol treatment for panic disorder, *Amer J Psychiatry* **152**(7):1084–1086.

Bernadt MW, Silverstone T, Singleton W (1980) Beta adrenergic blockade in phobic subjects, *Br J Psychiatry* **137**:452–457.

Black DW, Wesner R, Bowers W, et al (1993) A comparison of fluvoxamine, cognitive therapy and placebo in the treatment of panic disorder, *Arch Gen Psychiatry* **50**:44–50.

Bourin M, Malinge M (1995) Controlled comparison of the effects and abrupt discontinuation of buspirone and lorazepam, *Progress in Neuropsychopharmacology and Biological Psychiatry* **19**(4):567–575.

Brady KT, Sonne SC, Roberts JM (1995) Sertraline treatment of comorbid post-traumatic stress disorder and alcohol dependence, *J Clin Psychiatry* **56**(11):502–505.

Braun P, Greenberg D, Dasberg H, et al (1990) Core symptoms of post-traumatic stress disorder unimproved by alprazolam treatment, *J Clin Psychiatry* **51**:236–238.

Brown TA, Barlow DH, Liebowitz MR (1994) The empirical basis of generalized anxiety disorder, *Amer J Psychiatry* **151**(9): 1272–1280.

Charney DS, Woods SW, Goodman WK, et al (1986) Drug treatment of panic disorder: the comparative efficacy of imipramine, alprazolam, and trazodone, *J Clin Psychiatry* **47**(12):580–586.

Cross-National Collaborative Panic Study Second Phase Investigators (1992) Drug treatment of panic disorder: comparative efficacy of alprazolam, imipramine, and placebo, *Brit J Psychiatry* **160**:191–202.

Cumming S, Hay P, Lee T, et al (1995) Neuropsychological outcome from psychosurgery for obsessive-compulsive disorder, *Australia N Zealand J Psychiatry* **29**(2):293–298.

Davidson J, Kudler H, Smith R, et al (1990) Treatment of post-traumatic stress disorder with amitriptyline and placebo, *Arch Gen Psychiatry* **47**:259–266.

Dominguez RA, Mestre SM (1994) Management of treatment-refractory obsessive-compulsive disorder patients, *J Clin Psychiatry* **55**(suppl):86–92.

Dubovsky SL (1990) Generalized anxiety disorder: new concepts and psychopharmacologic therapies, *J Clin Psychiatry* **51**(suppl 1):3–10.

Friedman MJ (1991) Biological approaches to the diagnosis and treatment of post-traumatic stress disorder, *J Traumatic Stress* **4**:67–91.

Geracioti TD Jr (1995) Venlafaxine treatment of panic disorder: a case series, *J Clin Psychiatry* **56**(9):408–410.

Goodman WK, Delgado PL, Price LH, et al (1990) Comparison of fluvoxamine and desipramine in OCD, *Arch Gen Psychiatry* **47**:577–585.

Greist JH, Jefferson JW, Kobak KA, et al (1995) Efficacy and tolerability of serotonin transport inhibitors in obsessive-compulsive disorder: a meta-analysis, *Arch Gen Psychiatry* **52**(1):53–60.

Jefferson JW (1995) Social phobia: a pharmacologic treatment overview, *J Clin Psychiatry* **56**(suppl)(5):18–24.

Jenike MA, Baer L, Greist JH (1990) Clomipramine versus fluoxetine in obsessive-compulsive disorder: a retrospective comparison of side effects and efficacy, *J Clin Psychopharmacol* **10**:122–124.

Jenike MA, Baer L, Summergrad P, et al (1990) Sertraline in obsessive-compulsive disorder: a double-blind comparison with placebo, *Am J Psychiatry* **147**:923–928.

Lecrubier Y, Puech AJ, Azcona A, et al (1993) A randomized double-blind placebo-controlled study of tropisetron in the treatment of outpatients with generalized anxiety disorder, *Psychopharmacol (Berlin)* **112**(1):129–133.

Liebowitz MR, Gorman JM, Fyer AJ, et al (1988) Pharmacotherapy of social phobia: an interim report of a placebo-controlled comparison of phenelzine and atenolol, *J Clin Psychiatry* **49**:252–257.

Liebowitz MR, Schneier F, Campeas R, et al (1992) Phenelzine vs atenolol in social phobia: a placebo-controlled comparison, *Arch Gen Psychiatry* **49**:290–300.

Lydiard RB, Ballenger JC (1987) Antidepressants in panic disorder and agoraphobia, *J Affective Disorders* **13**:153–168.

Malazia, AL, Nutt, DJ (1995) The effects of flumazenil in neuropsychiatric disorders. *Clinical Neuropharmacology* **18**(3):215–232.

Mellman LA, Gorman TM (1983) Successful treatment of obsessive-compulsive disorder with ECT, *J Clin Psychiatry* **4**:131–132.

Modigh K, Westberg P, Eriksson E (1992) Superiority of clomipramine over imipramine in the treatment of panic disorder: a placebo-controlled trial, *J Clin Psychopharmacol* **12**:251–261.

Nutt DJ, Bell C (1995) Benzodiazepines in the treatment of anxiety. In: Hypnotics and Anxiolytics. Baillière's Tindall Ltd, London. Chapter 4:391–411.

■ Bibliography

Nutt DJ, Horvath R, Coupland NJ. (1995) The role of monoamine oxidase inhibitors in the treatment of anxiety. In: Hypnotics and Anxiolytics. Baillières Clinical Psychiatry. Ed. Byres C, Baillière's Tindall Ltd, London. Chapter 5...413–425.

Ontiveros A, Fontaine R (1990) Social phobia and clonazepam, *Can J Psychiatry* **35**:439–441.

Pato MT, Pigott TA, Hill JL, et al (1991) Controlled comparison of buspirone and clomipramine in obsessive-compulsive disorder, *Am J Psychiatry* **148**:127–129.

Pecknold JC, Swinson RP, Kuch K, Lewis CP (1988) Alprazolam in panic disorder and agoraphobia: results from a multi-center trial. III. Discontinuation effects, *Arch Gen Psychiatry* **45**:429–436.

Petracca A, Nisita C, McNair D, et al (1990) Treatment of generalized anxiety disorder: preliminary clinical experience with buspirone, *J Clin Psychiatry* **51**(suppl 9):31–39.

Piccinelli M, Pini S, Bellantuono C, et al (1995) Efficacy of drug treatment in obsessive-compulsive disorder: a meta-analytic review, *Br J Psychiatry* **166**(4):424–443.

Pigott TA, Pato MT, L'Heureux F, et al (1991) A controlled comparison of adjuvant lithium carbonate or thyroid hormone in clomipramine-treated OCD patients, *J Clin Psychopharmacol* **11**:242–248.

Rickels K, Downing R, Schweizer E, et al (1993) Antidepressants for the treatment of generalized anxiety disorder: a placebo-controlled comparison of imipramine, trazodone, and diazepam, *Arch Gen Psychiatry* **50**:884–895.

Rickels K, Schweizer E (1990) The clinical course and long-term management of generalized anxiety disorder, *J Clin Psychopharmacol* **10**:101S–110S.

Rickels K, Schweizer E, Csanalosi I, et al (1988) Long-term treatment of anxiety and risk of withdrawal: prospective comparison of clorazepate and buspirone, *Arch Gen Psychiatry* **45**:444–450.

Rickels K. Schweizer E, Weiss S, et al (1993) Maintenance drug treatment for panic disorder. II. Short- and long-term outcome after drug taper, *Arch Gen Psychiatry* **50**:61–68.

Schneier FR, Liebowitz MR, Davies SO, et al (1990) Fluoxetine in panic disorder, *J Clin Psychopharmacol* **10**:119–121.

Shader, RI, Greenblatt DJ (1993) Use of benzodiazepines in anxiety disorders, *NE J Med* **328**(19):1398–1405.

Sheehan DV, Raj BA, Sheehan KH, et al (1990) Is buspirone effective for panic disorder?, *J Clin Psychopharmacol* **10**(1):3–11.

Sheehan DV, Zak JP, Miller JA, et al (1988) Panic disorder: the potential role of serotonin re-uptake inhibitors, *J Clin Psychiatry* **49**(suppl):23–29.

Silver JM, Sandberg DP, Hales RE (1990) New approaches in the pharmacotherapy of post-traumatic stress disorder, *J Clin Psychiatry* **51**(suppl):33–38.

Tesar GE, Rosenbaum JF, Pollack MH, et al (1991) Double-blind placebo-controlled comparison of clonazepam and alprazolam for panic disorder, *J Clin Psychiatry* **52**(2):69–76.

Vallejo J, Olivares J, Marcos T, et al (1992) Clomipramine versus phenelzine in obsessive-compulsive dis: a controlled clinical trial, *Br J Psychiatry* **161**:665–670.

Van der Kolk BA, Dreyfuss D, Michaels M, et al (1994) Fluoxetine in post-traumatic stress disorder, *J Clin Psychiatry* **55**(12):517–522.

Van Vliet IM, den Boer JA, Westenberg HG (1994) Psychopharmacological treatment of social phobia: a double-blind, placebo-controlled study with fluvoxamine, *Psychopharmacol* (Berlin) **115**(1–2):128–134.

Wheadon DE, Bushnell WD, Steiner M (1993,December) A fixed-dose comparison of 20, 40 or 60 mg of paroxetine to placebo in the treatment of obsessive-compulsive disorder, *Proceedings of the American College Neuropsychopharmacology*, Maui, Hawaii.

Zitrin CM, Klein DF, Woerner MG, et al (1983) Treatment of phobias: I. Imipramine and placebo, *Arch Gen Psychiatry* **40**:125–138.

17. Treatment strategies – selected personality disorders

Coccaro EF, Still JL, Herbert JL, et al (1990) Fluoxetine treatment of impulsive aggression in DSM-III-R personality disorder patients, *J Clin Psychopharmacol* **10**:373.

Cowdry RW, Gardner DL (1988) Pharmacotherapy of borderline personality disorder: alprazolam, carbamazepine, triflouperazine and tranylcypromine, *Arch Gen Psychiatry* **45**:111–119.

Deltito JA, Stam M (1989) Pharmacological treatment of avoidant personality disorder, *Comprehensive Psychiatry* **30**:498–504.

Frankenburg FR, Zanarini MC (1993) Clozapine treatment of borderline patients: a preliminary study, *Comprehensive Psychiatry* **34**(6):402–405.

Gitlin MJ (1993) Pharmacology of personality disorders: conceptual framework and clinical strategies, *J Clin Psychopharmacol* **13**(5):343–353.

Hymowitz P, Frances A, Jacobsberg L, et al (1986) Neuroleptic treatment of schizotypal personality disorder, *Compr Psychiatry* **27**:267–271.

Kernberg OF, Selzer MA, Koenighsberg HW, et al (1989) *Psychodynamic Psychotherapy of Borderline Patients*. New York: Basic Books, Inc.

Kutcher S, Papatheodorou G, Reiter S, et al (1995) The successful pharmacological treatment of adolescents and young adults with borderline personality disorder: a preliminary open trial of flupenthixol, *J Psychiatry and Neurosci* **20**(2):113–118.

Liebowitz MR, Quitkin FM, Stewart JW, et al (1988) Antidepressant specificity in atypical depression, *Arch Gen Psychiatry* **45**:129.

Marin DB, De Meo M, Frances AJ, et al (1989) Biological models and treatments for personality disorders, *Psychiatr Ann* **19**:143.

Markovitz PJ, Calabrese JR, Schulz SC, et al (1991) Fluoxetine in the treatment of borderline and schizotypal personality disorders, *Amer J Psychiatry* **148**:1064–1067.

Norden MJ (1989) Fluoxetine in borderline personality disorder, *Prog Neuropsychopharmacol Biol Psychiatry* **13**:885.

Schulz SC (1986) The use of low dose neuroleptics in the treatment of "schizo-obsessive" patients, *Am J Psychiatry* **143**(10):1318–1319.

Siever LJ, Bernstein DP, Silverman JM (1991) Schizotypal personality disorder: a review of its current status, *J Pers Disord* **5**:193–208.

Soloff PH (1990) What's new in personality disorders: an update in psychopharmacologic treatment, *J Pers Disord* **4**(3):233–243.

Stein DJ, Hollander E, Anthony DT, et al (1992) Serotonergic medications for sexual obsessions, sexual addictions, and paraphilias, *J Clin Psychiatry* **53**:267–271.

Stein DJ, Hollander E, Josephson SC (1994) Serotonin re-uptake blockers for the treatment of obsessional jealousy, *J Clin Psychiatry* **55**(1):30–33.

Stone MH (1990) Treatment of borderline patients: a pragmatic approach, *Psychiatr Clin North Am* **13**:265–285.

18. Treatment strategies – eating disorders

Ayuso-Gutierrez JL, Palazon M, Ayuso-Mateos JL (1994) Open trial of fluvoxamine in the treatment of bulimia nervosa, *Int'l J Eating Disorders* **15**(3):245–249.

Biederman J, Herzog DB, Rivinus TM, et al (1985) Amitriptyline in the treatment of anorexia nervosa: a double-blind, placebo-controlled study, *J Clin Psychopharmacol* **5**(1):10.

Fairburn CG (1988) The current status of the psychological treatments for bulimia nervosa, *J Psychosom Res* **32**:635–645.

Goldbloom DS, Olmsted MP (1993) Pharmacotherapy of bulimia nervosa with fluoxetine: assessment of clinically significant attitudinal change, *Amer J Psychiatry* **150**:770–774.

Gwirtsman HE, Guze BH, Yager J, et al (1990) Fluoxetine treatment of anorexia nervosa: an open trial, *J Clin Psychiatry* **51**:378.

Halmi KA, Eckert E, LaDau TJ, et al (1986) Anorexia nervosa: treatment efficacy of cyproheptadine and amitriptyline, *Arch Gen Psychiatry* **43**:117.

Hughes PL, Wells LA, Cunningham CJ, et al (1986) Treating bulimia with desipramine: a double-blind placebo-controlled study, *Arch Gen Psychiatry* **43**:182–186.

Kennedy SH, Piran N, Warsh JJ, et al (1988) A trial of isocarboxazid in the treatment of bulimia nervosa, *J Clin Psychopharmacol* **8**:391–396.

Lam RW, Goldner EM, Solyom L, et al (1994) A controlled study of light therapy for bulimia nervosa, *Amer J Psychiatry* **151**(5):744–750.

Mitchell JE, Hoberman H, Pyle RL (1989) An overview of the treatment of the bulimia nervosa, *Psychiatr Med* **7**:317–332.

Pope HG, Jr, Keck PE, Jr, McElroy SL, et al (1989) A placebo-controlled study of trazodone in bulimia nervosa, *J Clin Psychopharmacol* **9**:254–259.

20. Treatment strategies – disorders associated with iatrogenic causes

Addonizio G, Susman VL, Roth SD (1987) Neuroleptic malignant syndrome: review and analysis of 115 cases, *Biol Psychiatry* **22**:1004–1020.

Casey DE (1987) Tardive dyskinesia. In Meltzer HY, ed. *Psychopharmacology: The Third Generation of Progress*, New York: Raven Press:1411–1419.

Casey DE (1989) Clozapine: neuroleptic-induced EPS and tardive dyskinesia, *Psychopharmacol* **99**:S47–S53.

Casey DE (1990) Tardive dyskinesia, *West J Med* **153**:535–541.

Davis JM, Janicak PG, Sakkas P, et al (1991) ECT in the treatment of NMS, *Convulsive Therapy* **7**(2):111–120.

Davis JM, Janicak PG, Sakkas P, et al (1991) Electroconvulsive therapy in treatment of the neuroleptic malignant syndrome, *Convulsive Ther* **7**(2):111–120.

Elkashef AM, Ruskin PE, Bacher N, et al (1990) Vitamin E in the treatment of tardive dyskinesia, *Am J Psychiatry* **147**(4):505–506.

Glazer WM, Morgenstern H, Schooler N, et al (1990) Predictors of improvement in tardive dyskinesia following discontinuation of neuroleptic medication, *Brit J Psychiatry* **157**:585–592.

Granacher RP, Baldessarini RJ (1975) Physostigmine, *Arch Gen Psychiatry* **32**:375–380.

Granato JE, Stern BJ, Ringel A, et al (1983) Neuroleptic malignant syndrome: successful treatment with dantrolene and bromocriptine, *Annals of Neurology* **14**:89–90.

Hermesh H, Molcho A, Aizenberg D, et al (1988) The calcium antagonist nifedipine in recurrent neuroleptic malignant syndrome, *Clin Neuropharmacol* **II**:552–555.

Jeste DV, Wyatt RJ (1982) Therapeutic strategies against tardive dyskinesia, *Arch Gen Psychiatry* **39**:803–816.

Johnson AL, Hollister LE, Berger PA (1981) The anticholinergic intoxication syndrome: diagnosis and treatment, *J Clin Psychiatry* **42**:313–317.

Miller DD, Sharafuddin MJA, Kathol RG (1991) A case of clozapine-induced NMS, *J Clin Psychiatry* **52**:99–101.

Miller PS, Richardson JS, Jyu CA, et al (1988) Association of low serum anticholinergic levels and cognitive impairment in elderly presurgical patients, *Am J Psychiatry* **256**:342–345.

Mori E, Yamadori A (1987) Acute confusional state and acute agitated delirium: occurrence after infarction in the right middle cerebral artery territory, *Arch Neurol* **44**:1139–1143.

Philbrick KL, Rummans TA (1994) Malignant catatonia, *J Neuropsychiatry and Clin Neurosci* **6**:1–13.

Sakkas P, David JM, Hau J, et al (1991) Pharmacotherapy of NMS, *Psychiatr Ann* **21**:157–164.

Shiloh R, Schwartz B, Weizman A, Radwan M (1995) Catatonia as an unusual presentation of posttraumatic stress disorder. *Psychopathology* **28**:285–290.

Thomas JI, Cameron DJ, Marianne FC (1988) A prospective study of delirium and prolonged hospital stay, *Arch Gen Psychiatry* **45**:937–940.